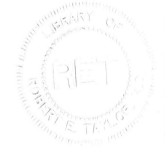

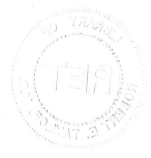

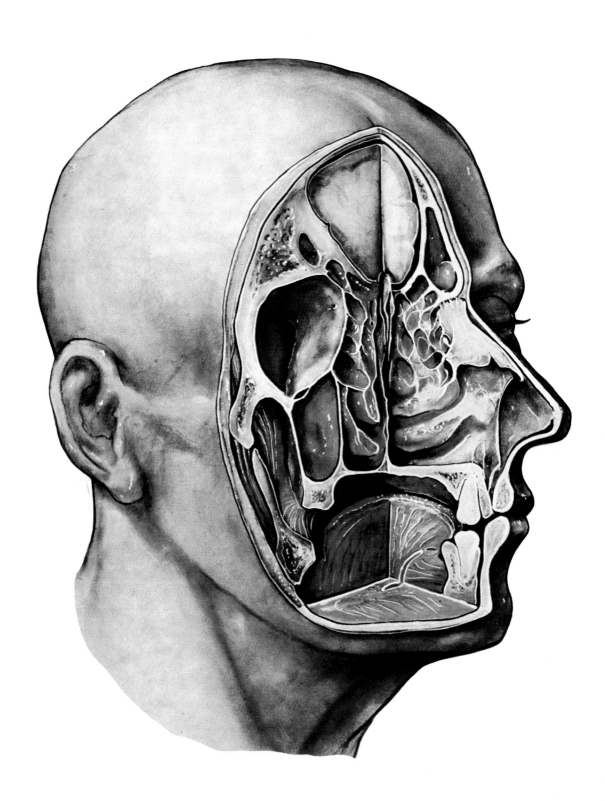

JOHN M. LORÉ, JR., M.D., F.A.C.S.

Professor and Chairman of the Department of Otolaryngology,
School of Medicine, State University of New York at Buffalo;
Head of the Department of Otolaryngology, Buffalo General
Hospital and Buffalo Children's Hospital; Head of the
Division of Otolaryngology, Edward J. Meyer Memorial Hospital;
Consultant, Veterans Administration Hospital and Deaconess Hospital;
Chief of the Combined Head and Neck Service, Buffalo General Hospital;
and Consultant, Head and Neck Services,
Roswell Park Memorial Institute, Buffalo, New York.
Formerly Director of Surgery, Good Samaritan Hospital, Suffern, New York.

Illustrated by

ROBERT WABNITZ

Director of Medical Illustration,
University of Rochester Medical Center, Rochester, New York

An Atlas Of

HEAD and NECK

SURGERY *Second Edition*

VOLUME I

W. B. SAUNDERS COMPANY

PHILADELPHIA • LONDON • TORONTO

W. B. Saunders Company: West Washington Square
Philadelphia, PA 19105

1 St. Anne's Road
Eastbourne, East Sussex BN21 3UN, England

1 Goldthorne Avenue
Toronto, Ontario M8Z 5T9, Canada

Vol. I: ISBN 0-7216-5796-6
Vol. II: ISBN 0-7216-5797-4

An Atlas of Head and Neck Surgery — Volume I

Print No.:   9   8   7   6   5   4

THIS ATLAS IS DEDICATED TO MY FATHER

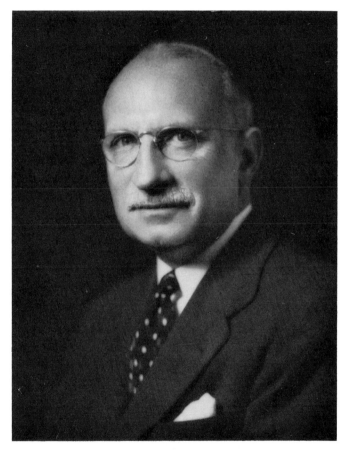

JOHN M. LORÉ, M.D., F.A.C.S.
1892–1950

whose energy and devotion both in his chosen field in medicine —
otolaryngology — and in his dedicated aim in medical education — a
new medical center for his medical school, New York University
— were and still are an inspiration. His desire for, cooperation in
and plans for a consolidated surgical training program in the field
of head and neck surgery provided the impetus for this Atlas.

PROLEGOMENA

In the completion of the "Atlas of Head and Neck Surgery" the author is to be commended on a job well done. It is indeed the culmination of an arduous task by one who is peculiarly qualified to effect its accomplishment.

Dr. Loré first completed a formal residency training in Otorhinolaryngology during which time a keen interest in the broad field of head and neck surgery was acquired. It was then realized that if one were to attain the fulfillment of an ideal, a broad basic knowledge relative to the principles and practice of general surgery and its allied specialties was necessary. Accordingly an extensive formal residency training in general surgery was obtained. During this time one year was spent in the experimental surgical research laboratory and another devoted to the surgical aspects of tumor therapy. Dr. Loré is certified by the American Board of Otolaryngology and the American Board of Surgery respectively, which I believe to be the ideal requisites for anyone specializing in surgery of the head and neck. This background, coupled with the talent for original creative thought, provides the basic reason for the ability of the author to complete this unique effort.

In a careful review of the text and illustrated material it soon becomes apparent that this is probably the most complete work relative to techniques in surgery of the head and neck that has been compiled. The illustrations are numerous, detailed, and follow each other in a clear, well correlated sequence. The text is appealing because of its simplicity, clarity, brevity and completeness. Particularly pleasing is the repetition of the illustrated page wherever required to conform with the continuation of the page of text. This obviates the necessity of "turning back" to compare the text with the illustrations. Furthermore, the necessity for the "compleat" head and neck surgeon to have an intimate knowledge of the related specialties and sub-specialties, as stressed by the author in the preface, is amply emphasized by the contents of the Atlas.

I have no doubt that many will find much to disagree with relative to the various niceties of surgical techniques that are employed. It would be most surprising if it were otherwise. However, I do not believe that there will be much, if any, disagreement relative to the basic surgical principles upon which each operation is based. Nor do I believe that there will be much dissension of opinion to the statement that the "Atlas of Head and Neck Surgery" fulfills a need of long standing and that it represents the completion of a monumental task of which Dr. Loré and the publishers should be justifiably proud.

JOHN L. MADDEN, M.D.

In his preface, Dr. Loré has postulated that all branches and specialties of surgical science are based upon and are outgrowths of the broad fundamental principles of *general surgery*. Listed among the American specialty boards there will be found nevertheless some surgical specialties which require no more than "a year's approved internship" (sic) before entering upon the special training that finally leads to certification. Other surgical specialty boards respectively require from one to three years' preliminary "general surgical" internships or residencies, but only one (the Board of Thoracic Surgery) requires full prior certification by the American Board of Surgery.

From the practical standpoint, there must obviously be some limitation in the requirements of preliminary general surgical training prior to entrance upon a course of special preparation for certification in some of the more circumscribed and limited surgical specialties. On the other hand, such limitations can hardly be applied reasonably to training for any branch of surgery which deals with entry into and manipulations within such anatomic areas as the abdominal, thoracic, cranial or pharyngeal cavities and the deep tissues of the extremities or of the face and neck.

Any surgeon who undertakes major surgery for neoplasms of the head and neck (in peace time the chief form of major surgery in this area) must in all conscience be prepared by sufficiently broad training and experience to cope with the varied problems incident to surgical entry (whether necessary or fortuitous) into such contiguous anatomic regions as the cranial cavity above and the thoracic cavity below.

The unfortunate and often tragic consequences of too limited surgical ability in this regard are several. To begin with, the possibilities of surgery may not even be considered in certain cases of advanced though nevertheless resectable growths and, therefore, there may be a preemptory assignment of too high a proportion of cases to the "inoperable" and therefore (by implication) to the "incurable" classification. The same limited perspective also may lead to "backing out" of an operation already in progress for the reason that the disease is ruled to be "inoperable" because it is found to be more extensive than was expected preoperatively. Examples of such untoward extensions may be those which involve the bony walls of the orbit, cribriform plate, the superior and/or bony posterior walls of the antral cavity, invasion of the common or internal carotid arteries, the superior mediastinum or a pleural cavity, and even the axilla. Surely no one could reasonably maintain that the technical ability to cope with such problems can be attained except by full preliminary training in general surgery. It is my opinion that comprehensive surgery of the head and neck for cancer cannot flourish other than as a sub-specialty of general surgery in which the most reliable verification of proficiency is certification by the American Board of Surgery. Proficiency in this sub-specialty can then be developed and maintained only by its continued active practice.

HAYES MARTIN, M.D.

PROLEGOMENA

The development of head and neck surgery as a specialty has become a significant aspect of American surgery. The basic concept of regional surgery is dramatically exhibited in the host of anatomical structures, physiological functions and organs contained in this area. An intermingling of otolaryngologists, general surgeons, plastic surgeons, oncologists and maxillofacial surgeons creates a lively academic and technical interest in the problems in the region of the head and neck.

There has been an increasing need for the organization and classification of the material encountered in this region. As the subject has matured, illustrative documentation of the surgical procedures applicable to this area in a single volume has become essential.

Dr. John M. Loré, Jr. has created a splendid compendium of illustrations of the essential surgical procedures and techniques in the region of the head and neck. The generous and artistic illustrations give the work appealing authenticity. Beyond this is the succinct presentment of essential diagnostic procedures, basic surgical techniques, congenital abnormalities and a solid exhibition of extirpative procedures for cancerous growths about the head and neck, and the pertinent fundamental plastic and rehabilitative procedures relating to these techniques. The simplicity of this work matches its significance and will prove to be a milestone in this work.

JOHN J. CONLEY, M.D.

PREFACE

Eleven years have passed since the publication of the first edition of this atlas. The convictions expressed in the preface of the first edition are reiterated here and, in addition to them, the grave importance of the cooperation of the various disciplines involved in surgery of the head and neck —both in the management of patients and in the training of residents—is emphasized. The combined efforts, contributions, cooperation and sharing of patient problems and management must be part of every aim in medicine and surgery, especially in head and neck surgery in which there is so much overlap among the various disciplines.

Fortunately, during the past five years, a definite cooperative trend among the prime disciplines of general surgery, otolaryngology, plastic and reconstructive surgery and oral surgery has been developing. A number of various types of combined head and neck services at universities known to the author are participants in this trend—the State University of New York at Buffalo, Northwestern University, the University of Virginia and Yale University—and others are surely in existence. However, even more important than these services is the emergence of a spirit of cooperation which has been spread as seeds throughout the surgical community. Unfortunately, among the fruitful seeds are still the weeds which attempt to choke out the wheat because of inherent parochialism, insecurity, jealousy and greed of power or whatever. Regardless of the type of arrangement of a combined venture, its success or failure depends not so much on signed documents as on a spirit of equal cooperation, understanding and trustworthiness. To *insist* that a combined head and neck service lies solely within one discipline or is a subspecialty of general surgery is to lead the entire endeavor to certain doom.

Flexibility should be tolerated. For example, if need be, a multidiscipline head and neck service could be established within one department and thus achieve an objective similar to that of a head and neck service which involves more than one department. It is interesting to note that during the past decade otolaryngology has made significant strides and at present is believed by many to be the prime discipline in the complete training of the head and neck surgeon.

The problem does not appear to lie among the various head and neck surgeons of different backgrounds but rather with certain autocratic and political forces who attempt to control a major portion of surgery—the so-called "umbrella of general surgery," an antiquated and obsolete concept. However, it is the conviction that general surgery serves as the foundation and the specialties as the superstructure. Therefore it appears that the concept of regional surgery of the head and neck will be the end-result.

It was not so long ago that mutual scorn and distrust between several disciplines were so intense that any exchange of ideas was tantamount to proclaimed heresy. Now, it is changing toward a mood of basic ecumenicalism. The two head and neck societies, the Society of Head and Neck Surgeons and the American Society for Head and Neck Surgery, have had a joint meeting in 1973—an event which might well have been unthinkable a few years ago. Both societies have opened their memberships to capable surgeons in the various disciplines with similar standards and requirements. It is believed that this cooperation is leading to a more complete exchange of ideas and that this can be achieved without the destruction of some of the good points of a competitive climate.

As we proceed along the common pathway, a number of questions are encountered. For example:
1. What does the field of head and neck surgery encompass?
2. What is the need in quality and quantity of surgeons well trained in this field?
3. Should all residents in general surgery, otolaryngology and plastic and reconstructive surgery be trained as head and neck surgeons?
4. What should this training entail?
5. Should there be a cooperative effort among the various disciplines or boards, and if so, how best is this objective achieved?
6. Should there be a certificate of competency issued by the various boards involved?
7. Is some type of basic framework for residency training desirable, or rather, should there be an individual solution to the training problem at the various larger centers?

These queries cannot be answered or solved overnight, and yet a few responses are possible at present.

The field and training in head and neck surgery should have a broad base and be flexible. Individual surgeons and groups of surgeons may have their own specific interests; there is no criticism of this action. Nevertheless, it is important that the trainee develop a versatility in the changing world of medicine and surgery, and hence it is believed that to have a lasting and firm foundation head and neck surgery should encompass four categories:
1. Malignant and benign tumors.
2. Reconstructive surgery.
3. Congenital lesions.
4. Infectious surgical diseases.

Thus it is quite obvious that such training crosses and encompasses a number of specialties as we know them today. The old boundaries are no longer valid nor practical, and the new boundaries are far more flexible.

It must be emphasized that the various surgical specialties, as well as general surgery, are not in existence for their own benefit but rather for the promotion of ultimate excellence in patient care.

Another point appears quite clear. There is not a need for a large number of head and neck surgeons, but rather a need for a moderate number (how many??) of well trained head and neck surgeons. For example, many of the procedures outlined in this atlas are not intended for the occasional operator with limited background, but are intended as a reminder or review for those well educated in the overall field of head and neck surgery. For the latter audience, this atlas may be a source of material in the ever-continuing field of medical education.

During the past six years as a program director, the author has realized a number of problems. First of all, not all residents in either otolaryngology, general surgery or plastic surgery need be, nor should be, trained as head and neck surgeons per se. Secondly, a solid block of time in general surgery (two to four years) followed by a solid block of time in otolaryngology (three years) has certain drawbacks. There is a psychological problem of a candidate being a senior resident in general surgery and then starting at the bottom in otolaryngology. This is no small matter. Another problem is that of graded training in both fields. It would seem much easier to train a resident in physical diagnosis in both specialties at an early stage in his career. The same comparison goes for the senior levels in which major surgery will be performed. It is at this stage of one's training that senior responsibility in both specialties should be achieved, almost side by side, and certainly not separated by several years, as is the case in the solid block concepts.

At any rate, it appears worthwhile to outline an integrated step-wise plan for head and neck surgical training, which recently has been passed by both the American Board of Otolaryngology and the Conference Committee on Graduate Education in Surgery, representing the American Board of Surgery, the American College of Surgeons and the Council of Medical Education of the American Medical Association. This experimental program, applicable to certain selected candidates with approval on an individual basis, exists at the State University of New York at Buffalo with instruction in otolaryngology, general surgery and plastic surgery.

This concept was originally planned with the cooperation of John R. Paine, then Chairman of the Department of Surgery. Glenn Leak played an integral part in the original outline. With the untimely passing of both of these friends, G. Worthington Schenk, Jr., now Chairman of the Department of Surgery, gave his support and effort to achieve the final approval of this plan. The program entails a five-year residency which, in step-wise fashion, integrates in graded responsibility the basic aspects of otolaryngology and general surgery and the principles of plastic surgery. The years in training would alternate between general surgery and otolaryngology, with plastic surgery training incorporated within general surgery, and additional reconstructive surgery within otolaryngology. Senior resident levels in both general surgery and otolaryngology would be reached in the final two years. Not all residents in either of these two fields would be included in the program—only one or two at the most in any one year. Nor is this program intended to be the only avenue of training in head and neck surgery.

In summary, the second edition of this atlas is directed to the ecumenical approach in both patient care and resident training in the field of head and neck surgery.

REFERENCES

Baker, H. W.: Head and neck surgery: The pursuit of excellence. Amer. J. Surg., 122:433–436, 1971.

Beahrs, O. H.: The next plateau. Amer. J. Surg., 114:483–485, 1967.

Bordley, J. E.: Problems facing otolaryngology today. Ann. Otol., 80:783, 1971.

Chase, R. A.: I'm against a rigid core curriculum prior to specialty training in plastic surgery. Plast. Reconstr. Surg., 46:384–388, 1970.

Chase, R. A.: The "core knowledge" principle and erosion of specialty barriers in surgical Training. Ann. Surg., 171:987–990, 1970.

Eckert, C. (panel member): Panel discussion: Head and neck surgical training. Medical Society of the State of New York Convention, February 1972.

Fitz-Hugh, G. S. (panel member): Panel discussion: Head and neck surgical training. Medical Society of the State of New York Convention, February 1972.

James, A. G.: Board to Death. Amer. J. Surg., 116:477–481, 1968.

Klopp, C. T.: Presidential address. Tenth annual meeting of Society of Head and Neck Surgeons. Amer. J. Surg., 108:451–455, 1964.

Loré, J. M., Jr.: Editorial. Head and neck surgery. Surg. Gynec. Obstet. 118:117–118, 1964.

Loré, J. M., Jr.: Future of head and neck surgery. A combined head and neck service: An ecumenical approach. Arch. Otolaryng. 87:659–664, 1968.

Loré, J. M., Jr.: Head and neck surgery: The problem. Arch. Otolaryng. 78:842–843, 1963.

Loré, J. M., Jr.: Head and neck surgery: Proposed head and neck training program. Arch. Otolaryng. 79:112–113, 1964.

MacComb, W. S.: Future of the head and neck cancer surgeon. Amer. J. Surg., *118*:651–653, 1969.

McCormack, R. M. (panel member): Panel discussion: Head and neck surgical training. Medical Society of the State of New York Convention, February 1972.

Sisson, G. A.: Otolaryngology, maxillofacial surgery embark on challenging course. From the Department of Otolaryngology and Maxillofacial Surgery, Northwestern University, Evanston, Illinois.

Southwick, H. W.: Presidential address. Eleventh annual meeting of the Society of Head and Neck Surgeons. Amer. J. Surg., *110*:499–501, 1965.

Wullstein, H. L.: A concept for the future of otorhinolaryngology. Ann. Otol., 77:805–814, 1968.

ACKNOWLEDGMENTS

As with the first edition, my prime indebtedness is to my wife Chalis, who single-handedly transcribed the changes in the first edition and all the new text for this expanded second edition. In addition to the manuscript, she typed the bibliography with some help in classification from my daughters Margaret and Joan.

The medical artist and illustrator is the same skilled and dedicated one — Robert Wabnitz. Without him, this atlas simply would not be. His persistence in accuracy and consistent drive for detail is obvious in the artwork. To him, also, am I deeply indebted.

Again I am thankful to my mother for her encouragement and prayers.

For his revisions and statistics relative to temporal bone resection, I am thankful to John S. Lewis, M.D.

I wish to thank William R. Nelson, M.D., who has contributed a new section on pre- and postoperative care. He has been kind enough to condense a much larger treatise on this aspect of head and neck surgery which he originally produced in booklet form.

Gratitude is extended to James Upson, M.D., for his review of the section on surgery of degenerative vascular lesions and to John Bozer, M.D., as a consultant internist.

I also wish to thank a number of photographers at the various hospitals affiliated with the Medical School at the State University of New York at Buffalo. They are Sheldon Dukoff and Charles Jackson, of the Edward J. Meyer Memorial Hospital; Joseph A. Dommer and Doug Hanes, of Buffalo General Hospital; and Harold C. Baitz, Theodore A. Scott and their secretary, Mrs. Alfred Davis, of the Medical Illustration Service of the Veterans Administration Hospital, Buffalo, New York. Although many of their photographs do not appear in the atlas, they served as a guide for the artwork and the text.

Thanks also go to Joan R. Bilger, R.N., of the Edward J. Meyer Memorial Hospital, for help in preparing some of the photographic arrangements and supplying other technical data; and to Bette Stinchfield, my secretary at the Buffalo General Hospital, for aid in obtaining some of the reference material.

During the time between editions, many new techniques and modifications have reached the surgical arena, a significant number of changes have occurred and friends have lent their ideas and methods; however, one bit of philosophical admonition comes to mind — *primum non nocere* — first, do no harm. I know not the originator of this phrase, but to Julius Pomerantz, a senior fellow physician from Good Samaritan Hospital, Suffern, New York, I am indebted. It is to my residents who have also contributed unwittingly to this endeavor that I often pass on this thought in the management of our patients.

A great debt of gratitude is due the entire staff of the W. B. Saunders Company for their unparalleled aid in publishing this atlas. Their continuing help both as publisher and personal friends makes an otherwise burdensome task possible; their skill in the art of publication makes it all worthwhile.

JOHN M. LORÉ, JR.

PREFACE
TO THE FIRST EDITION

The purpose and intent of this atlas is to encompass in one volume related regional procedures of the head and neck. It is actually a plea for a broader training program to reunite with basic general surgery the many surgical specialties and subspecialties concerned in this area. Surely, there will always be a need for such specialty groups alone but there is an even greater need for the amalgamation and dissemination of their skills in the total treatment of problems of the head and neck. The foundation upon which this concept is built is the basic principle that general surgery is the mother and nurturer of all major surgery. The specialties are the fruits. Hence, general surgery as well as the specialties of otolaryngology, plastic and reconstructive surgery, maxillofacial surgery, neurosurgery, oral surgery and thoracic surgery is involved. Disease knows not the man-made barriers that have been set up.

Each field can contribute to the others. One has only to reflect on the importance of mirror laryngoscopy before and after thyroid surgery. Adequate examination of the larynx is felt to be a sine qua non for any surgeon who performs a thyroidectomy just as a sigmoidoscopy should be performed by the surgeon who performs the abdominoperineal resection. For anyone who does major surgery in the neck, extension of resectability must not be hampered by a lack of familiarity with thoracic surgery when the disease has extended below the clavicles. This principle holds true for both malignant disease and trauma. Major surgery on the larynx sooner or later will involve the cervical esophagus and basic knowledge of bowel surgery will enhance the armamentarium of the surgeon and aid in his decision when selecting the most suitable type of esophageal reconstruction. Procedures on the nose, except the very simplest, can be refined and well selected only when the surgeon borrows from the otolaryngologist, the plastic and reconstructive surgeon and the general tumor surgeon.

The skills and tricks of one field are often applicable to another field. In the definitive treatment of malignant tumors the details of an elaborate reconstruction procedure are of little avail unless the primary disease has been handled correctly with full knowledge of the natural history of the disease. By the same token, radical surgical treatment is incomplete if a suitable and adaptable reconstructive procedure or prosthesis has been omitted purely through a lack of versatility. Obstructive vascular disease affecting the intracranial circulation amenable to surgical correction may have its center of trouble located either in the chest or neck or in both regions. The selection of the best-suited vascular procedure is enhanced by a working knowledge of general vascular surgery.

With anticipation of the criticism that such a concept would lead to a Jack-of-all-trades, master of none, one need but read the history of surgery. Many of the great surgeons of yesterday were first primarily general surgeons; with this basic knowledge they contributed lasting ideas both in the specialty fields and in general surgery. Billroth was the master of gastrectomy and at the same time contributed to cleft palate repair by fracturing the hamulus of the pterygoid process, thus releasing the tensor veli palatini muscle. King, a general surgeon, made a significant contribution in the treatment of bilateral abductor cord paralysis of the larynx. Such examples are not intended to detract from the innumerable contributions by the surgical specialists which in their own fields outnumber these examples. Nor is the concept that is portrayed in this atlas intended to lessen or minimize in any way the need for the specialist. Actually it supports the specialist and re-emphasizes the natural evolution of surgery.

John Henry Cardinal Newman in his classic *The Idea of a University* advocated a liberal education which would serve as the background for future endeavors. He pointed out that any student able "to think and to reason and to compare and to discriminate and to analyze, who has refined his taste, and formed his judgment will not indeed at once be a lawyer, or a pleader, or an orator, or a statesman or a physician . . . but he will be placed in that state of intellect in which he can take up any one of the sciences or callings . . . with an ease, a grade, a versatility, and a success to which another is a stranger." So in the art and science of surgery, a liberal basic foundation is necessary. From such a foundation and broad outlook, the field of head and neck surgery seems to have drifted. Reunification of all groups interested in the field of surgical problems related to the head and neck is the intention, hope and aim of this Atlas of surgical techniques.

JOHN M. LORÉ, JR.

ACKNOWLEDGMENTS
IN THE FIRST EDITION

I am deeply grateful to my wife, Chalis, for her sacrifice, patience and able skill as an executive secretary. She has typed and retyped the manuscript under considerable duress.

My children, John III, Peter, Margaret and Joan, have all felt the pressures and sacrifices resulting from the loss of many happy hours together which have been missed because of the time consumed in the preparation of this work.

I am indebted to my mother for her encouragement and prayers.

Professionally, my indebtedness extends from books, journals and other collections of the surgical literature, through various opinions voiced at surgical meetings (the authors of which I regret to say have slipped my memory), to my recent and past teachers and associates. All education is a compendium, and even more so surgical education. Hence many of the steps in this atlas are the ideas, thoughts and work of surgeons under whom I have trained or worked. I owe much to my father and to John J. Conley who were my early teachers. A great many of the surgical procedures and techniques concerned with the treatment of tumors of the head and neck either originated with or were developed by Hayes Martin and other surgeons on the Head and Neck Service of Memorial Hospital. In the basic background of general surgery which forms an integral part of this atlas, I owe a debt of great magnitude to John L. Madden, Director of Surgery at Saint Clare's Hospital.

To make the decision after my father's death to continue surgical training in general surgery after completion of the first phase in otolaryngology presented a crisis. Two men convinced me and gave me advice of immeasurable value. They are Michael Deddish, M.D., and Alexander Conte, M.D. Without them I never would have completed my surgical training and never would have come to realize the benefits of a multifaceted surgical background.

John S. Lewis, M.D., who is mainly responsible for the present technique of temporal bone resection in cancer of the middle ear, has kindly contributed to that section of the atlas.

Edward Scanlon, M.D., has been kind in lending his original experiences and thoughts in colon transplants for reconstruction of the esophagus. These ideas have been of considerable aid and have been a guide to personal experiences in this problem. Again to Alexander Conte my thanks for supplying original photographs of his technique of cervical esophageal reconstruction.

During the two years of pressure to complete this work, my surgical partner, Louis J. Wagner, M.D., has unselfishly covered our practice to allow me the necessary undisturbed time. From him, I have also learned a number of operative steps which have been successful in the solution of some technical problems.

When this atlas was in its infancy, it was only through the cooperation of John L. Madden and the administration of Saint Clare's Hospital, specifically the late Mother M. Alice, O.S.F., and her successor Sister M. Columcille, O.S.F., that actual work began. At Saint Clare's Hospital I met Robert Wabnitz, the sole illustrator of this volume, who since then has spent many hours in the operating room making sketches and at the drawing board completing the art work. Without his skill as an artist and his knowledge of anatomy, the illustrations would have been impossible. Both he and I are grateful to the University of Rochester where he now heads the Medical Illustration Department for allowing him time to complete this work. If it were not for the skill in its reproduction, the best of art work would be for naught. The W. B. Saunders Company has excellently completed this endeavor. I am deeply indebted to the staff of the Company for their advice, suggestions and patience. I am grateful to my colleague William J. McCann, M.D., for initiating this most fortunate association with the Saunders Company.

I wish also to acknowledge the cooperation of the Administrator and Assistant Administrator of Good Samaritan Hospital, Sister Miriam Thomas and Sister Joseph Rita, as well as the Operating Room Supervisor, Miss Martha Henry, and the entire nursing staff for their help and vision in the treatment and care of the patients with many of these operative and postoperative problems. I would be remiss if I did not add the aid of the administration and staff of Tuxedo Memorial Hospital.

My thanks to Anthony Paul for drawing many of the lead lines and some of the labels and to David Hastings for his care in photographing the x-rays in Chapter I.

JOHN M. LORÉ, JR.

CONTENTS

1. SECTIONAL RADIOGRAPHIC ANATOMY

Sagittal Section Through the Midportion of the Maxillary Sinus
  and Orbit
Sagittal Section Through the Lateral Wall of the Nose, Lateral Border
  of the Tongue and Lamina of the Thyroid Cartilage Showing Its
  Superior and Inferior Cornua
Sagittal Section Through the Floor of the Nose and the Body
  of the Tongue
Sagittal Section Through the Middle of the Skull
Frontal Section in the Region of the Second Molar Teeth
Frontal Section Just Beyond the Third Molar Teeth
Frontal Section in the Region of the Anterior Faucial Pillar and Tonsil

The following seven radiographic plates are part of a series of sagittal and frontal sections of the head and neck made almost thirty-five years ago by John M. Loré, Sr. Their purpose at that time was to study the anatomy primarily in relation to deep infections of the neck. Since then such infections have become almost a surgical curiosity, yet the basic anatomy portrayed by this technique is believed to be of considerable value to both the surgeon and the radiologist. Both the actual relationship of bony structures and that of soft tissue are well depicted in the original x rays with some interpretation in the facing color illustration.

The technique of their preparation began with cadaver sections, for the most part one-half inch thick. The sections were fixed in formaldehyde and allowed to dry a little so that there would be some separation of the various structures in the specimens. Radiographs were then made of the sections. In the original presentation of this material, read at the New York Academy of Medicine, Section on Otolaryngology, December 21, 1938 and published in Laryngoscope, June, 1939, Dr. Loré, Sr., acknowledged assistance in this work thus: "For the material, the late Professor Senior and his successor, Professor Sheehan, of the Anatomy Department of the Medical School of New York University, have been more than generous. For the X-ray work, Dr. Frederick Law, of the Manhattan Eye, Ear, Nose and Throat Hospital, and the X-ray department of St. Vincent's Hospital have been most helpful and unstinting in their aid."

More recently the color plates have been developed with the aid of Robert Wabnitz. Each plate alone and all as a group should aid in the understanding of sinus surgery, both limited and radical, as well as fractures of the facial bones and related skull fractures.

SAGITTAL SECTION THROUGH THE MIDPORTION OF THE MAXILLARY SINUS AND ORBIT

The posterior relations of the maxillary sinus to the floor of the middle cranial fossa are clearly depicted. The roof of the maxillary sinus forms the floor of the orbit and the floor of the maxillary sinus forms the roof of the alveolar ridge. Within this latter structure are seen the upper teeth protruding almost into the sinus cavity. This anatomy is important in minor operations on the maxillary sinus as well as in partial or total resections of the maxilla for carcinoma. The course of the internal carotid artery and the carotid canal in the base of the skull is seen, with the jugular foramen slightly posterior. Temporal bone resection reaches almost this depth, being somewhat lateral to this.

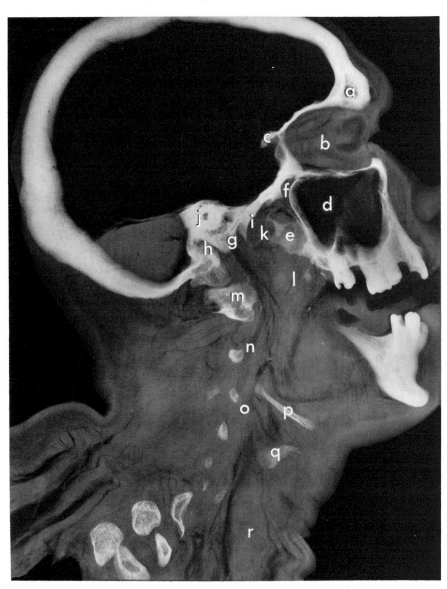

a. Frontal sinus
b. Optic nerve
c. Anterior clinoid process
d. Maxillary sinus
e. Lateral pterygoid plate of sphenoid bone
f. Pterygomaxillary fissure

g. Carotid canal
h. Jugular foramen
i. Foramen spinosum (for middle meningeal artery)
j. Petrous portion of temporal bone
k. Upper and lower heads of external pterygoid muscle

Plate 1   Sectional Radiographic Anatomy

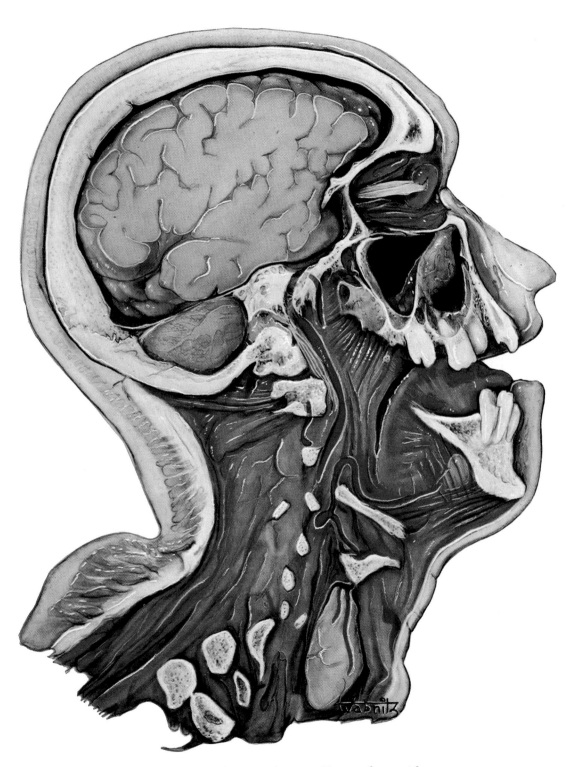

l. Deep and superficial head of internal pterygoid muscle
m. First cervical vertebra or atlas
n. Internal carotid artery
o. External carotid artery
p. Hyoid bone
q. Portion of thyroid cartilage
r. Thyroid gland

SAGITTAL SECTION THROUGH THE LATERAL WALL OF THE NOSE, LATERAL BORDER OF THE TONGUE AND LAMINA OF THE THYROID CARTILAGE SHOWING ITS SUPERIOR AND INFERIOR CORNUA

The continuity of the posterior ethmoid sinus cells to the sphenoid sinus is shown. The section includes the medial wall of the orbit which is the lateral wall of the ethmoid sinus and incidentally very thin. With the major portion of the middle turbinate excluded, the underlying maxillary sinus is visible.

The main extrinsic tongue muscle—the genioglossus—is easily seen with its attachment to the mandible. Also noteworthy are the relationships of the hyoid bone, thyroid cartilage and cricoid cartilage.

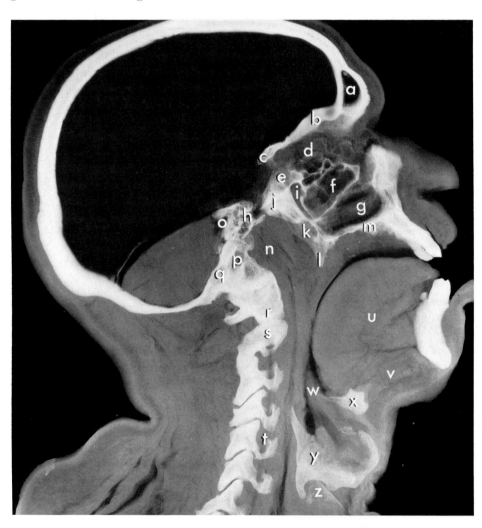

a.	Frontal sinus	**j.**	Pterygoid canal
b.	Orbital plate of frontal bone forming floor of anterior cranial fossa	**k.**	Medial pterygoid plate of sphenoid bone
c.	Anterior clinoid process	**l.**	Hamulus of pterygoid
d.	Ethmoid sinus or labyrinth	**m.**	Hard palate and floor of nose
e.	Sphenoid sinus	**n.**	Longus capitis muscle
f.	Underlying maxillary sinus	**o.**	Internal auditory meatus
g.	Inferior turbinate	**p.**	Hypoglossal canal
h.	Carotid canal leading to foramen lacerum	**q.**	Jugular bulb
i.	Pterygopalatine fossa	**r.**	First cervical vertebra or atlas
		s.	Second cervical vertebra or axis

4

Plate 2   Sectional Radiographic Anatomy

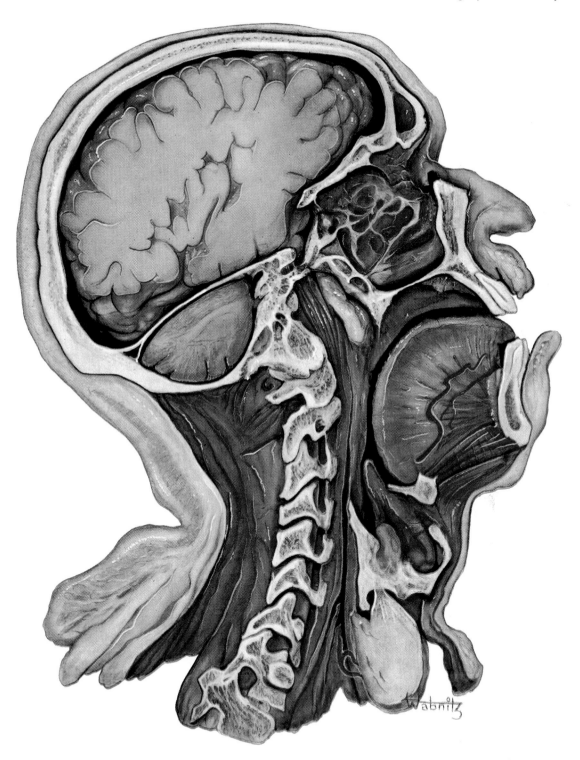

t. Vertebral artery
u. Lingual artery within genioglossus muscle
v. Geniohyoid muscle

w. Epiglottis
x. Hyoid bone
y. Thyroid cartilage
z. Cricoid cartilage

SAGITTAL SECTION THROUGH THE FLOOR OF THE NOSE AND
THE BODY OF THE TONGUE

Except for the superior turbinate, the structures of the lateral wall of the nose are well visualized. The prevertebral space is seen extending from the base of the skull inferiorly toward the thorax. Note the relationship of the ethmoid sinus to the floor of the anterior cranial fossa and its continuity posteriorly with the sphenoid sinus. Within the sphenoid sinus is the cradle for the pituitary gland, the sella turcica.

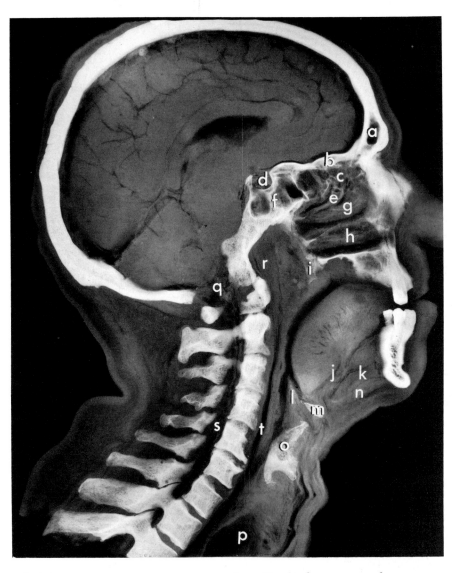

a.	Frontal sinus	**k.**	Genioglossus muscle
b.	Cribriform plate of ethmoid	**l.**	Epiglottis
c.	Ethmoid sinus or labyrinth	**m.**	Hyoid bone
d.	Pituitary gland	**n.**	Geniohyoid muscle
e.	Uncinate process of ethmoid bone	**o.**	Thyroid cartilage
f.	Sphenoid sinus	**p.**	Trachea
g.	Middle turbinate	**q.**	Foramen magnum
h.	Inferior turbinate	**r.**	Longus capitis muscle
i.	Pterygoid process of sphenoid bone	**s.**	Spinal cord
j.	Lingual artery within genioglossus muscle and hyoglossus muscle	**t.**	Prevertebral space

Plate 3   Sectional Radiographic Anatomy

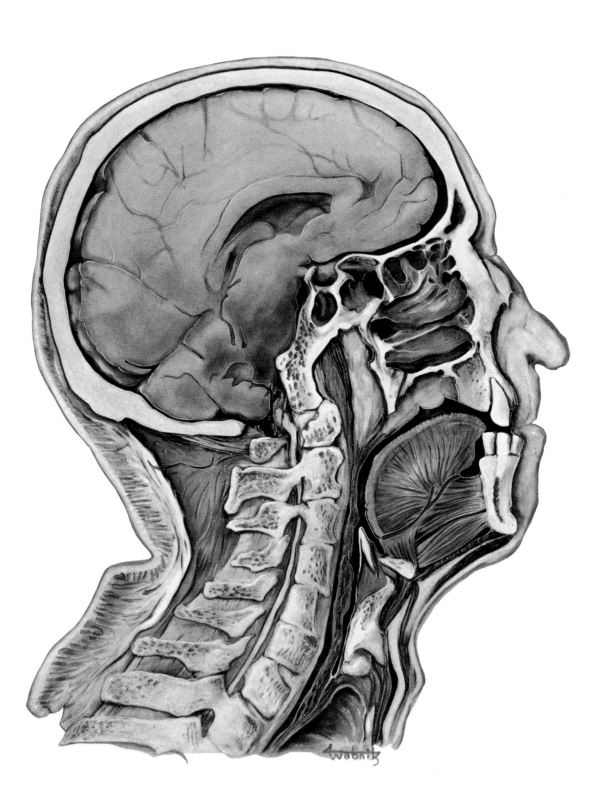

The relationship of the nasal septum to the anterior wall of the sphenoid sinus is visualized, demonstrating the route of the trans-septal approach to the pituitary. The surface anatomy at the base of the tongue and the interior of the larynx is seen. At the entrance to the cervical esophagus, the lower-most fibers of the inferior pharyngeal constrictor muscle —the cricopharyngeus—are hypertrophied with an **S** type curve to the lumen. This explains some of the difficulty that may be encountered during the introduction of the esophagoscope. The tendency of the so-called postcricoid carcinoma of the larynx to esophageal spread is explained by this view.

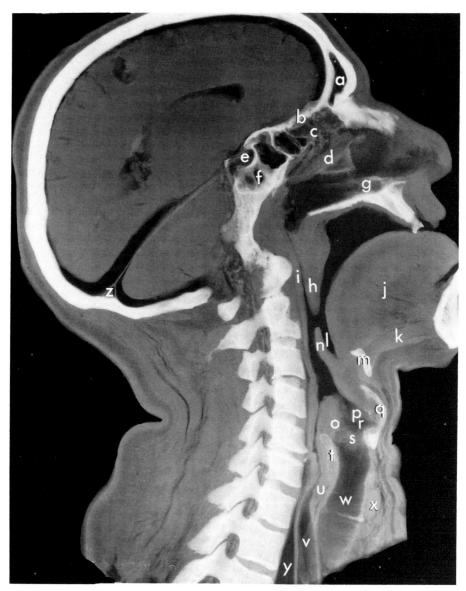

a.	Frontal sinus	**j.**	Genioglossus muscle
b.	Cribriform plate of ethmoid	**k.**	Geniohyoid muscle
c.	Ethmoid sinus or labyrinth	**l.**	Vallecula
d.	Perpendicular plate of ethmoid	**m.**	Hyoid bone
e.	Pituitary	**n.**	Epiglottis
f.	Sphenoid sinus	**o.**	Arytenoid
g.	Vomer bone	**p.**	Ventricular band
h.	Soft palate and uvula	**q.**	Thyroid cartilage
i.	Superior pharyngeal constrictor muscle	**r.**	Ventricle

Plate 4   Sectional Radiographic Anatomy

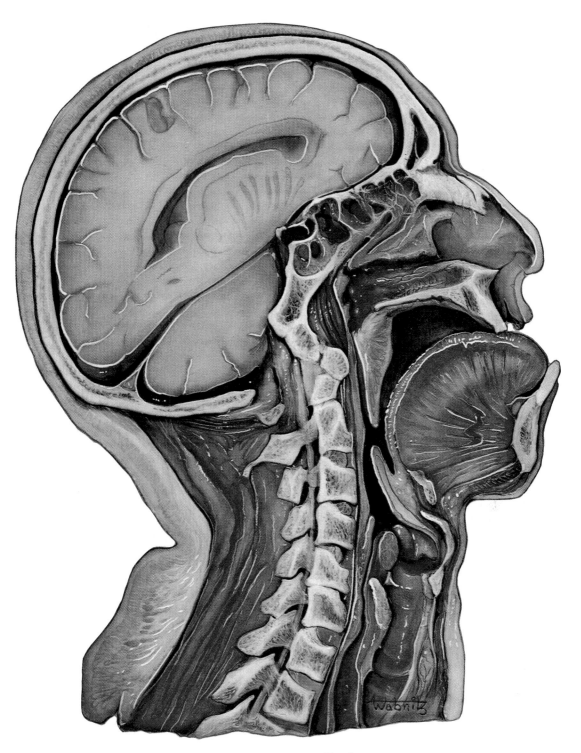

s. True vocal cord
t. Posterior aspect of cricoid cartilage
u. Cricopharyngeus portion of inferior constrictor muscle of pharynx
v. Lumen of cervical esophagus
w. Trachea
x. Thyroid isthmus
y. Prevertebral space
z. Straight sinus

Note the thin wall forming the boundary between the ethmoid sinus and the orbit. The variable relationship of the floor of the maxillary sinus to the floor of the nose is represented. Between the sublingual gland and the submaxillary gland is the mylohyoid muscle originating from the mylohyoid line on the mandible. Fractures of the infraorbital rim usually occur through the thinned area of the infraorbital foramen, always involving to a greater or a lesser degree the maxillary sinus itself.

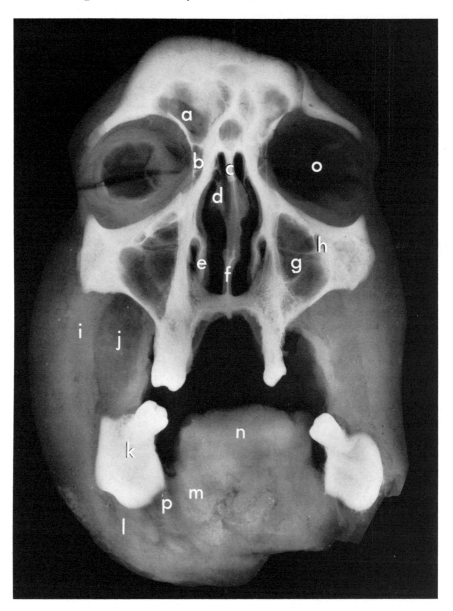

a.	Frontal sinus	**i.**	Masseter muscle
b.	Anterior ethmoid sinus	**j.**	Buccal fat pad
c.	Perpendicular plate of ethmoid	**k.**	Mandible
d.	Middle turbinate	**l.**	Submaxillary salivary gland
e.	Inferior turbinate	**m.**	Sublingual salivary gland
f.	Vomer bone	**n.**	Tongue
g.	Maxillary sinus	**o.**	Orbit
h.	Infraorbital foramen	**p.**	Mylohyoid muscle

Plate 5   Sectional Radiographic Anatomy

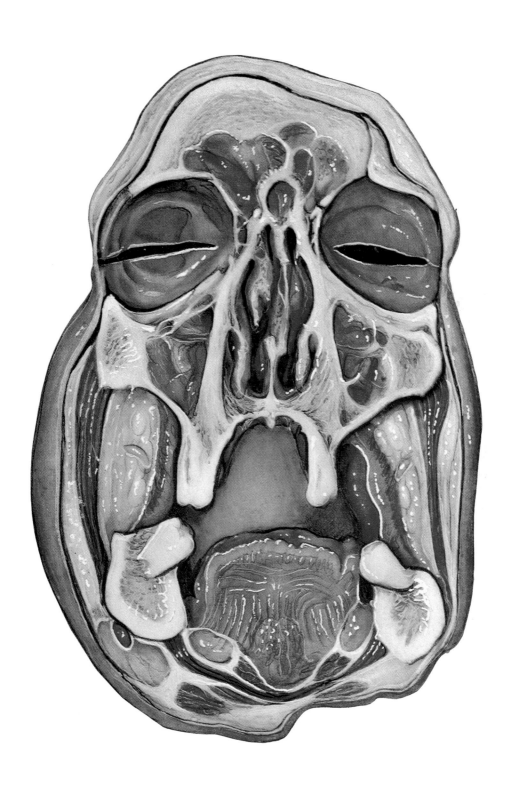

FRONTAL SECTION JUST BEYOND THE THIRD MOLAR TEETH

As in the previous section, the thin bony boundary between the ethmoid sinus and orbit is depicted. The conservative approach to the ethmoid sinus for drainage purposes and moderate exenteration is just above and lateral to the attachment of the middle turbinate. This is easily seen on the right side of the section. Also visualized is the hamulus of the pterygoid process around which courses the tensor veli palatini. It is this process which is fractured in cleft palate repair. For extensive carcinoma of the maxillary sinus, inclusion of the ethmoid sinus en bloc is clearly shown to be the aim of the radical resection including the orbital contents. The relationship of the floor of the maxillary sinus to the floor of the nose is demonstrated, as is the roof of the maxillary sinus to the orbit in blowout fractures.

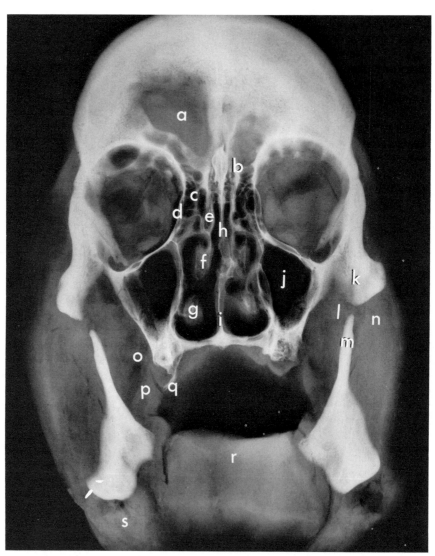

a. Frontal sinus
b. Cribriform plate of ethmoid
c. Ethmoid sinus
d. Medial wall of orbit formed by lacrimal bone and lamina papyracea of ethmoid bone
e. Superior turbinate
f. Middle turbinate
g. Inferior turbinate
h. Perpendicular plate of ethmoid
i. Vomer bone
j. Maxillary sinus
k. Body of malar bone
l. Temporalis muscle
m. Ascending ramus and coronoid process of mandible
n. Masseter muscle
o. External pterygoid muscle

Plate 6   Sectional Radiographic Anatomy

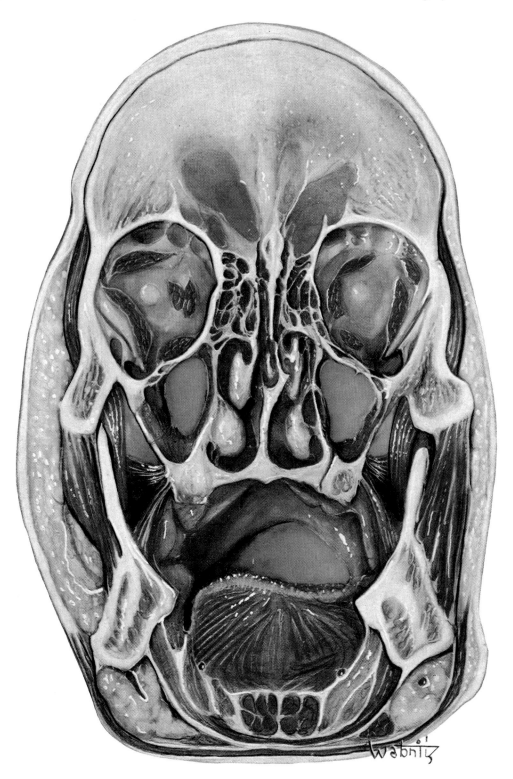

p. Internal pterygoid muscle
q. Hamulus of pterygoid process of sphenoid bone

r. Tongue
s. Submaxillary salivary gland with external maxillary artery

FRONTAL SECTION IN THE REGION OF THE ANTERIOR FAUCIAL PILLAR AND TONSIL

This section demonstrates the structures that are encountered laterally and posteriorly in radical resection of the maxilla and ethmoid sinus for carcinoma. The zygomatic arch is vividly depicted as vulnerable in fractures of the facial bones. Extensive carcinoma of the soft palate involving the tonsil usually requires resection of the pterygoid process of the sphenoid with at least the internal pterygoid muscle. Hemimandibulectomy is seen also to be warranted by the proximity of the mandible to the structures involved.

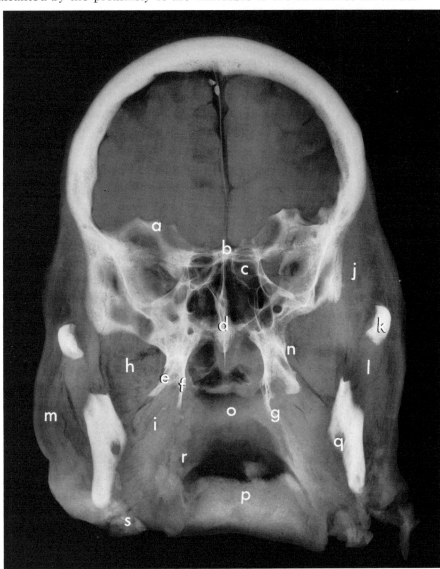

a. Orbital plate of frontal bone
b. Cribriform plate of ethmoid
c. Posterior ethmoid cells
d. Rostrum of sphenoid bone
e. Lateral pterygoid plate of sphenoid bone
f. Medial pterygoid plate of sphenoid bone
g. Hamulus of pterygoid process
h. Upper and lower heads of external pterygoid muscle
i. Internal pterygoid muscle

j. Temporalis muscle
k. Zygomatic arch
l. Masseter muscle
m. Parotid gland
n. Internal maxillary artery
o. Soft palate
p. Tongue
q. Mandibular canal
r. Anterior faucial pillar and tonsil
s. Submaxillary salivary gland

Plate 7   *Sectional Radiographic Anatomy*

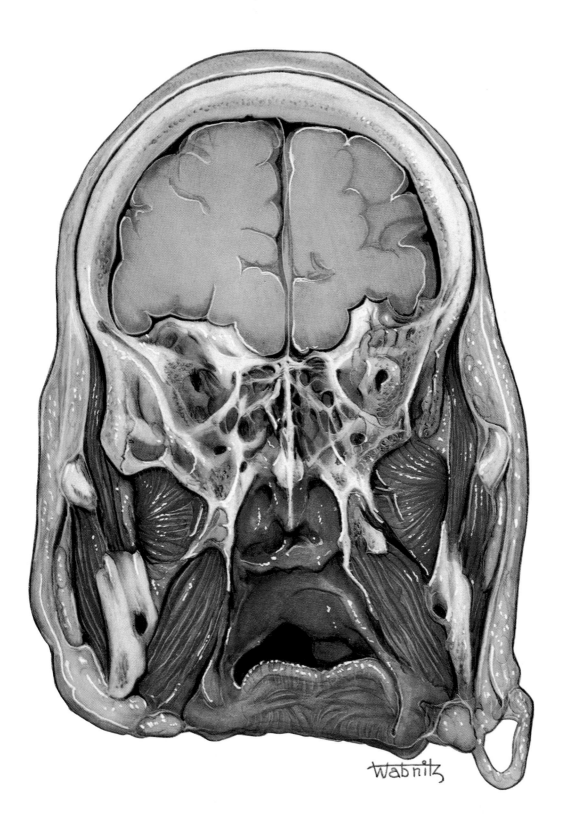

BIBLIOGRAPHY

Gardner, E., Gray, D. J., and O'Rahilly, R.: Anatomy: A Regional Study of Human Structure. 3rd ed. Philadelphia, W. B. Saunders Company, 1969.

Loré J. M.: Deep infections of the neck. Applied anatomy. Laryngoscope *49*: 448–470, 1939.

Quiring, D. P., and Warfel, J. H.: The Head, Neck and Trunk. 2d ed. Philadelphia, Lea and Febiger, 1950.

2. BASIC TECHNIQUES

CARDIORESPIRATORY RESUSCITATION

Cardiac "arrest" and respiratory "arrest" go hand in hand and sometimes it is uncertain which is the initiating culprit, especially relative to head and neck problems. The patient with myocardial infarction usually has his initiating factor on the cardiac side whether it be ventricular fibrillation standstill or collapse, while the patient aspirating blood and heavily sedated usually has his initiating factor on the respiratory side. Synergistic effects are also very possible. Suffice it to say that successful resuscitation requires management of both aspects.

Prevention and recognition of predisposing factors is of paramount importance. Hypertensive patients, whether treated or not, have a propensity to lethal cardiac arrhythmias and arrest on induction of anesthesia. Ten per cent of all cardiac arrests occur on induction. Direct laryngoscopy is also associated with a high incidence of arrhythmias.

Critical time is four minutes.

*Diagnosis**

Type	Heartbeat	EKG	Signs
1. Cardiac standstill	Absent	Flat	Breathing absent
2. Ventricular fibrillation	Uncoordinated	Erratic	Pulse absent
3. Cardiovascular collapse	Rhythmic; ineffective	May be near normal	Pupils dilated

Always continue heart-lung resuscitation without interruption during diagnosis.

*(After Gordon, Palich, and Fletcher, 1965.)

CARDIORESPIRATORY RESUSCITATION (*Continued*)

If at all possible, the following steps are performed simultaneously:

Airway

Neck slightly extended.
Head further extended maximally in relation to neck.
Oropharyngeal airway.
Ambu bag assistance or mouth-to-mouth air exchange.
12 per minute for adults
20 per minute for young children
If this fails, endotracheal tube or bronchoscope.
Anesthesia machine.
Oxygen.
If after five effective exchanges, spontaneous respirations are still absent, pulse is absent and pupils are dilated, commence cardiac "massage."

CLOSED VERSUS OPEN CARDIAC MASSAGE OR COMPRESSION

There is little doubt at this point in time that closed cardiac massage is just as effective — maybe more so — as open cardiac massage except in the patient in the operating room undergoing open thoracotomy, in the patient with a severe chest injury or possibly in the postoperative open thoracotomy patient.

CLOSED MASSAGE RESUSCITATION
(After Kouwenhoven, Jude, and Knickerbocker, 1960)

A 1. Ideally two persons are involved. One person continues respiratory assistance at the rate of one breath between five cardiac compressions.
2. The other person compresses the heart by placing the heel of one hand over the lower half of the sternum (avoiding the xiphoid process) with the heel of the other hand over the first hand (avoid using fingers — avoid pressure on ribs and abdomen).
   a. Elbows straight.
   b. Use weight of body with 60 to 100 lbs. pressure;
   c. depress sternum 4 to 5 cm for 60 to 80 times per minute with smooth regular rhythm — 50 per cent compression and 50 per cent relaxation.
3. Intracardiac epinephrine, 0.5 mg or 0.5 to 1.0 cc (1:1000), intravenously — if no response within two minutes.
4. Place board under patient and continue resuscitation.
5. EKG, check pupils, blood pressure and peripheral pulse.
6. Intravenous cutdown with three-way stopcock.
7. Five to 15 minutes — intravenously and repeat every 10 minutes if necessary:
   a. Sodium bicarbonate (3.75 gm in 50 cc) — combats acidosis and may improve cerebral blood flow.
   b. Calcium gluconate (10 cc of 10 per cent solution) or calcium chloride — increases myocardial tone and cardiac output.
   c. Neosynephrine (20 mgm per 500 cc) by drip.
   d. Procainamide if indicated (100 to 500 mgm slowly) as per EKG toxicity.
8. External defibrillation — a weak ventricular fibrillation usually requires epinephrine to convert to sinus rhythm. Always continue cardiac and respiratory resuscitation during defibrillation.

Plate 8   *Basic Techniques*

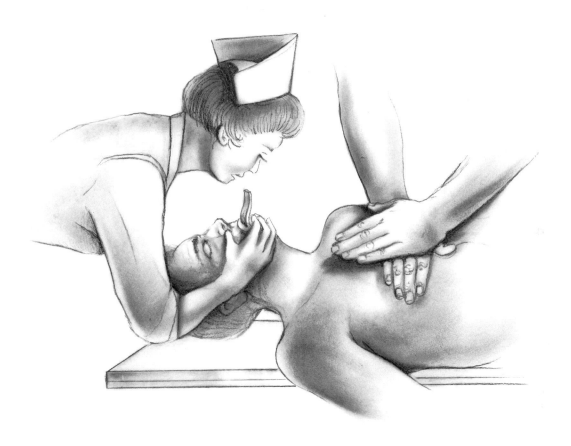

9. Hypothermia—if a lapse period occurs over four minutes or if response is slow and protracted.
10. Continue efforts up to one and one-half hours.
11. Have extra personnel if available; keep record.
12. Feel the peripheral pulse. If there is no response in the peripheral pulse within a minute and the patient is in the operating room, one should then perform open cardiac massage. At this time a check for pulmonary emboli can be done since this may be the cause of the cardiac arrest initially. The Trendelenburg technique (1908) is used by opening the right pulmonary artery and removing any thrombus, and then with a clamp one can check the left pulmonary artery. If feasible, cardio-pulmonary by-pass is initiated for more leisurely removal of pulmonary emboli.

OPEN MASSAGE RESUSCITATION

The supportive measures are the same as under closed massage resuscitation.

Technique

A   An inframammary incision is made. This will be in the region of the fourth or fifth interspace. Clamping vessels at this stage is unnecessary.

B   The pleural cavity is immediately entered, exposing the pericardium medially and the lung laterally.

C   If a suitable rib retractor is available, it is used to open the thoracotomy incision further. A triangular wedge of wood is satisfactory. Using fingers of both hands, compression begins. The rate of massage is between 45 and 60 beats per minute. Pressure by the thumb is to be avoided since rupture of the heart muscle may occur. Adequate time is allowed for the filling phase of the heart. From time to time the massage is interrupted to observe whether the heart beat has returned.

D   If preferred, the pericardium may be opened longitudinally and the massage continued from within the pericardial sac. Injury to cardiac muscle and coronary vessels is to be avoided.

E   Following resuscitation, the wound is inspected for bleeding, especially from the internal mammary and intercostal vessels. A large catheter is inserted through a dependent intercostal space near the anterior axillary line and connected to an underwater drainage bottle. Pericostal sutures of 1-0 chromic catgut in double strands are inserted, avoiding the intercostal neurovascular bundle and the lung expanded by positive pressure.

F   If available, a rib approximator is used, while the intercostal sutures are tied. The intercostal muscles may be approximated with either interrupted or continuous sutures. The remainder of the wound is closed in layers. The catheter is secured with an encircling suture of 2-0 silk.

G   The underwater drainage bottle is kept below the level of the patient and upon return to the recovery room it is secured to the floor (plate 12).

Plate 9   Basic Techniques

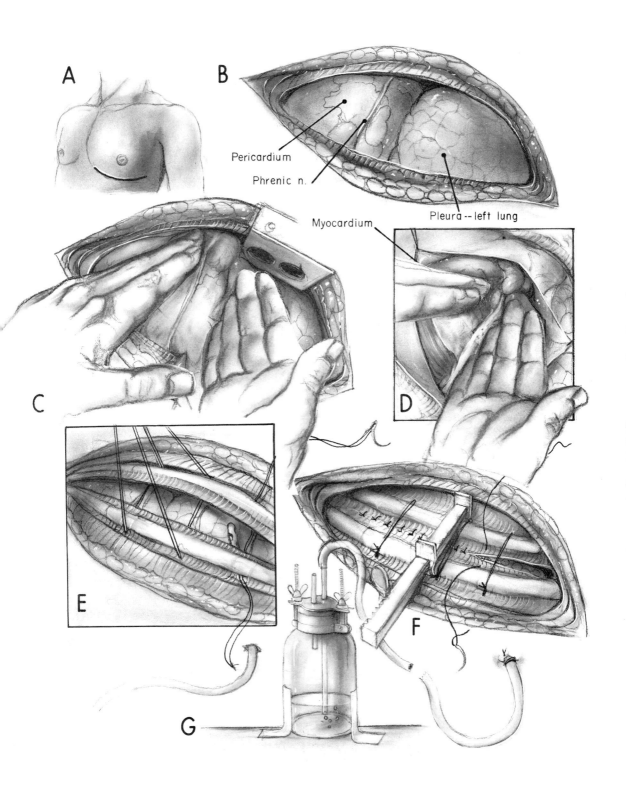

Pericardium

Phrenic n.

Pleura -- left lung

Myocardium

A

B

C

D

E

F

G

THORACENTESIS

Indications

1. For rapid decompression of a pneumothorax or tension pneumothorax.
2. For aspiration of intrapleural fluid.
3. For diagnosis.

Highpoints

1. Insert needle at upper border of selected rib.
2. Use second anterior interspace for pneumothorax.
3. Use seventh or eighth interspace at posterior axillary line for intrapleural fluid or according to x-ray localization.
4. In pneumothorax a single aspiration may suffice, but it is usually safer to replace the needle with an intercostal catheter connected to underwater drainage. This is mandatory in a tension pneumothorax or persistent air leak. If a large leak is present, as evidenced by almost continual bubbling of air through the underwater seal bottle, two or more large catheters may be necessary, each connected to a separate set of underwater drainage bottles.
5. When a tension pneumothorax associated with severe respiratory distress exists, it may be lifesaving to insert any type of needle, knife or sharp instrument into the chest without syringe or any other equipment.

A For pneumothorax or tension pneumothorax the patient is preferably supine. A 15 to 18 gauge needle is inserted in the second anterior interspace (**X**) along the midclavicular line. This location will avoid the internal mammary vessels. If the patient is in acute distress and sitting in an upright position, it is better not to have the patient lie down. The needle is guided along the superior edge of the third rib to avoid the intercostal vessels. In an emergency, no anesthesia is necessary; if time permits local anesthesia is used intradermally with infiltration down to the parietal pleural level.

For aspiration of fluid, the sitting position at the side of the bed resting over a bed stand elevated to breast height is ideal. The site of insertion of the needle depends on the x-ray findings; however, the classic location is through the seventh or eighth interspace at the posterior axillary line.

B A 20 cc or 50 cc syringe with an interposed three-way stopcock is ideal. Rubber tubing or a catheter may be connected to the stopcock if a hydrothorax is present. This facilitates removal of the fluid. In a tension pneumothorax, the barrel of the syringe may be pushed out by the increased intrathoracic pressure. When the proper depth of insertion is reached a straight hemostat immediately clamps the needle at the skin surface, preventing the needle from going any further into the intrapleural space.

INSERTION OF INTERCOSTAL CATHETER

Indications

1. For prolonged underwater drainage.
2. In an emergency tension pneumothorax when other equipment is not available.

Highpoints

Similar to those under thoracentesis.

C A #11 blade knife is inserted in the selected interspace hugging the superior edge of the rib to avoid the neurovascular intercostal bundle.

D With a curved Kelly clamp, the incision is widened both horizontally and vertically.

E Using the Kelly clamp as a guide in the stab wound, a multiholed #26 to #30 French plain rubber catheter is inserted in the thoracic cavity. A straight hemostat is used to grasp the catheter and pass it in through the stab wound.

Plate 10   Basic Techniques

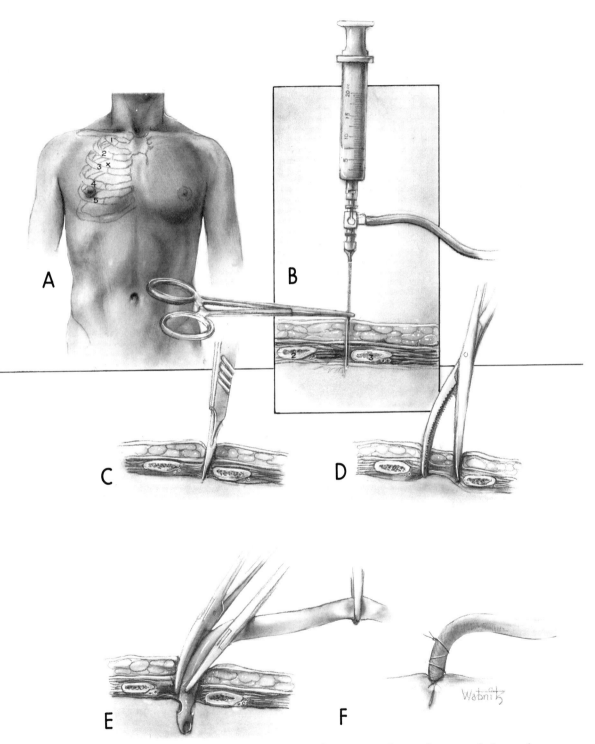

F Silk sutures close the stab wound tightly and are wound snugly around the catheter to help hold it in place. A small dressing of petrolatum and plain gauze with supporting adhesive completes the dressing. The catheter is unclamped after it is connected to the tubing from the underwater drainage system (see plate 12).

G When a large bore trocar with cannula is available, an intercostal catheter is easily inserted. The technique is similar to the method described in the previous plate. The trocar is kept close to the superior border of the rib. A clamp is placed on the catheter before insertion.

H As the cannula is withdrawn, the catheter is inserted.

I After a sufficient length of the catheter has been inserted — at least until all the holes are within the thoracic cavity — the trocar is gradually removed. When the catheter is visible at the skin margin, a clamp grasps the catheter to prevent it from being withdrawn. After the trocar is completely removed, the catheter is connected to the underwater drainage system as shown in plate 12. In infants and children similar results can be achieved by inserting a plastic tubing through the lumen of a large bore needle which has been inserted into the pleural space. The needle can then be removed by withdrawing it along the tubing. Such smaller tubing, however, may become plugged.

J Pictured is a simple self-contained intercostal catheter with an attached needle (after Algird, 1966).

Plate 11   Basic Techniques

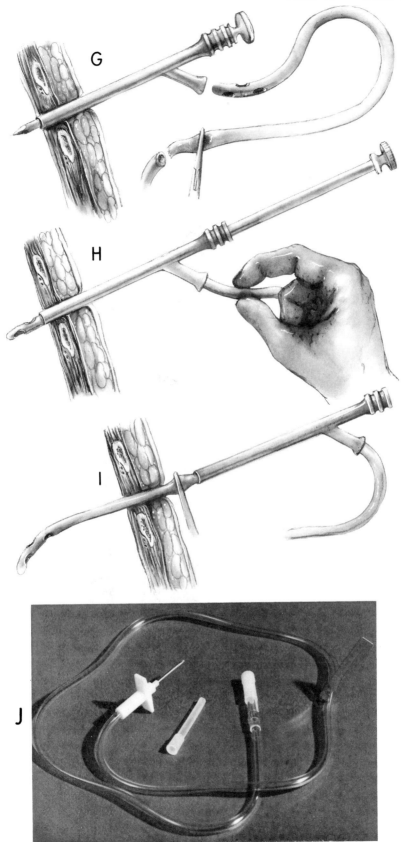

OPEN THORACOTOMY FOR EMPYEMA DRAINAGE

Although thick, purulent empyema of the pleural space is uncommon following head and neck surgery, when this complication does occur open thoracotomy is necessary. Rarely, it may follow deep abscesses of the neck which extend into the mediastinum and then perforate into one or both pleural cavities. Perforation of the esophagus causing mediastinitis may likewise cause empyema, and in addition to drainage of the mediastinum (plate 324) open thoracotomy then becomes necessary.

Highpoints

1. Local anesthesia.
2. Most dependent point should be drained.
3. Resect section of rib and make large opening in pleura.
4. Resect neurovascular bundle.
5. Underwater drainage system not used.

K   An incision is made over the selected rib removing about a 6 cm section of the rib (see plate 334, steps *E*, *F*, *G* and *H*). An elliptical incision is then made in the posterior periosteum and pleura, removing a portion of the periosteum and pleura and making an opening which is larger than would seem necessary since there is a marked tendency for the wound to close too rapidly. It is likewise recommended to excise the dependent neurovascular bundle to minimize pain and delayed hemorrhage resulting from pressure of the drainage tubes.

L   One or two large (1.0 to 1.5 cm in diameter) rubber or plastic tubes with multiple holes are then inserted into the empyemic cavity for drainage. Sutures are either passed through or tied securely around the tubes to prevent their loss in the pleural cavity.

Frequent changes of dressings are necessary. If the pus is thick, the tubes may be irrigated with saline and changed as necessary. As the cavity becomes smaller, the tubes are replaced by a catheter and drainage is continued until the cavity has a volume capacity of less than 5 cc. Prolonged drainage is usually the case and premature removal is to be avoided.

Plate 11   Basic Techniques

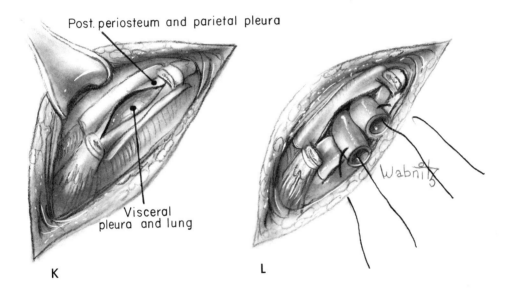

Post. periosteum and parietal pleura

Visceral
pleura and lung

K

L

Wabnitz

INTERCOSTAL CATHETER SUCTION DRAINAGE
WITH UNDERWATER SEALS

To facilitate sealed chest drainage, a variety of devices is available which eliminates the cumbersome multiple drainage bottles depicted. Yet, it is worthwhile to describe the older multiple bottle technique if these devices are not available and also to aid in the understanding of the basic mechanical principles involved.

Highpoints

1. Be certain nursing personnel understand:
   a. Bottles are not elevated or removed from floor.
   b. Bottle stoppers are not removed.
   c. Fluid is not emptied.
   d. Tubing is not disconnected.
   e. All connections and stoppers are taped securely.
2. Tubing should be "milked" from time to time to prevent plugging.
3. Kinks and loops in tubing and catheter should be avoided.

A   The intercostal catheter, #26 to #30 French with multiple holes, is usually connected to a single bottle which acts as a water seal and drainage bottle. The bottle is securely taped to the floor. This arrangement usually suffices for the minor pleural leaks complicating head and neck surgery. The long glass tube extends 1 to 2 cm below the level of the water, acting as a water seal so that air will not be sucked back into the thoracic cavity. Bubbling of air out through the tube into the water indicates that the pleural leak is still present. The water column in the glass tube should rise and fall with respirations whether there is a pleural leak or not. If it does not, it indicates that the tubing is plugged. The catheter is removed 24 hours after there is no further evidence of air leak or evidence of significant drainage. A large curved clamp is kept in a conspicuous location for emergency clamping of the catheter close to the chest in the event of accidental break in the system.

B   A three-bottle system connected to a source of suction facilitates more rapid expansion of the lung when there is a known or persistent air leak. In such cases two intercostal tubes are used, one being placed upward toward the apex where it is secured to the parietal pleura. Each tube is then connected to separate underwater seal bottles. Bottle 1 collects any fluid draining from the thoracic cavity and serves as a measure for this drainage. This bottle should be emptied only by the physician, and then only when the intercostal catheter is clamped. Bottle 2 serves as the underwater seal and prevents the patient from sucking air back into the pleural space if the suction fails. It also indicates the presence or absence of a pleural leak by the presence or absence of bubbling. The long glass tube is 1 to 2 cm below water level. Bottle 3 is the negative pressure control bottle. By adjusting the depth of the long tube in the water, the amount of negative pressure is controlled. Usually 8 to 10 cm of water is ideal. The normal intrapleural negative pressure is −8 to −15 cm of water and if necessary the negative pressure in Bottle 3 may be increased to −15 cm. The source of suction can be any pump or apparatus or wall suction which is able to make the air tube bubble in Bottle 3 even though the source of suction is much more powerful. Bottle 3 adjusts it exactly.

C   In the event a three-holed stopper is not available, this arrangement using a **Y** connector duplicates the physical principles of Bottle 3. The only drawback is the danger of kinking of the tubing.

The principles outlined under the use of a single bottle system apply to the three-bottle system, including the indications for discontinuance.

D   Pictured is a pleural-evac device for self-contained sealed underwater chest drainage which replaces the previously described bottle system.

Plate 12　Basic Techniques

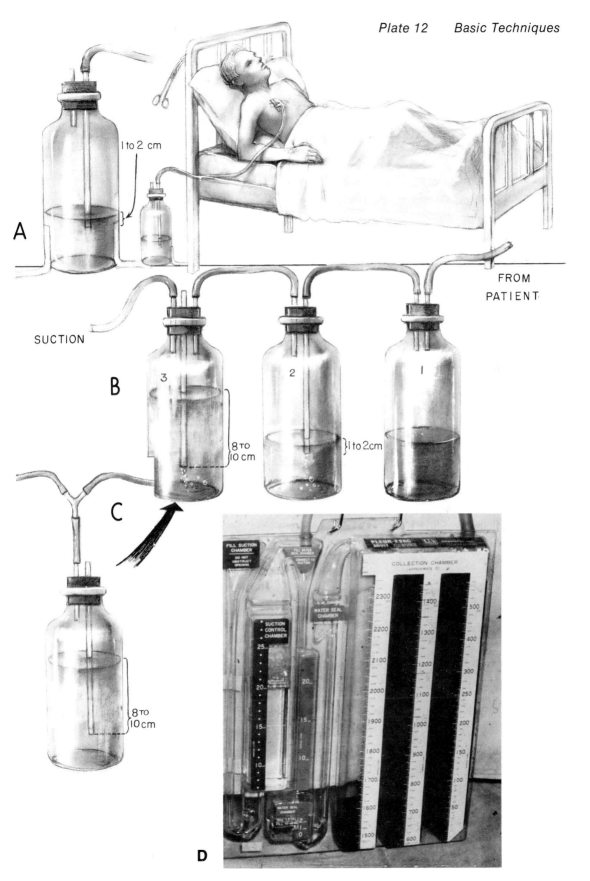

A

1 to 2 cm

B

SUCTION

3

2

1

8 TO 10 cm

1 to 2 cm

FROM PATIENT

C

8 TO 10 cm

D

FILL SUCTION CHAMBER

DO NOT OBSTRUCT OPENING

FILL WATER

PLEUR-EVAC

COLLECTION CHAMBER

WATER SEAL CHAMBER

SUCTION CONTROL CHAMBER

25

20

15

10

20

15

10

WATER SEAL CHAMBER

0

2300

2200

2100

2000

1900

1800

1700

600

1500

1400

1300

1200

1100

1000

900

800

700

600

500

400

300

250

200

150

100

50

NEEDLE ASPIRATION (After Martin, 1934)

Indications

Needle aspiration is an ancillary method of diagnosis which is not to be used indiscriminately. Its success depends on both the surgeon and the pathologist knowing its restrictions and limitations. Only after a complete head and neck examination, including laryngoscopy, nasopharyngoscopy and careful bimanual examination of the oral cavity, should it be considered as an aid in determining the nature of a mass in the head or neck. Its main use is for tumefactions in the neck when metastatic disease is suspected or when a primary lesion cannot be found. When successful, it is superior to open biopsy since the latter method is more likely to spread disease if only a section of the mass is removed or may distort the natural surgical planes if the entire mass is removed. Needle aspiration has questionable value in thyroid nodules themselves and is not used by the author except for diffuse massive enlargement of the thyroid gland resembling undifferentiated carcinoma. However, it is of distinct value when enlarged cervical nodes accompany a thyroid mass. When aspiration of such nodes reveals thyroid tissue, the diagnosis of metastatic cancer of the thyroid is virtually certain realizing the extremely low incidence of normal thyroid tissue in cervical lymph nodes. In similar fashion, squamous cells discovered in a lymph node aspiration lead the surgeon to suspect metastatic squamous cell carcinoma from an unrecognized primary. The other more common sites of unrecognized primary lesions are the palatine tonsils, base of tongue, nasopharynx and pyriform sinus. In a lymphoma, needle aspiration usually cannot facilitate a definitive diagnosis — only a suggestion and then open biopsy is necessary. Obviously, a pulsatile mass should not be aspirated.

In tumors of the salivary glands, needle aspiration is used in selective situations, especially when a positive diagnosis of a malignant tumor would significantly change the operative approach. A needle core biopsy might be preferred. The usual technique for diagnosis in the absence of cervical lymph nodes is the removal of the entire salivary gland or lobe and then frozen section. Open incisional biopsy of such tumors is condemned because of the danger of spreading disease. Nevertheless, there are situations when this becomes necessary.

A With a local anesthetic injected into the overlying skin and using a #11 blade, a small stab wound is made in the skin directly over the mass. The skin only is entered — not the mass itself. The stab wound should be placed so that it can easily be included in the standard neck dissection incision if operation becomes necessary.

B A large bore needle (#17 is ideal) with stylet is inserted through the stab wound into the mass with the index finger holding the stylet in place. The purpose of the stab wound and stylet is to facilitate ease of insertion and to avoid picking up cells from the skin and other overlying tissue.

C With the stylet in place, the needle is moved back and forth in the mass a few millimeters, first in the same plane as the original insertion and then a few degrees to either side. This step is repeated with the stylet removed.

D Negative pressure is then applied with a specially designed locking syringe with a metal plunger similar to those used in the old direct transfusion sets. This is known as a Hayes Martin needle aspiration syringe and is manufactured with a special locking device to hold the barrel in position to facilitate negative pressure. If this type syringe is not available, an ordinary glass 30 cc syringe can be used. The needle with syringe under negative pressure is again moved back and forth a few times and then needle and syringe are briskly removed together. With this technique, the material in the needle is deposited on the end of the barrel of the syringe.

E The aspirate on the barrel of the syringe is spread on one or more slides as a thin film. Any material left in the needle is sprayed out over another slide and smeared. The slides may be placed face to face, and the material spread by sliding the slides across one another. The slides may be either immediately fixed in alcohol and ether or air dried, according to the wishes of the pathologist.

Plate 13   *Basic Techniques*

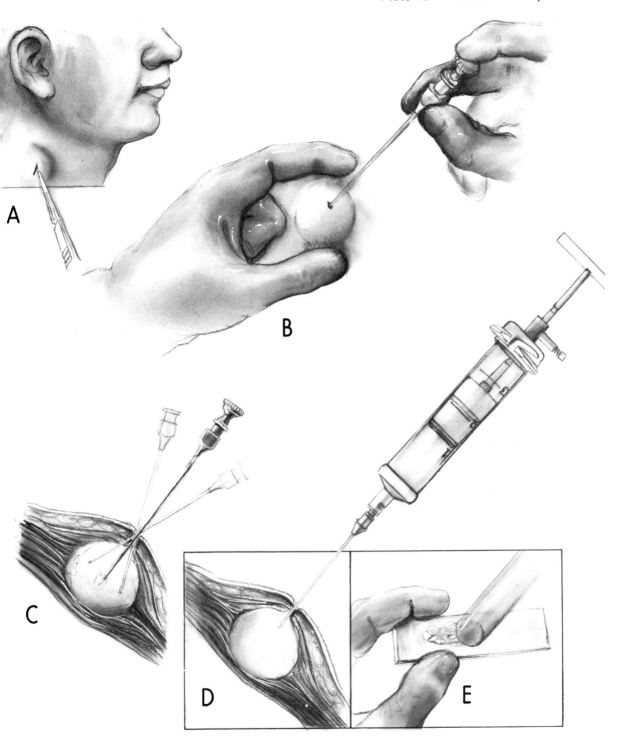

If any sizable particles are adherent to the inner wall of the syringe, these are removed with a "rake" or swab, placed on filter paper and fixed in formalin for block paraffin section. If the pathology is malignant, the needle tract and site of puncture is excised at the time of definitive surgery. If there is any question regarding an inflammatory process, some of the material is sent for culture.

Z-PLASTY

A
D
A Z-plasty is the transposition of two opposing triangular skin flaps, thereby reversing the initial "Z" incision. The central arm of the initial Z is thus rotated and the distance between points 1 and 2 are increased (*A'* and *D'*). The most useful angle formed by each lateral arm to the central arm is 60 degrees. The central arm corresponds to the scar contracture which is to be changed in *direction, lengthened* and *tension released.* The length of each lateral arm equals the length of the central arm. Variations in the angle will vary the direction of the resulting central arm and the length gained. An extended description of the Z-plasty follows since it has wide application in reconstruction procedures in head and neck surgery.

TECHNIQUE OF BASIC Z-PLASTY

Highpoints

1. Optimal flap angle is 60 degrees. This will rotate scar or incision 90 degrees (*A* and *A'*).
2. Be sure resultant rotated scar is in or in line with natural skin crease. The base ends of the lateral arms should be in the line of the natural crease (*A* and *A'*).
3. Realize effect of changes of flap angle to gain in length of scar line and the degree of rotation of scar line. The smaller the angle, the less the gain in length and the less amount of rotation (*H* and *I*, p. 37).
4. The smaller the flap angle, the greater the danger of tip necrosis (points X and Y of *A*); the larger the flap angle, the more tension on surrounding tissue.
5. Care with placement of sutures to avoid strangulation of blood vessels.
6. Each lateral arm should be the same length as the central arm in the classic Z-plasty.
7. As a check for correct planning of the classic Z-plasty with 60 degree flap angles, an imaginary line (natural skin crease) connecting the base ends (points X[1] and Y[1] of *A'*) of both lateral arms should pass through the midpoint of the central arm.
8. It may be advantageous to have a set of dividers and protractor in the sterile field.

A
A'
The scar, web or linear contracture extends along the line X–Y (central arm). An incision or excision of a small amount of skin is made along the line X–Y. From points X and Y two other incisions (lateral arms), each of equal length to line X–Y are made to X[1] and Y[1] respectively at a 60 degree angle (flap angle) (range is 30 to 90 degrees). Points X[1] and Y[1] are along the natural skin crease.

B
The flaps formed by X and Y are widely undermined with extreme care to preserve both arteries and veins. Small skin hooks or fine nylon sutures are used to handle the flaps. Trauma must be minimum. The transposition is begun by rotation of Y to Y[1].

C
X is rotated to X[1]. Sutures of 5-0 or 6-0 nylon are usually used. These sutures are placed slightly obliquely to relieve tension along central arm after closure.

D
D'
Rotation completed. The scar line (central arm) has been rotated 90 degrees and the distance between point 1 and 2 has been increased 75 per cent. These geometrical figures refer to a flap angle of 60 degrees.

Plate 14   Basic Techniques

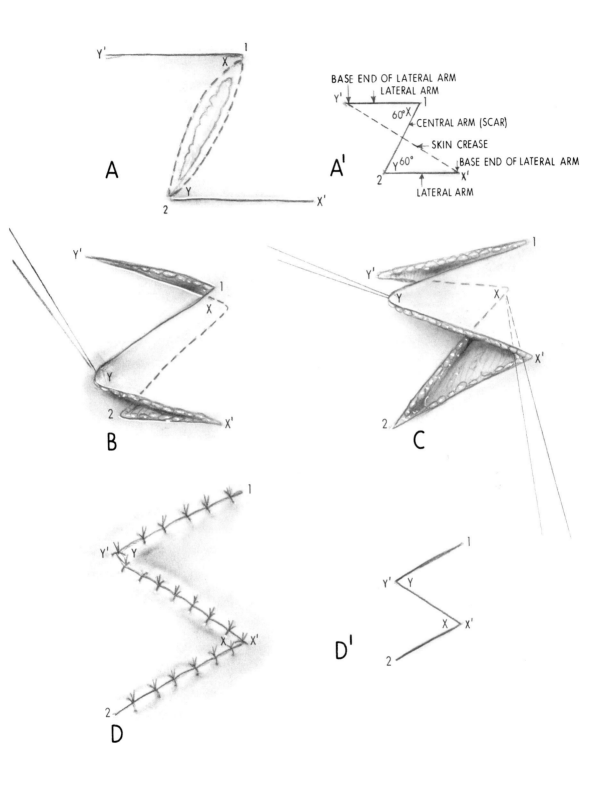

A

A'

BASE END OF LATERAL ARM
LATERAL ARM
Y'   1
60° X
CENTRAL ARM (SCAR)
SKIN CREASE
Y 60°   BASE END OF LATERAL ARM
2   X'
LATERAL ARM

B

C

D

D'

Z-PLASTY (*Continued*)

TECHNIQUE OF BASIC Z-PLASTY (*Continued*)

Geometrical Considerations

    1. If a parallelogram is outlined around the corners of the Z-plasty, some interesting theoretical measurements are obtained:

E
F
G

The short diagonal (points 1 and 2 in step *E*) of the parallelogram before the Z-plasty (which is the length of the scar contracture) between points 1 and 2 becomes the long diagonal of the parallelogram after the Z-plasty (points 1′ and 2′ in step *F*). These diagonals approximately maintain their respective lengths when rotated, hence the distance gained in any classic Z-plasty between points 1 and 2 corresponds to the long diagonal minus the short diagonal (*G*). Expressed in another way, the total length desired between points 1 and 2 after the Z-plasty can be easily achieved by constructing a parallelogram before the Z-plasty whose long diagonal is equal to the final desired length and the direction of the final or resultant central arm.

The shaded triangle in step *E* corresponds to one rotated flap of a Z-plasty, the base being the dotted line which is shown transposed in step *F*. The nonshaded triangle is the corresponding flap in the Z-plasty, the dotted line being the base. Points *A* and *B* refer to the tips of the respective triangular flaps which are transposed.

    2. The flap angle can be varied from a range of 20 to 90 degrees, with the most variable range around 60 degrees. The smaller the flap angle, the less percentage rate of increase in the length of the release (McGregor, 1962):

        30 degree angle yields 25 per cent increase in length

        45 degree angle yields 50 per cent increase in length

        60 degree angle yields 75 per cent increase in length

Plate 15   Basic Techniques

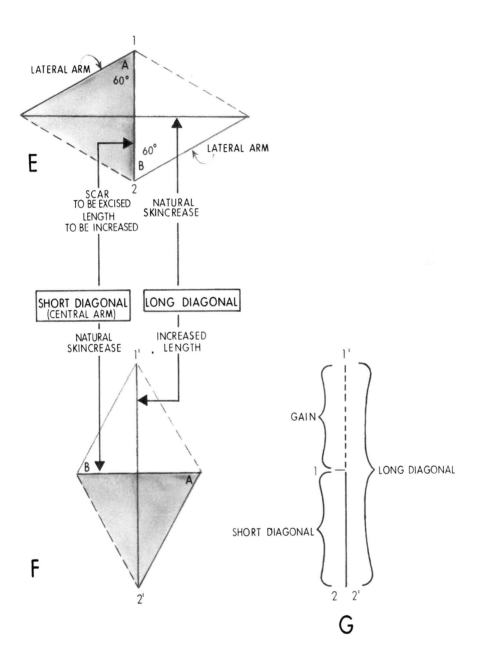

E

LATERAL ARM

A
60°

60°
B

LATERAL ARM

SCAR
TO BE EXCISED
LENGTH
TO BE INCREASED

NATURAL
SKINCREASE

SHORT DIAGONAL
(CENTRAL ARM)

LONG DIAGONAL

NATURAL
SKINCREASE

INCREASED
LENGTH

F

B
A

GAIN

LONG DIAGONAL

SHORT DIAGONAL

G

35

Z-PLASTY (*Continued*)

TECHNIQUE OF BASIC Z-PLASTY (*Continued*)

H
I
Also to be realized is the smaller the flap angle, the less number of degrees the central arm or "scar" line is rotated. This is important in planning the resultant arm to lie in a natural skin crease (dotted line).

Variations of flap angle result in various positions of the resultant central arm which is the long diagonal of the parallelogram. This demonstrates how a Z-plasty is varied so that the resultant central arm can rest along a natural skin crease. This is further shown in the following steps.

J
K
L
First select the length of the central arm which may equal the entire length of the scar or a part thereof. If the scar is long, multiple Z-plasties are necessary (*S* and *T*, p. 41). The midpoint of the central arm should lie on the natural skin crease (*J*) and the base end of each lateral arm must be located on the natural skin crease (*K*). Each lateral arm is equal in length to the central arm. A protractor can be of aid in determination of these measurements. *L* demonstrates the final result. (To achieve a more pleasing result, the lateral arms can be slightly curved.)

The smaller the flap angle, especially less than 30 degrees, the greater the danger of tip necrosis.

The larger the flap angle, especially over 90 degrees, the greater the tension on the surrounding tissue with too much borrowing from each side. These larger angles tend to result in larger dog-ears at the base of the triangle.

Clinically a 60 degree flap angle has been shown to be the largest angle which will allow transposition of triangular flaps while achieving the greatest increase of length along the central arm or line of contracture. With this angle the central arm is rotated 90 degrees.

3. As the central arm length is increased, greater is the percentile increase in length.
4. Depending on the relative position of scar to natural skin crease, the two flap angles may be of unequal size (step *Q*, p. 41). This is also referred to half Z when one of the angles is 90 degrees.

Plate 16   Basic Techniques

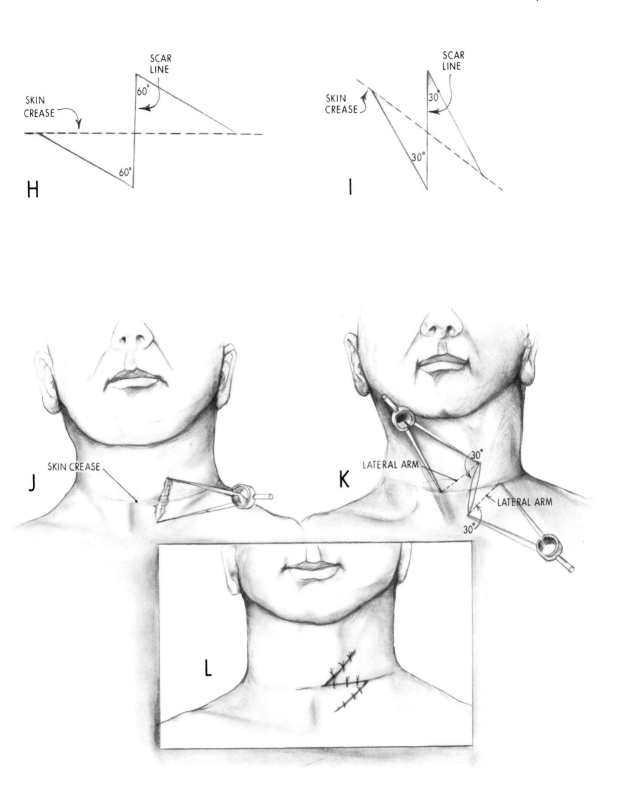

SCAR
LINE

SKIN
CREASE

60°

60°

H

SCAR
LINE

SKIN
CREASE

30°

30°

I

SKIN CREASE

J

LATERAL ARM

30°

LATERAL ARM

30°

K

L

37

Z-PLASTY (Continued)

Examples of Purposes and Accomplishments

    1. Change of direction of linear scars or webs or linear contractures.

M
N   a. From vertical to horizontal in scars of neck. The size of the Z-plasty is large for clarity's sake. In actual practice multiple Z-plasties with a long scar are preferred (*S* and *T*, p. 41) or a slight curvature of the lateral arms.

O
P   b. Scar across nasolabial fold converted to lie in and along the natural skin crease of the nasolabial fold.

Plate 17   Basic Techniques

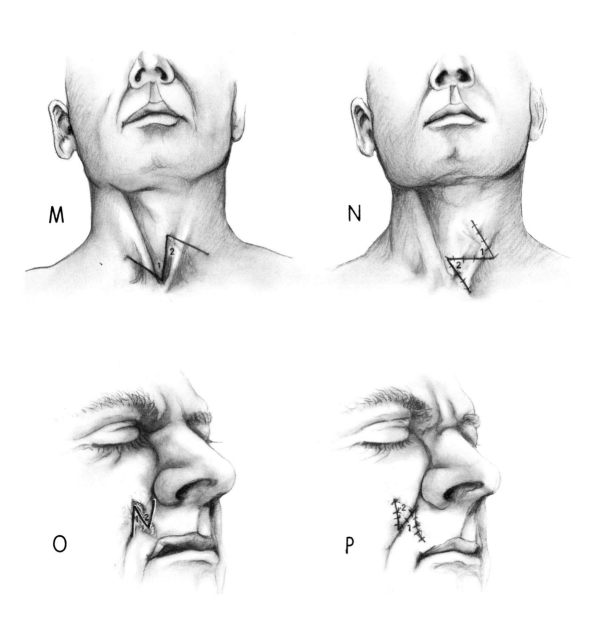

TECHNIQUE OF BASIC Z-PLASTY (*Continued*)

Examples of Purposes and Accomplishments (Continued)

Q 2. Increase the length between the ends of the original scar contracture, e.g., lengthening of the contracted tissue causing upward distortion of the upper lip.

R 3. Release and redistribution of tension along linear contracture, e.g., breaks up unsightly scars of cheek and thus returns some elasticity aiding in normal facial expression. This is accomplished either by multiple Z-plasties (steps *S* and *T*), by opposing Z-plasties (see plate 19, steps *U* and *V*) or by W-plasty (see plate 20, steps *X* and *Y*).

Types and Modifications of Z-Plasty

1. *Single Z-Plasty* (*M* and *N*).   The single or basic Z-plasty has multiple applications as previously described. By and large, however, it is limited to relatively short scars. It can be useful in longer scars only when the surrounding tissue is very loose, as, for example, in the neck.

2. *Half Z-Plasty* (*Q* and *R*).   This actually is a variant of the angles of a basic Z-plasty. It simply means that an incision is made at right angles to a wound into which is transposed one triangular flap (step *Q*). This is useful in the elongation of wound, especially the short side of a curved defect (step *R*).

3. *Multiple Z-Plasty* (*S* and *T*, *S′* and *T′*) (Limberg, 1963; Morestin, 1914; Davis, and Kitlowski, 1939).   Multiple Z-plasties are two or more Z-plasties in either a continuous series or interrupted series with a number of other modifications. Of necessity the arms are usually short, as used in the face or neck. This technique is useful for large scars of the cheek where, as in the latter case, the surrounding tissue is tight or has lost its elasticity. A single Z-plasty in a long scar would be impractical and almost devastating on the cheek.

Continuous Types (Entire Scar Excised)

S Depicted is a series of continuous Z-plasties in which all the arms are equal, all the angles 60 degrees and all the lateral arms parallel. The entire scar contracture is excised in a continuous line. The lengthening of the scar contracture is obvious.

S¹ Depicted is a similar type of continuous Z-plasties except that the lateral arms are independent with a space between each Z.

Interrupted Types (Portions of Scar Excised)

T Depicted is a series of multiple Z-plasties of equal size similar to those in S¹ except that intervening portions of the linear scar between each Z is not excised. The length of the remaining portion of the scar varies according to the desired result.

T¹ This series of interrupted multiple Z-plasties differ from those in T in that two are opposite. This is the so-called opposing Z-plasties.

Plate 18   Basic Techniques

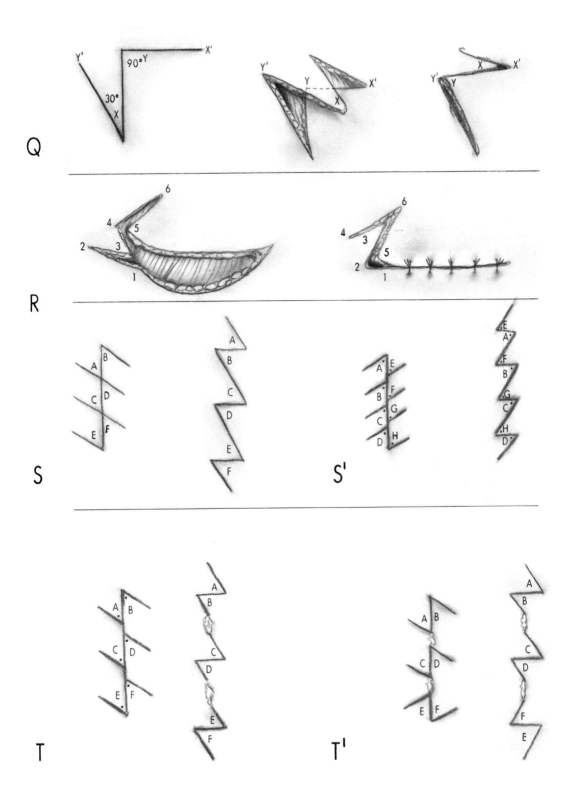

Q

R

S

S'

T

T'

TECHNIQUE OF BASIC Z-PLASTY (*Continued*)

U   Depicted in steps *U* and *V* is an example of the excision and reconstruction of a
scar on the side of the cheek. This technique is very useful in upsetting the tension of
V   contractures especially on the cheek (after Converse, 1964).

Plate 19   Basic Techniques

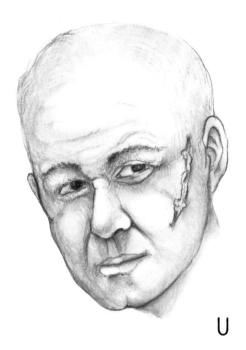

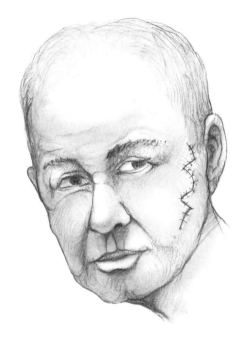

U

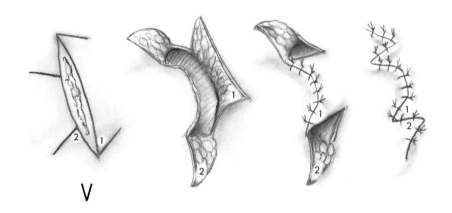

V

TECHNIQUE OF BASIC Z-PLASTY (*Continued*)

W   4. *S-Plasty.* The lateral arm of a basic Z-plasty may curve in a convex arc. This aids in preserving the blood supply, especially in burn scars in which the blood supply is compromised. The full application of this modification is in the neck where a large S-plasty is performed. This is possible because of the laxity of the surrounding tissue.

X   5. *W-Plasty* (Borges, 1959). This is a method of excising a scar to break up a
Y   straight line by removing small interdigitating triangles on either side of the scar line. It is useful in depressed linear scars of the cheek when no lengthening of the line of contracture is necessary. The W-plasty, unlike the Z-plasty, does not gain length. A metal template or bent flap metal strip modeled to correspond to small equal triangles is useful to mark the area for the line of excision (step *X*). McGregor has demonstrated a modification of the W-plasty for the closure of an oval wound (step *Y*).

Limitations and Complications

1. Dog-ears are apt to form near base of transposed flaps. If these require excision, they cannot be excised toward the base but rather away from the base (see plate 21, steps *D*, *E*, and *F*).
2. When an angle formed by a scar with a natural skin crease is progressively less than 50 degrees, the angle of the tip of the transposed flap of the Z-plasty becomes less than 30 degrees and hence reduces practicability of the Z-plasty.
3. A word of caution regarding the use of an extensive Z-plasty in the primary closure of a wound for a malignant lesion. Margins must be free of disease for fear of implantation of tumor cells along the transposed flaps.
4. Tip necrosis. Wilkinson and Rybka have shown experimentally that glue or tapes prevent tip necrosis.
5. Too much lateral tension with larger flaps in tight surrounding tissue.
6. Strangulation of blood supply with suture.

NYLON SUTURES FOR MUCOSAL REPAIR

Although nylon suture material has been shown to result in minimal tissue reaction and is utilized almost exclusively in repairs of mucous membrane of the oral cavity and oropharynx, its use involving the mucosa in laryngeal and hypopharyngeal surgery has been found to be not as satisfactory. The problem is that loose loops, ends and knots of nylon are sites for the collection of debris, mucus and food. If the sutures are totally buried, nylon is ideal; otherwise an absorbable material is usually recommended.

Plate 20   Basic Techniques

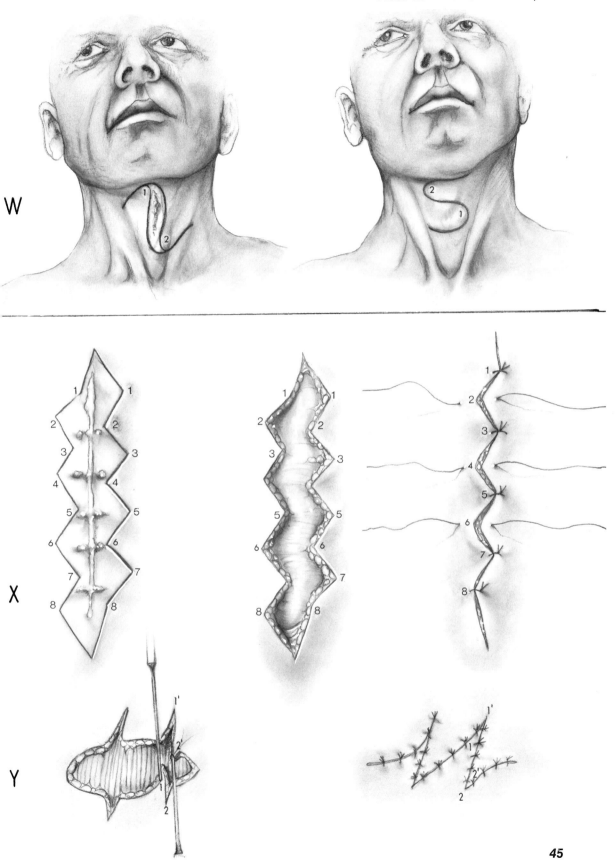

W

X

Y

DERMABRASION

Dermabrasion is a form of surgical planing of the skin using abrasive devices which removes the epidermis and the superficial layer of the dermis. A new epidermis regenerates from the cutaneous adnexa consisting of the sweat glands and pilosebaceous structures. It is used to smooth irregularities of the skin surface.

Indications

1. Acne scars.
2. Traumatic scars.
3. Superficial tattoos.
4. Superficial nevi.
5. Burn scars when combined with split thickness skin grafting.
6. Small multiple irregular shallow epidermal lacerations.

Anesthesia

Local or general infiltration. Epinephrine is not injected in any form because of the danger of cardiac arrhythmia.

Highpoints

1. Extensive areas should be treated in hospital.
2. Iverson high speed dermabrader is preferred, using the various sized emery paper cylinders rather than wire brush.
3. Proceed slowly, especially over bony prominences.
4. Do not abrade eyelids or lower anterior neck.
5. Preoperative skin care with germicidal soap. Cleaning the skin with ether will remove sebaceous material deep in acne scars. Be careful not to allow ether to reach the eyes.
6. Copious use of saline during procedure and afterward.
7. Keep loose gauze clear of revolving parts of equipment.
8. Repeat abrasion usually should be spaced 10 to 12 months apart.
9. Surgical excision of deep scars is combined with dermabrasion.
10. "Feather" the edges of the area to be abraded to avoid sharp depression at the edges.
11. Deep pits are marked with methylene blue.

A Iverson dermabrader with guard in position. The inside of the cheek may be supported by packing the buccal space with gauze to add support to the soft tissues. The area to be abraded has been outlined with a suitable dye. The depth is gauged primarily by experience. As the epidermis is removed and dermis exposed, small bleeding sites will appear which are the dermal papillae. Next will be seen parallel ridges of collagen. It is wise to terminate the procedure at this level. If one proceeds deeper, adipose tissue will be detected. If deep scars remain, they are best excised at the conclusion of the abrasion. This is the purpose of first marking with methylene blue. This is especially necessary if local infiltrative anesthesia is used, since the pockets of the scars may be partially obliterated. At the margins the planing must be feathered so that there is a gradual sloping area to normal skin; otherwise, a sharp depressed edge will result.

Dickinson has demonstrated the advantage of immediate use of dermabrasion for small multiple irregular shallow epidermal lacerations.

B Close-up view of Iverson dermabrader with small cylinder covered with emery paper sleeve.

Postoperative dressing consists of Furacin impregnated gauze or antibiotic oint-
(*Text continued on page 48.*)

Plate 21   Basic Techniques

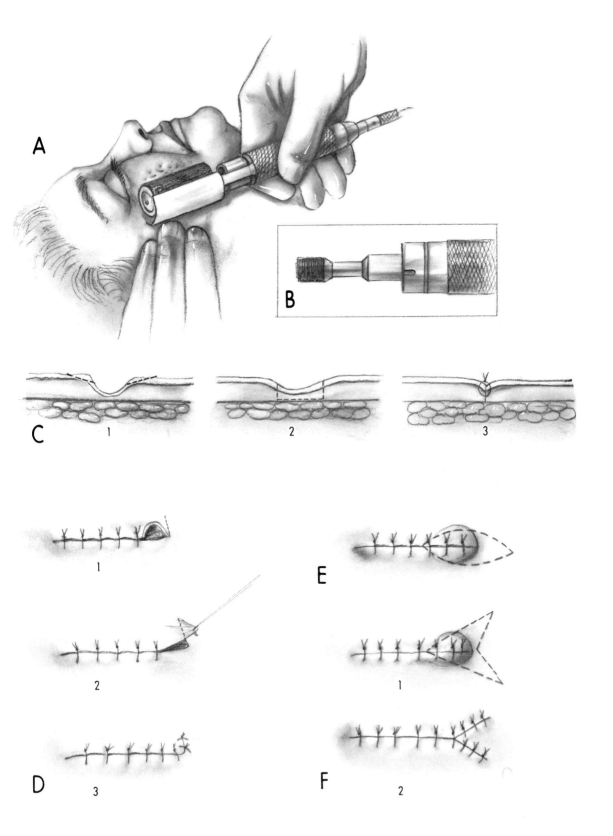

DERMABRASION (*Continued*)

ment covered with Telfa or Adaptex and an outer fluffed gauze held in place with Kling. This outer pressure dressing may be removed in 24 to 48 hours while the inner dressing is left in place for seven to 10 days. It is important that this inner dressing not be forcibly removed earlier since this would injure the regenerating epithelium.

Approximate regeneration periods:

1 week — Complete epithelialization
1 month — Pigment begins to reappear
6 months — Epidermis approaches normal thickness (dermis does not reach preoperative thickness)

Complications

1. *Hyperpigmentation.* Patients should be told to avoid excessive sunlight — use sun protective creams, ascorbic acid and cortisone.
2. *Milia.* These are small white cysts which arise from the epidermal appendages as the epidermis regenerates, i.e., pilosebaceous structure and sweat glands. If these small cysts do not disappear spontaneously as they usually do, they may require uncapping and pressure to remove their contents.
3. *Erythema.* This reddish hue always occurs immediately after dermabrasion and usually gradually disappears. Again, overexposure to sunlight is to be avoided.
4. *Hypertrophic scars* result with too deep dermabrasion or dermabrasion in which there is a paucity of cutaneous adnexa as in the eyelids and lower anterior neck.

C Depicted are the steps associated with the dermabrasion and then the excision of a deep scar.

1. The epidermis alongside the depressed scar is feathered by dermabrasion down to the dotted lines.
2. The remaining deep scar which is excised along the dotted lines.
3. Approximation of the edges of the resected scar.

EXCISION OF DOG-EARS

Most dog-ears can be handled initially by flattening and lengthening the ellipse of skin to be excised. If this is impractical or dog-ears are present, one of the following techniques can be utilized.

D The dog-ear has resulted from unequal lengths of each side of the repair.

1. The dotted line is the back cut.
2. A back cut has been performed and the excess skin along the longer skin edge is excised on the dotted line.
3. Completed closure.

E A dog-ear is excised by resection of a longer and flatter ellipse of skin.

F A dog-ear is excised using the V (step 1) to Y (step 2) principle (see plate 128, steps J and K). Dog-ears can also be prevented by modified W-plasty as depicted on plate 20, steps X and Y.

Plate 21 Repeated   Basic Techniques

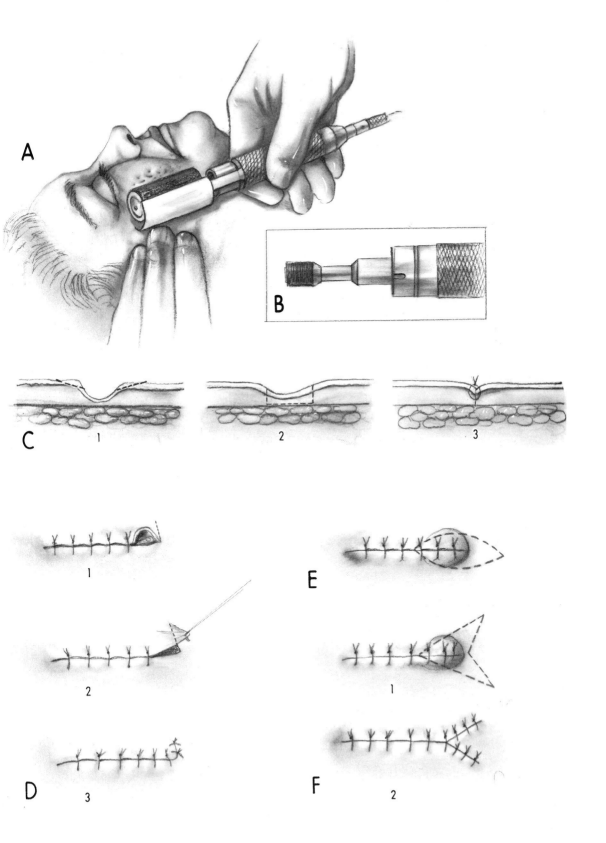

BONE AND CARTILAGE GRAFTS

Highpoints

1. Preserve periosteum with cortical bone graft or perichondrium on at least one surface.
2. Excise a larger section of graft than is necessary. This will allow sufficient latitude for choice of best configuration of graft. The use of a template or model made from plastic or stiff paper is a great aid in shaping the graft.
3. Cartilage grafts are more apt to absorb.

A   Location of incisions for rib (1), iliac crest (2) and costochondral cartilage (3) grafts.

Rib Graft

A-1 An inframammary incision is made extending toward the posterior axillary line. The greater the curve that is desired for the graft, the more posterior the incision. The pectoralis major and minor muscles are transected. Depending on the extent posteriorly, the latissimus dorsi muscle may be sectioned. The attachments of the serratus anterior muscle are separated from the selected rib, which is usually the sixth or seventh. The presenting periosteum is preserved intact.

B   With the periosteum of the rib exposed, an incision is made through the periosteum along the superior margin and another incision along the inferior margin of the rib. The periosteum is sectioned at either end.

C   Cross section of rib graft with intact periosteum on anterior surface.

D   Using an Alexander rib periosteal elevator, the periosteum along the superior and inferior surfaces of the rib is separated. The neurovascular bundle is included in the inferior periosteal flap and preserved at the donor site.

E   A Doyen elevator completes the periosteal separation posteriorly. If this is carefully performed, the pleural cavity is not entered. When the pleural cavity is inadvertently opened, it is necessary to employ underwater drainage (plate 12), or close the chest slightly with the lung fully expanded.

F   With rib rongeurs, the rib is sectioned at either end. The periosteum on the anterior surface of the rib has been preserved intact with the rib graft. The wound is closed in layers approximating the sectioned muscles over the bed of the removed rib.

Iliac Graft

A-2 An incision is made along the anterior extent of the crest of the ilium including the anterior superior spine. The anterior attachments of the external and internal oblique abdominal muscles are sectioned close to the bone. A portion of the tensor fasciae latae may also require transection. The periosteum is left intact with the graft if the cortex is used.

G   Depending on the length and width of the defect to be grafted, a somewhat larger section of iliac crest is removed with a Stryker saw.

Costochondral Graft

A-3 An oblique incision is made over the broadest expanse of the seventh, eighth and ninth costochondral cartilages. The anterior rectus sheath and the rectus abdominis muscle are transected and separated exposing the underlying perichondrium, which is left intact.

H   An area is outlined representing a much larger graft than is required. This is cut to the desired depth, avoiding a through and through incision of the cartilage.

(Text continued on page 52.)

50

Plate 22   **Basic Techniques**

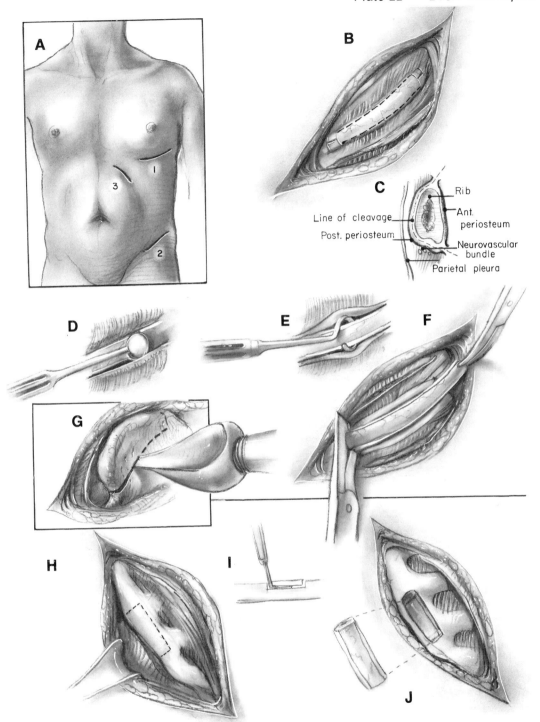

C

Rib

Ant. periosteum

Line of cleavage

Post. periosteum

Neurovascular bundle

Parietal pleura

I   A rectangular block is then excised with the aid of a right angle knife (Beaver Blade #64).

J   The excised block of cartilage with anterior layer of perichondrium intact. The wound is closed in layers.

     Not depicted is the technique for obtaining cancellous bone. This is procured from the iliac bone either through burr holes or plugs or sections of cortical bone first removed. The cancellous bone can then be obtained either with a curet or in strips or blocks depending on its use. The use of curetted cancellous bone is shown in the reconstruction of the mandible using a metal trough to hold the bone in place (see plate 196, step *H*).

SKIN INCISION

All skin incisions in the neck, with few exceptions, should follow the natural skin creases. This is important from a functional as well as a cosmetic point of view. Adequate exposure is accomplished by the development of upper or lower skin flaps, which include the platysma muscle. After adequate skin flaps are elevated, the deeper fascial incision may be changed as the exposure dictates.

Skin incisions for operations in the superior cervical regions should be 3 to 5 cm below the horizontal ramus of the mandible to avoid injury to the mandibular branch of the facial nerve. For operations in the inferior cervical region, the skin incision usually should at least be 2 to 3 cm above the clavicle, since incisions placed lower will tend to drop over the clavicle in time and become unsightly. An exception is the upper incision for a deltopectoral flap which lies close to the level of the clavicle.

If a single horizontal incision following a natural skin crease does not give adequate exposure as, for example, in a thyroglossal cyst which lies at the level of the thyroid gland or in a branchial fistula, multiple horizontal incisions in stepladder fashion solve the problem admirably. A skin incision made along the anterior border of the sternocleidomastoid muscle is entirely unnecessary except in an extreme emergency. Even in an emergency tracheostomy, the horizontal incision is always used.

There are exceptions to any rule of thumb. The exposure for a radical neck dissection is the main exception. Although multiple horizontal incisions can be used in this operation, the exposure and time consumed raises some questions (see plate 230, skin incisions of radical neck dissection).

Another exception may be a total laryngectomy for malignant disease in an individual with a long, thin neck, in whom two horizontal incisions may extend too far laterally and thus enter an area of later metastatic spread. This exemplifies a basic principle in operations for malignant disease: i.e., avoid skin incisions for cosmetic purposes and the use of skin flaps for reconstructive purposes in and from regions to which metastatic disease may later spread. Scars in such areas will delay an early detection of metastases and often make later radical surgery difficult.

PRE- AND POSTOPERATIVE CARE

By William R. Nelson, M.D.

In this brief treatise, specific problems are mentioned and procedures described which are somewhat different from those encountered and utilized in routine general surgical and ear, nose and throat patient management. Adequate preoperative evaluation and preparation are of the utmost importance in these patients often afflicted with disabling medical disease. After surgery, these individuals need unusual care. Wound healing may well depend upon the surgeon's detailed knowledge of the complication which might arise and of specific peculiarities of tissues in the head and neck region.

PREOPERATIVE CARE

A   The *sine qua non* of preoperative preparation is proper evaluation of the disease for which surgery is planned. This includes radiographic and pathologic studies, a positive biopsy in a tumor patient being mandatory. In the event that an unusual neoplasm has been diagnosed (such as a soft-part sarcoma, atypical lymphoma or uncommon variety of salivary tumor), it is often wise to ask the attending pathologist to seek consultation on the tissue slides. A second opinion from an experienced tumor pathologist may alter the surgical approach. Chest x-rays are essential in the research for metastatic disease or concomitant bronchogenic carcinoma, the latter being a frequent second neoplasm in any patient with head and neck mucosal cancer.

   Barium studies of the laryngopharynx and hypopharynx are often quite revealing as regards the extent of neoplasm in these regions. On the other hand, simple soft tissue studies may be even more important in studying lesions of the larynx and nasopharynx. Laminography is useful in the analysis of invasion by laryngeal cancer and may be significant in determining operability in paranasal sinus neoplasms. Of course, angiography is most essential in blood vessel problems, and can be helpful in neoplasms such as carotid body tumors, juvenile nasopharyngeal angiofibromas and parathyroid adenomas.

B   The usual supportive and diagnostic measures must be instituted preoperatively in patients with surgical diseases of the head and neck. Careful medical evaluation and therapy are important since cardiovascular, pulmonary or hepatic dysfunction commonly accompanies the surgical problem, especially in the case of mucosal cancer.

C   Cultures of infected lesions should be made well in advance of surgery, for these problems may require both local and systemic control measures. The irrigation or power spraying of the oral cavity (with half hydrogen peroxide and half saline solution) will often clear up necrotic tissue and exudate on the surface of a tumor. If systemic antibiotics are to be given (and this is wise in sizable resections involving mucosa or bone), they should be started 24 hours preoperatively. One per cent neomycin mouthwash or gargle three times a day may also be used when combined with mechanical cleansing (Hawk, personal communication).

   This regimen is now being used routinely in all procedures in which the upper respiratory–digestive tract is entered. It is used two to three days preoperatively and continued postoperatively, the duration being determined by the conditions in each situation. It is believed that this has significantly reduced the incidence of fistula formation; however, the surgeon should be aware that neomycin absorption may result in oto- or nephrotoxicosis.

D   Cigarette smoking must be stopped well ahead of scheduled procedures. Often, dramatic clearing of excessive secretions will occur and postoperative tracheobronchial difficulties will be less severe. Positive pressure breathing (with or without added drugs for bronchodilatation and mucous liquefaction) may be a great aid to those individuals with pulmonary and tracheobronchial disease.

53

PREOPERATIVE CARE (*Continued*)

E   The alcoholic patient should be "dried out" for at least a week before surgery, as postoperative delirium tremens yields a high mortality. Most alcoholics will be evasive about their liquor consumption! The families of suspected alcohol addicts should be questioned prior to the final scheduling of surgery so that plans for adequate preoperative hospitalization can be made. High caloric feedings, vitamin therapy and tranquilization will be of help during the "drying out" phase.

F   Nasopharyngeal or nasogastric tube feedings may be advisable preoperatively in patients plagued with nutritional deficiencies and swallowing problems when immediate surgery is not planned. This approach is of little value unless a preoperative period of several weeks is available in which to restore depleted protein stores. Wound healing may not be delayed in the starved individual, but convalescence is certainly shortened when the patient's preoperative nutritional status is more nearly normal. Preoperative feedings could be used in cancer patients undergoing preoperative radiation therapy.

G   Whole blood transfusions may be required preoperatively and generous amounts of blood should be held in readiness for any radical surgical procedure. Coagulation studies may be in order when bleeding tendencies are suspected, especially in patients with hepatic dysfunction.

H   The anesthesiologist should be consulted well in advance when airway, cardiac, alcoholic, hepatic and other systemic problems are present. Prior to the scheduled procedure, the surgeon and the anesthesiologist should have completed detailed plans regarding type of intubation (oro- or nasotracheal), tracheostomy, cardiac monitoring and optimum positioning of anesthetic equipment. In some instances of partial airway obstruction, a careful attempt to intubate the patient may be made transorally by the anesthesiologist (with the surgeon standing in readiness to perform tracheostomy under local anesthesia in the event the transoral method fails). This is permissible in selected cases since tracheostomy may interfere with exposure in laryngectomy and other procedures in and around the larynx.

I   Adequate skin preparation is required also, and germicidal soap cleansing plus sufficient shaving must be ordered. These procedures must widely encompass the area of surgery. In clean, healthy skin, germicidal soap preparation the night before surgery and again in the operating room is sufficient. Some patients, especially senile individuals, require careful skin cleansing twice daily for three to four days ahead of time. The ear should be thoroughly soaped and the external canal gently cleansed with a cotton-tipped applicator on two or more occasions prior to parotid surgery and other procedures carried out in the ear area. Skin and bone graft donor areas should be well prepared in advance. Shaving can be performed the night before surgery in many instances, but the face and anterior neck should be shaved in the early morning on the day of surgery in most adult males.

J   It is vitally important for the surgeon to discuss frankly and honestly with his patients the possibilities of loss of any function during an operative procedure. If total laryngectomy is to be performed, the patient should be enlightened about the physiologic and anatomic changes to be incurred, and must be encouraged about esophageal speech possibilities. In situations in which there is some doubt as to the extent of surgery, the possibilities of postoperative functional loss must be outlined. It is always best to give each patient some hope that such losses will not be incurred. Any person awaiting surgery should be given a lucid description of planned tracheostomy, feeding tube or wound drainage tube utilization. In general, simple explanations of planned procedures are helpful, but too detailed a discussion of the surgical technique may frighten an already apprehensive patient. Preoperative visits by previously operated patients may or may not be wise, depending on the disfigurement or dysfunction present and the preoperative patient's own personality and state of anxiety. After surgery—when the individual is recuperating—a visit by one of these veteran patients may be extremely helpful. The "Lost Chord Club" must be contacted about each new laryngectomy case so that plans for visits by these laryngectomees can be set up. Speech therapy must be arranged through this organization or through a professional speech therapist.

Bowel Prep

There are many methods of preparing the colon for surgery, and the following outline is a popular approach to the problem:

1. The patient must be on a clear liquid diet for at least two to three days prior to the operation.
2. *Cathartics.* Thirty cc of 50 per cent magnesium sulfate solution daily will produce a prompt mechanical cleansing of the colon if begun three to four days prior to surgery. Other saline cathartics are equally effective. Of course, significant dehydration can develop in some individuals with this dose. Lesser doses can be utilized effectively along with antibiotic preparation, as will be mentioned later. Many authorities in the field of colon surgery use cathartics and liquid diet without antibiotics or sulfa preparations.
3. Sulfathalidine* may be used alone or with small doses of cathartics beginning four to five days prior to the operation. A modified regimen consists of an immediate dose of 4 gm in the average patient, followed by 2 gm four times daily.
4. Neomycin is used by many physicians in order to produce a "rapid" bowel prep. This technique utilizes 1 gm of the drug every hour for four doses, followed by 1 gm every four hours (for 24 to 72 hours).
5. Enemas actually are not necessary if effective cathartics are used.

The advantages of one approach over the other certainly are not easy to prove. Proper mechanical cleansing seems to be the most important means of preparing the patient's large bowel for surgery.

---

*This drug has recently been recalled by the manufacturer since it is anticipated that the Food and Drug Administration will withdraw its approval.

PRE- AND POSTOPERATIVE CARE (*Continued*)

POSTOPERATIVE CARE

The postoperative orders for typical, all-inclusive care after head and neck surgery might be outlined as follows:

A   Careful monitoring of vital signs. Head should be elevated to 60 to 90 degrees when blood pressure has stabilized. (Among the rare exceptions would be a situation in which the common or internal carotid artery has been ligated; in this case a flat or slightly head-down position would be imperative). The head-up position decreases postoperative edema and seems to greatly improve respiratory function. Early ambulation should be ordered when the patient's condition warrants. (Syncope should be watched for in the elderly!)

B   Tracheostomy Care (plate 23)
Oxygen should be given through a loosely applied funnel (not by catheter into tracheostomy tube) as necessary. A mist collar (with oxygen) is better. Suctioning should be carried out frequently in the early stage, and a sterile, open-ended catheter must be inserted well below the inner tip of the tracheostomy tube. (The person performing this procedure must use sterile gloves or a sterile hemostat.) Deeper suctioning is occasionally necessary.

At times counterclockwise rotation of the tracheostomy tube can facilitate the introduction of the suction catheter into the left main stem bronchus. Ordinarily with deep suctioning, the catheter passes into the right main stem bronchus since the right bronchus is in more of a direct line with the trachea than the left bronchus.

Y-tube attachment is imperative so that brief, intermittent spells of suctioning can be utilized, each lasting a few seconds (no longer than the person handling the catheter can comfortably hold his or her breath). The catheter should be gently twisted during each insertion and withdrawal to prevent trauma to any one area of tracheal mucosa. The thumb should be repeatedly placed over the open end of the **Y**-tube and removed as the procedure is carried out. Prolonged and continuous suctioning is to be avoided. Hyperventilation with 100 per cent oxygen is recommended for two or three minutes prior to suctioning.

Sterile normal saline solution must be instilled with an eyedropper or syringe (if a needle is used, it must fit tightly!) into the trachea in 1 to 2 cc amounts every two to four hours and removed by suctioning to prevent dry tracheitis. (Detergents such as dilute solution of sodium lauryl sulfate or enzymes such as Dornavac can be very helpful locally in cases of severe dry tracheitis with crusting.)

The inner tube of the tracheostomy should be removed carefully and cleaned at least every four hours. The entire tube should be removed, cleaned and replaced every day or two after the tracheostomy has been well established (usually in five to six days). Large crusts may require forceps removal (with entire tube out if a solid tract is present). Extreme care must be taken when changing a tracheostomy tube in an infant. At least with the first change it should be done in the operating room with a bronchoscope and an endotracheal tube available.

A cuffed tracheostomy tube is helpful when positive pressure breathing is required, using a low leak technique to minimize injury to the trachea and thus prevent tracheal stenosis; otherwise, the traditional noncuffed tube with inner cannula is desirable. The disposable, cuffed, plastic tube (without inner cannula) has become popular with many thoracic surgeons in patients requiring very brief tracheostomies. This tube has not been generally satisfactory in our hands because of its large, outer diameter (requiring a very large tracheal wall opening), and the lack of an inner tube for cleansing purposes. The tracheostomy must never be discontinued until it is certain that the patient has a satisfactory airway. Mirror laryngoscopy must always be performed to evaluate the subglottic, glottic and supraglottic airway. In spite of some criticism of this method, half and full corking can be safely carried out in the process of "weaning" the patient from a tracheostomy. However, one must be certain that the tracheostomy tube is not filling the lumen of the trachea when corking is attempted!

Plate 23   Basic Techniques

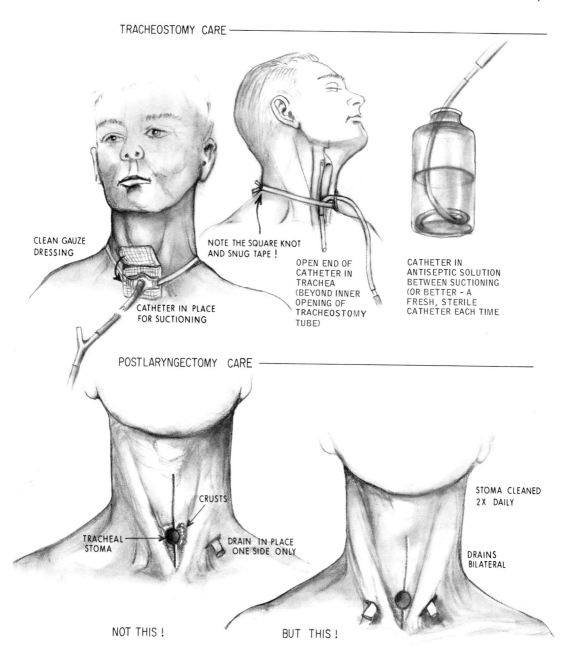

TRACHEOSTOMY CARE

CLEAN GAUZE
DRESSING

CATHETER IN PLACE
FOR SUCTIONING

NOTE THE SQUARE KNOT
AND SNUG TAPE !

OPEN END OF
CATHETER IN
TRACHEA
(BEYOND INNER
OPENING OF
TRACHEOSTOMY
TUBE)

CATHETER IN
ANTISEPTIC SOLUTION
BETWEEN SUCTIONING
(OR BETTER - A
FRESH, STERILE
CATHETER EACH TIME

POSTLARYNGECTOMY CARE

CRUSTS

TRACHEAL
STOMA

DRAIN IN PLACE
ONE SIDE ONLY

STOMA CLEANED
2X DAILY

DRAINS
BILATERAL

NOT THIS !

BUT THIS !

By gradually decreasing the size of the tracheostomy tube (from the standard #7 for men to #6 or #5), the surgeon can then cork with ease and finally remove the tube, *assuming the swallowing function is satisfactory!*

The patient must be able to pull the cork at any time if breathing becomes difficult. Of course, the corked, inner cannula must be removed and cleansed, just as previously described, until final discontinuance of the tracheostomy. After oral or laryngopharyngeal surgery has been performed along with a tracheostomy, the feeding tube may be removed when the patient is swallowing with ease. The tracheostomy tube must be left in place as a "safety valve" in case aspiration occurs. The surgeon must then carefully test the swallowing function to be certain that ingested liquid is not being aspirated before final termination of the tracheostomy.

POSTOPERATIVE CARE (*Continued*)

Following partial laryngectomy, removal of the tracheostomy tube may be necessary to initiate the act of swallowing. Close observation for aspiration is necessary, and if significant, the tracheostomy tube is reinserted.

C   Laryngectomy stomata need similar care (plate 23). The entire laryngectomy tube must be removed and replaced at least twice daily (by the surgeon, a member of the house staff or other trained personnel) and carefully cleansed. At this time the suture line is meticulously cleared of crusts of mucus (if necessary with cautious peroxide application to loosen any dried material). Antibiotic ointment is then applied to the skin-mucosal edge prior to tube reinsertion. Most patients are allowed to go without the laryngectomy tubes for increasing periods of time during the waking hours, after the first two to three days. Many surgeons prefer to keep the tube in place at night until it is certain that a large, rigid stoma has been developed. Plastic "buttons" or stoma rings are helpful in preventing stenosis when stomata are small and in treating stenosis (by dilation with larger and larger rings). A "bib" of porous gauze (without cotton filling), moistened frequently with water, should be placed loosely over the stoma at all times.

D   Narcotics are usually unnecessary in aged patients following procedures which include radical neck dissection; however, analgesics for headache and tranquilizers for anxiety or restlessness are important. Small doses of narcotics may be required by younger individuals. In the alcoholic, large doses of tranquilizers may be necessary.

Care must be used to avoid oversedation with respiratory depressions in any patient who might aspirate. Serious consequences have been observed, e.g., in patients with a posterior nasal hemorrhage with a posterior pack who have been oversedated.

E   High dose antibiotic therapy is advisable following extensive resection involving mucosa or bone. Recently, the time-honored penicillin-streptomycin combination has given way to single agents such as Cloxacillin, cephalothin and many others. Intravenous doses are used initially, followed as soon as possible by oral or feeding tube administrations. The preoperative cultures and antibiotic sensitivity studies will be helpful in determining the postoperative drug of choice.

F   The oral cavity *must be* carefully irrigated at least four times daily when suture lines are present. (Tube feedings should replace oral intake during the postoperative healing phase in all except the smaller, intraoral resection cases.) Peroxide-saline solution administered by power atomizer, Asepto syringe or Water Pik is useful in keeping the operative site clean. Aspiration of the irrigating solution is best managed by a tonsil tip attached to a portable or wall suction apparatus (plate 24). The patient should be placed in a sitting position for this treatment to prevent the aspiration or swallowing of the irrigating solution. In addition, brief suture line applications of gauze soaked in hydrogen peroxide or the now-scarce zinc peroxide paste are extremely helpful in clearing infection, especially when anaerobic organisms have invaded an area of wound disruption or necrosis. Neomycin mouthwash, 1 per cent three times a day, is used in procedures which enter the upper respiratory-digestive tract. Again, be cautious of oto- and nephrotoxicity.

G   Daily dressings are advisable to prevent wound contamination by saliva and tracheal secretions. Of course, stents over grafts are kept in place for periods varying from four to five days for mucosal defect skin grafts, to six to seven days for skin defect grafts. Pressure dressings may or may not be required, depending on the presence or absence of vacuum tube wound drainage. This latter technique may obviate the necessity of *any* wound coverage. Both pressure dressings and vacuum tube drainage may be advisable when pharyngeal wound closures are under tension (beneath neck dis-

(*Text continued on page 60.*)

Plate 24   *Basic Techniques*

CARE OF INTRAORAL SURGICAL WOUNDS ──────────────────────

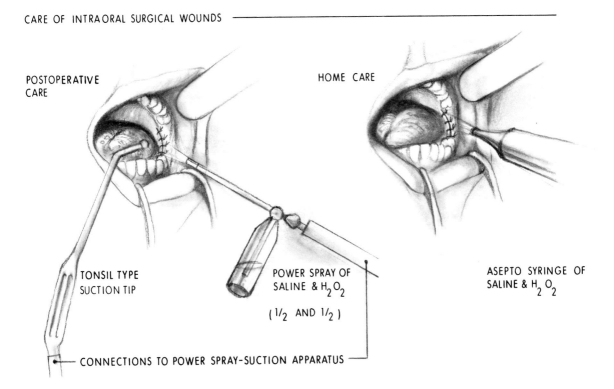

POSTOPERATIVE
CARE

HOME CARE

TONSIL TYPE
SUCTION TIP

POWER SPRAY OF
SALINE & H_2O_2

($1/2$ AND $1/2$)

ASEPTO SYRINGE OF
SALINE & H_2O_2

─── CONNECTIONS TO POWER SPRAY-SUCTION APPARATUS ───

section flaps). Antibiotic ointment may be applied over exposed suture lines. Some would prefer a quick-drying liquid adhesive administered by spray to these skin closures.

The technique of pressure dressings is pictured in plate 25. Kling or Kerlix is a useful material for application over fluffed gauze when pressure is desired. Elastoplast should be applied for additional support supplemented with adhesive strips. The entire head should be covered, especially when *parotid* or upper neck wounds are being dressed. The ear must be adequately padded and care taken not to fold the ear lobe forward while applying the dressing.

Fluid accumulation can be prevented and skin flaps made to adhere nicely to deeper structures with the use of properly managed vacuum wound catheters. Two multiholed rubber catheters (16F in adults), attached by a Y-tube to a GOMCO pump (on "low"), will give excellent results following neck dissection. A single, smaller catheter (14F) is all that is required for parotidectomy or other smaller skin-flap wounds. The Hemo-Vac apparatus (*if the large-sized plastic catheters and large, bellows-type bag are used*) is convenient and handy, but early clotting within these catheters must be watched for. The catheters should be disconnected from suction when fluid withdrawal has ceased or has dropped to minute amounts. These tubes should then remain in place to function as ordinary drains to prevent additional fluid accumulation. They can be gradually shortened. A word of caution regarding these tubes—they must not cross the carotid vessels nor be located too close to any major vessel since there is danger of pressure necrosis leading to carotid artery blowout. One or two 3-0 catgut sutures loosely placed can be utilized to keep the tubes in the desired location.

All tubes and drains are possible sources of ascending infection and appropriate precautions should be taken. (A sump-type drain with an air inlet tube is used by some, but in our hands this has not been as successful as the closed vacuum method.) The neck wound should be carefully examined daily for any evidence of fluid accumulation. Prompt evacuation is imperative. Late accumulations often herald the development of pharyngeal suture line disruptions. (Foul-smelling, mucus-containing material is usually diagnostic of such a complication.) In this case, the overlying skin flaps should be widely laid open and irrigations promptly started after adequate drainage of any pockets. Loosely and temporarily applied saline peroxide or zinc peroxide paste packs after each irrigation will clear up any anaerobic infection and stimulate granulation tissue formation. These should be changed frequently.

Carotid artery exposure (which is usually prevented by muscle flap coverage or dermal graft [plates 372 and 373] during the operation) necessitates extremely vigorous local wound care. Ligation may become necessary if granulation does not quickly cover the vessel! The appearance of a pale, avascular area in the arterial wall indicates an impending rupture. If the wound is not infected, proximally and distally, an elective arterial by-pass graft could be performed through clean surgical fields (refer to Chapter 21).

In the presence of *Pseudomonas aeruginosa* (*Bacillus pyocyaneus*) infections, characterized by a blue-green pus with a rather sweet, musty, pungent odor, acetic acid, 1 to 3 per cent, is very efficacious.

Dressings for thyroidectomy, maxillectomy and smaller procedures will not be discussed because of space limitations.

H   *Tube Feedings.* By the use of nasoesophageal or nasogastric tubes, gastrostomies are circumvented. Faulty tracheal insertions of a feeding tube must be watched for. Patients with tracheostomies and those who have undergone extensive head and neck procedures may not demonstrate the usual coughing when a feeding tube is accidentally placed into the trachea. Proper positioning is indicated by a lateral

Plate 25   Basic Techniques

HEAD AND NECK SURGICAL DRESSINGS

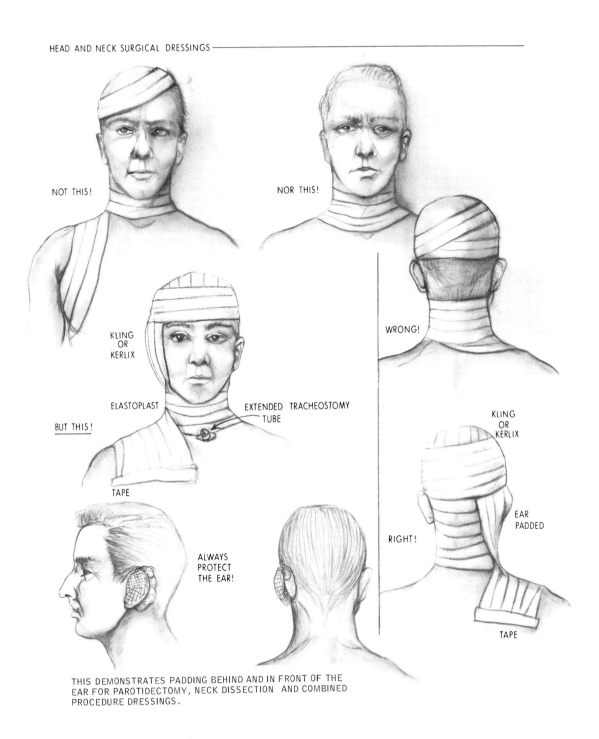

NOT THIS!

NOR THIS!

KLING
OR
KERLIX

ELASTOPLAST

BUT THIS!

EXTENDED TRACHEOSTOMY
TUBE

WRONG!

TAPE

KLING
OR
KERLIX

ALWAYS
PROTECT
THE EAR!

RIGHT!

EAR
PADDED

TAPE

THIS DEMONSTRATES PADDING BEHIND AND IN FRONT OF THE
EAR FOR PAROTIDECTOMY, NECK DISSECTION AND COMBINED
PROCEDURE DRESSINGS.

POSTOPERATIVE CARE *(Continued)*

pharyngeal position of the tube as seen through the open mouth (see plate 26). Often the feeding tube must be inserted by the anesthesiologist, especially when a laryngectomy is being carried out. Here, the tube insertion must be completed prior to pharyngeal wall closure to prevent possible perforation of the suture line. Some surgeons are now leaving out the feeding tube in a laryngectomy in the hopes of decreasing the incidence of fistula formation. In any event, do *not* reinsert an accidentally removed feeding tube in the immediate postoperative period prior to wound healing since the reinserted tube can disrupt the suture line. Cervical esophagostomy or pharyngotomy is useful when prolonged feedings are required. Some use this method even with standard radical neck dissection and total laryngectomy for greater patient comfort. With the existence of a planned fistula or a fistula resulting from wound breakdown, direct insertion of the feeding tube into the pharynx or esophagus through such a fistula can be employed. To avoid a carotid artery blowout, extreme care must be taken so that such an arrangement does not place the feeding tube across or near the carotid vessels.

High caloric liquid feedings are best administered by tube after the first postoperative day when nausea and gastric atony have subsided. Clear surgical liquids may be given in the interim. The nurse- or patient-administered funnel-gravity method is best, and has distinct advantages over the time-honored drip method which may result in gastric distension (in a sleeping or lethargic patient who is unattended). The patient must be cautioned to immediately indicate to the nurse when his stomach feels "full." Sterilized or thoroughly cleaned equipment is essential in preventing bacterial contamination, one of the common causes of diarrhea in tube-fed patients. Graduated daily increases in caloric content to the point of tolerance are advisable. Many patients will develop gastric distress and diarrhea with high caloric feedings; 1500 to 2000 calories per 24 hour period is about the average maximum. Two hundred fifty to 300 cc every three hours of a balanced feeding high in protein (omitting the 3 A.M. dose) is a good schedule, with at least 90 cc of water being added after each feeding (and on request). If long-term feedings are required, blenderized foods may be utilized in larger increments four to six times daily. (Commercial feeding mixtures, such as Sustagen or Gevral Protein, are convenient for tube feedings and can be easily prepared by adding water. These preparations should be diluted in order to cut the caloric intake.) Some surgeons prefer only the use of ordinary liquids, e.g., juices, meat broth and teas rather than blenderized or commercial mixtures.

Complications

Hypernatremia may follow prolonged tube feedings in debilitated patients who are not given adequate amounts of water. This is the "solute-loading hypertonicity" described by Moore (1959). Thirst results and the conscious patient ordinarily requests water between feedings. Unconscious persons, therefore, are the usual victims of the "solute-loading" problem. Hypernatremia, azotemia and extracellular volume deficits follow. At least 7 cc of water per gram of dietary protein is essential in the prevention of this serious difficulty. Thoroughly crushed or powdered medications in water, or liquid analgesic preparations of various types, may be given per feeding tube. Therapeutic doses of vitamins B and C should be added to the tube feedings daily. Irrigation of these tubes after each feeding or medication is essential in preventing blockage by inspissated material. Replacement of a blocked feeding tube may be risky in patients with pharyngeal suture lines. Bleeding and perforation from a stress peptic ulcer should be watched for in postoperative head and neck patients.

These brief pre- and postoperative suggestions should serve as a guide in the management of patients undergoing head and neck surgery. Meticulous attention to the details of patient care will help to decrease morbidity and mortality in these surgical cases involving complex anatomic areas.

Plate 26   *Basic Techniques*

PUTTING IN THE FEEDING TUBE
(NASOESOPHAGEAL CATHETER FOR FEEDING)

CORK MUST BE USED!

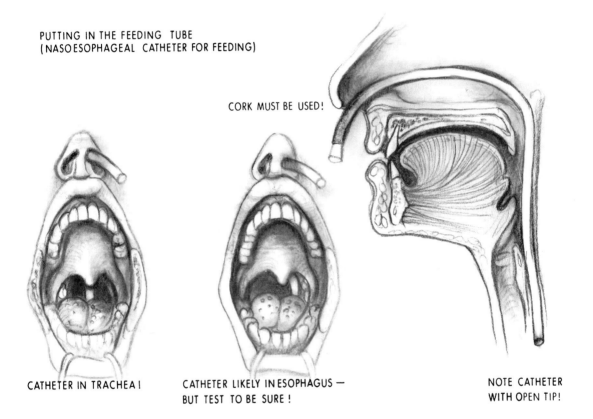

CATHETER IN TRACHEA!

CATHETER LIKELY IN ESOPHAGUS —
BUT TEST TO BE SURE!

NOTE CATHETER
WITH OPEN TIP!

BIBLIOGRAPHY

Alford, B. R.: Rubella—La Bête Noire de la Médecine. Laryngoscope 78:1623–1659, 1968.

Algird, J. R.: A technique for thoracentesis utilizing a disposable catheter unit. Cancer 19:281–283, 1966.

Bernstein, L.: Z-Plasty in head and neck surgery. Arch. Otolaryng. 89:574–584, 1969.

Borges, A. F.: Improvement of antitension-lines scar by the "W-plastic" operation. Brit. J. Plast. Surg. 12:29–33, 1959.

Borges, A. F.: The W-plastic versus the Z-plastic scar revision. Plast. Reconstr. Surg. 44:58–62, 1969.

Borja, A. R., and Lansing, A. M.: Technique of selective pulmonary embolectomy without bypass. Surg. Gynec. Obstet. 130:1073–1076, 1970.

Breed, J. E.: Management of the patient with terminal illness. Illinois Med. J. 139:503–505, 1971.

Breen, K. J., Bryant, R. E., Levinson, J. D., and Schenker, S.: Neomycine absorption in man, Ann. Intern. Med. 76:211–218, 1972.

Bryce, D. P., and Crysdale, W. S.: Non-healing granuloma: A diagnostic problem. Laryngoscope 79:794–805, 1969.

Buchheit, W. A., Ronis, M. L., and Liebman, E.: Brain abscesses complicating head and neck infections. Trans. Amer. Acad. Ophthal. Otolaryng. 74:548–554, 1970.

Calcaterra, T. C.: Orolaryngeal histoplasmosis. Laryngoscope 80:111–120, 1970.

Carey, J. S., Mohr, P. A., Brown, R. S., and Shoemaker, W. C.: Cardiovascular function in hemorrhage, trauma and sepsis: Determinants of cardiac output and cardiac work. Ann. Surg. 170:910–921, 1969.

Catlin, D.: Cutaneous melanoma of the head and neck. Amer. J. Surg. 112:512, 1966.

Cole, S. L., and Corday, E.: Four-minute limit for cardiac resuscitation. J.A.M.A. 161:1454–1458, 1956.

Converse, J. M. (ed.): Reconstructive Plastic Surgery. Principles and Procedures in Correction, Reconstruction and Transplantation. Vol. I. Philadelphia, W. B. Saunders Company, 1964.

Cox, H. T.: Progressive post-operative cutaneous gangrene. Brit. J. Surg. 23:576, 1949.

Davis, J. S.: Present evaluation of the merits of the Z-plastic operation. Plast. Reconstr. Surg. 1:26–38, 1946.

Davis, J. S., and Kitlowski, E. A.: The theory and practical use of the Z-incision for the relief of scar contractures. Ann. Surg. 109:1001, 1939.

DeSanto, L. W.: Application of cryosurgery to otolaryngology. Minn. Med. 53:29–32, 1970.

Dickinson, J. T.: Maxillofacial injuries and soft tissue repair. Frederick T. Hill Seminar, Waterville, Maine, August 1972.

Dingman, R. O.: Some applications of the Z-plastic procedure. Plast. Reconstr. Surg. 16:246–263, 1955.

Dunbar, J. S.: Upper respiratory tract obstruction in infants and children. Caldwell Lecture, 1969. Amer. J. Roentgen. 109:227–246, 1970.

Eberle, R. C., and Conley, J. J.: Nerve suturing. Trans. Amer. Acad. Ophthal. Otolaryng. 73:274–278, 1969.

Eilert, J. B., Binder, P., McKinney, P. W., Beal, J. M., and Conn, J. Jr.: Polyglycolic acid synthetic absorbable sutures. Amer. J. Surg. 121:561–564, 1971.

Eller, J. J., and Walsh, W. R.: Dermal abrasion in the treatment of acne. GP 24:89–91, 1961.

Epstein, E.: Present status of dermabrasion. J.A.M.A. 206:607–610, 1968.

Everts, E. C.: Cervicofacial actinomycosis. Arch. Otolaryng. 92:468–474, 1970.

Farrior, R. T.: Implant materials in restoration of facial contour. Laryngoscope 75:934–954, 1966.

Farrior, R. T.: Synthetics in head and neck surgery. Arch. Otolaryng. 84:82–90, 1966.

Fell, T., and Cheney, F. W.: Prevention of hypoxia during endotracheal suction. Ann. Surg. 174:24–28, 1971.

Fischer, J. E., Turner, R. H., Herndon, J. H., and Riseborough, E. J.: Massive steroid therapy in severe fat embolism. Surg. Gynec Obstet. 132:667–672, 1971.

Flanagan, J. P., Gradisar, I., Gross, R. J., and Kelly, T. R.: Air embolus—A lethal complication of subclavian venipuncture. New Eng. J. Med. 281:488–489, 1969.

Fry, H.: Cartilage and cartilage grafts: The basic properties of the tissue and the components responsible for them. Plast. Reconstr. Surg. 40:426–439, 1967.

Gault, M. H., Dixon, M. E., Doyle, M., and Cohen, W. M.: Hypernatremia, azotemia and dehydration due to high-protein tube feeding. Ann. Intern. Med. 68:778–791, 1968.

Goldstein, J. C.: Cryotherapy in head and neck cancer. Laryngoscope 80:1046–1052, 1970.

Gordon, A. S., Palich, W. E., and Fletcher, E. E.: Emergency heart-lung resuscitation and external defibrillation. Scientific Exhibit at 39th Congress of International Anesthesia Research Society, Washington, D. C., March 1965.

Grabb, W. C., and Dingman, R. O.: The fate of amputated tissues of the head and neck following replacement. Plast. Reconstr. Surg. 49:28–32, 1972.

Graham, W. P., III, Noone, R. B., and Nicholas, G. G.: Cervical pharyngostomy: A simplified method of tube feeding. The Department of Surgery, Division of Plastic Surgery and the Harrison Department of Surgical Research, University of Pennsylvania, Philadelphia.

Greenfield, L. J., Bruce, T. A., and Nichols, N. B.: Transvenous pulmonary embolectomy by catheter device. Ann. Surg. 174:881–886, 1971.

Hagerty, R. F., Braid, H. L., Bonner, W. M., Jr., Hennigar, G. R., and Lee, W. H., Jr.: Viable and nonviable human cartilage homografts. Surg. Gynec. Obstet. 125:485–492, 1967.

Hall, J. E.: The physiology of respiration in infants and young children. Proc. Roy. Soc. Med. 48:761–764, 1955.

Hardaway, R. M., III: The problem of acute severe trauma and shock. Surg. Gynec. Obstet. 133:799–806, 1971.

Harkin, J. C., and Skinner, M. S.: Experimental and electron microscopic studies of nerve regeneration. Ann. Otol. 79: 218, 1970.

Hawk, J.: Personal communication, 1968.

Hellström, K. E., and Hellström, I.: Some aspects of the immune defense against cancer. Cancer 28:1266–1268, 1971.

Ivy, R. H.: Who originated the Z-plasty? Plast. Reconstr. Surg. 47:67–72, 1971.

James, P. M., and Myers, R. T.: Central venous pressure monitoring. Ann. Surg. 175:693–701, 1972.

Jesse, R. H.: Preoperative versus postoperative radiation in the treatment of squamous carcinoma of the paranasal sinuses. Amer. J. Surg. 110:552–556, 1965.

Jobe, R. P., and Briggs, R. M.: Marking the surgical specimen in skin neoplasm excision. Surg. Gynec. Obstet. 126: 1325–1326, 1968.

Johnson, J., and Kirby, C. K.: Surgery of the Chest. 2d ed. Chicago, Year Book Medical Publishers, Inc., 1958.

Jordan, W. S., Graves, C. L., and Elwyn, R. A.: New therapy for postintubation laryngeal edema and tracheitis in children. J.A.M.A. 212:585–588, 1970.

Jude, J. R., and Tabbarah, H. J.: Otolaryngological aspects of cardiac arrest. Ann. Otol. 79:889, 1970.

Jude, J. R., Kouwenhoven, W. B., and Knickerbocker, G. G.: A new approach to cardiac resuscitation. Ann. Surg. 154: 311–319, 1961.

Kaye, R. L., and Sones, D. A.: Relapsing polychondritis – Clinical and pathologic features in fourteen cases. Ann. Intern. Med. 60:653–664, 1964.

Ketcham, A. S., Hoye, R. C., Chretien, P. B., and Brace, K. C.: Irradiation twenty-four hours preoperatively. Amer. J. Surg. 118:691–697, 1969.

Kirimli, B., Kampschulte, S., and Safar, P.: Resuscitation from cardiac arrest due to exsanguination. Surg. Gynec. Obstet. 129:89–97, 1969.

Kornblut, A. D., and Shumrick, D. A.: Complications of head and neck surgery. Arch. Otolaryng. 94:246–254, 1971.

Kouwenhoven, W. B., Jude, J. R., and Knickerbocker, G. G.: Closed-chest cardiac massage. J.A.M.A. 173:1064–1067, 1960.

Lane, M., Moore, J. E., III, Levin, H., and Smith, F. E.: Methotrexate therapy for squamous cell carcinomas of the head and neck. J.A.M.A. 204:561–564, 1968.

Lichti, E. L., Turner, M., Henzel, J. H., and DeWeese, M. S.: Wound fluid zinc levels during tissue repair. Sequential determination by means of surgically implanted Teflon cylinders. Amer. J. Surg. 121:665–667, 1971.

Limberg, A. A.: Planning of Local Plastic Operations of the Body's Surface: Theory and Practice. Medgiz, Moscow, 1963.

Lindskog, G., and Liebow, A. A.: Thoracic Surgery and Related Pathology. New York, Appleton-Century-Crofts, 1953.

Loré, J. M., Jr.: Suction tubing and tip-holding forceps. Amer. J. Surg. 58:679, 1954.

Loré, J. M., Jr.: Tender grip forceps. Amer. J. Surg. 194:84–85, 1962.

Loré, J. M., Jr.: Treatment of recurrent tumors of the head and neck. Laryngoscope 78:1445, 1968.

Loré, J. M., Jr., Gordon, S. G., and Gordon, E. W.: Successful use of hypothermia following cardiac arrest in twelve-day-old infant. New York J. Med. 60:278–279, 1960.

Lundberg, G. D., Mattei, I. R., Davis, C. J., and Nelson, D. E.: Hemorrhage from gastroesophageal lacerations following closed-chest cardiac massage. J.A.M.A. 202:195–198, 1967.

Macgregor, F. C., Abel, T. A., Bryt, A., Lauer, E., and Weissmann, S.: Facial Deformities and Plastic Surgery—A Psycho-Social Study. Charles C Thomas, Publishers, Springfield, Ill., 1952.

Madden, J. L.: Atlas of Techniques in Surgery. New York, Appleton-Century-Crofts, 1958.

Madden, J. E., Edlich, R. F., Custer, J. R., Panek, P. H., Thul, J., and Wangensteen, O. H.: Studies in the management of the contaminated wound. IV. Resistance to infection of surgical wounds made by knife, electrosurgery, and laser. Amer. J. Surg. 119:222–224, 1970.

Marchetta, F. C., Sako, K., and Camp, F.: Multiple malignancies in patients with head and neck cancer. Amer. J. Surg. 110:537–541, 1965.

Marchetta, F. C., Sako, K., and Maxwell, W.: Complications after radical head and neck surgery performed through previously irradiated tissues. Amer. J. Surg. 114:835–838, 1967.

Martin, H.: Aspiration biopsy. Surg. Gynec. Obstet. 59:578–589, 1934.

Martin, H.: "Malignancies" and cancers. Amer. J. Roentgen. 38:479–482, 1937.

Martin, H.: Untimely lymph node biopsy. Amer. J. Surg. 102:17–18, 1961.

Marx, G. F., Steen, S. N., Arkins, R. E., Foster, E. S., Joffe, S., Kepes, E. R., and Schapira, M.: Clinical anesthesia conference: Endotracheal suction and death. New York J. Med. 68:565–566, 1968.

Masson, J. K., and Soule, E. H.: Embryonal rhabdomyosarcoma of the head and neck. Report on eighty-eight cases. Amer. J. Surg. 110:585–591, 1965.

Mauney, F. M., Jr., Ebert, P. A., and Sabiston, D. C., Jr.: Postoperative myocardial infarction: A study of predisposing factors, diagnosis and mortality in a high risk group of surgical patients. Ann. Surg. 172:497–503, 1970.

McCabe, B. F.: Hemorrhage in otolaryngologic surgery. Trans. Amer. Acad. Ophthal. Otolaryng. 72:23–24, 1968.

McGregor, I. A.: Fundamental Techniques of Plastic Surgery and Their Surgical Applications. E. & S. Livingstone, Ltd., Edinburgh, 1962.

McLaughlin, J. S.: Physiologic consideration of hypoxemia in shock and trauma. Ann. Surg. 173:667–679, 1971.

McNamara, J. J., Molot, M. D., Wissman, D., Collins, C., and Stremple, J. F.: Intravenous hyperalimentation. An important adjunct in the treatment of combat casualties. Amer. J. Surg. 122:70–73, 1971.

McNamara, J. J., Lamborn, P. J., Mills, D., and Aaby, G. V.: Effect of short-term pharmacologic doses of adrenocorticosteroid therapy on wound healing. Ann. Surg. 170:199–202, 1969.

Miller, D.: Three years experience with cryosurgery in head and neck tumors. Ann. Otol. 78:786, 1969.

Miller, D., and Metzner, D.: Cryosurgery for tumors of the head and neck. Trans. Amer. Acad. Ophthal. Otolaryng. 73:300–309, 1969.

Moore, F. D.: Metabolic Care of the Surgical Patient. Philadelphia, W. B. Saunders Company, 1959.

Moore, G. E.: The importance of biopsy procedures. J.A.M.A. 205:917–920, 1968.

Morestin, H.: De la Correction des Flexions Permanentes des Doigts. Rev. Chir. 50:1, 1914.

Neely, W. A., Berry, D. W., Rushton, F. W., and Hardy, J. D.: Septic shock: Clinical, physiological, and pathological survey of 244 patients. Ann. Surg. 173:657–666, 1971.

Nyberg, C. D., Samartano, J. G., and Terry, R. N.: Use of innovar as an anesthetic adjunct in oral surgery. J. Oral Surg. 28:175–180, 1970.

Oberleas, D., Lenaghan, R., Wilson, R. F., Seymour, J. K., Hovanesian, J., and

Prasad, A. S.: Effect of zinc deficiency on wound-healing in rats. Amer. J. Surg. *121*:566–568, 1971.

Olsen, N. R., and Newman, M. H.: Acrylic frontal cranioplasty. Arch. Otolaryng. *89*:774–777, 1969.

Olwin, J. H.: Tumor metastasis and anticoagulants. Surg. Gynec. Obstet. *132*: 1064–1066, 1971.

Pappelbaum, S., Lang, T. W., Bazika, V., Bernstein, H., Herrold, G., and Corday, E.: Comparative hemodynamics during open vs. closed cardiac resuscitation. J.A.M.A. *193*:659–662, 1965.

Pickard, R. E.: Tantalum radiography in otolaryngology. Arch. Otolaryng. *94*: 202–207, 1971.

Postlethwait, R. W.: Long-term comparative study of nonabsorbable sutures. Ann. Surg. *171*:892–898, 1970.

Pradier, R., Sako, K., De La Pava, S., and Marchetta, F. C.: Distant metastases and vascular invasion in patients with en bloc resections of head and neck cancer. Surg. Gynec. Obstet. *119*:17–18, 1964.

Puryear, G. H., Osborn, J. J., Beaumont, J. O., and Gerbode, F.: The influence of adjuvant ventilators in the respiratory effort of acutely ill patients. Ann. Surg. *170*:900–909, 1969.

Quarantillo, E. P., Jr.: Effect of supplemental zinc on wound healing in rats. Amer. J. Surg. *121*:661–664, 1971.

Riker, W. L.: Cardiac arrest in infants and children. Pediat. Clin. N. Amer. *16*: 661–669, 1969.

Rubin, L. R., Bromberg, B. E., and Walden, R. H.: Long term human reaction to synthetic plastics. Surg. Gynec. Obstet. *132*:603–608, 1971.

Rusca, J. A., Bornside, G. H., and Cohn, I., Jr.: Everting versus inverting gastrointestinal anastomoses: Bacterial leakage and anastomotic disruption. Ann. Surg. *169*:727–735, 1969.

Sake, K., Marchetta, F. C., Badillo, J., and Burke, E.: Results of cytologic studies of wound washings and use of a local cytotoxic agent in head and neck surgery. Amer. J. Surg. *102*:818–822, 1961.

Salyer, J. M.: Management of spontaneous pneumothorax or pneumomediastinum in the newborn. Surg. Gynec. Obstet. *131*:115–116, 1970.

Schechter, D. C.: Role of the humane societies in the history of resuscitation. Surg. Gynec. Obstet. *129*:811–815, 1969.

Schuman, B. M.: Tube feeding as part of the supportive care of the surgical patient. Henry Ford Hosp. Med. J. *19*:35–37, 1971.

Shoemaker, W. C., Mohr, P. A., Printen, K. J., Brown, R. S., Amato, J. J., Carey, J. S., Youssef, S., Reinhard, J. M., Kim, S. I., and Kark, A. E.: Use of sequential physiologic measurements for evaluation and therapy of uncomplicated septic shock. Surg. Gynec. Obstet. *131*: 245–254, 1970.

Sisson, G. A.: Problems and complications in head and neck surgery. Laryngoscope *70*:1142–1155, 1960.

Smith, R. O., Jr., Dickinson, J. T., and Cipcic, J. A.: Composite grafts in facial reconstructive surgery. Arch. Otolaryng. *95*:252–264, 1972.

Snow, J. B., Jr.: The classification of respiratory viruses and their clinical manifestations. Laryngoscope *79*:1485–1493, 1969.

Soroff, H. S. et al.: Metabolism of burned patients. *In* Artz, C. P. (ed.): Research in Burns. Philadelphia, F. A. Davis Company, 1962.

Stallings, J. O., Huffman, W. C., and Bernstein, L.: Skin grafts on bare bone. Plast. Reconstr. Surg. *43*:152–156, 1969.

Stevenson, T. W.: Release of circular constricting scar by Z flaps. Plast. Reconstr. Surg. *1*:39–42, 1946.

Straith, R. E., Lawson, J. M., and Hipps, C. J.: The subcuticular suture. Postgrad. Med. *29*:164–173, 1961.

Sweet, R. H.: Thoracic Surgery. Philadelphia, W. B. Saunders Company, 1950.

Thieme, E. T., and Fink, G.: A study of the danger of antibiotic preparation of the bowel for surgery. Surg. *67*:403–408, 1970.

Thompson, D. S., and Eason, C. N.: Hypoxemia immediately after operation. Amer. J. Surg. *120*:649–651, 1970.

Tisi, G. M., Twigg, H. L., and Moser, K. M.: Collapse of left lung induced by artificial airway. Lancet *1*:791–793, 1968.

Twigg, H. L., and Buckley, C. E.: Complications of endotracheal intubation. Amer. J. Roentgen. *109*:452–454, 1970.

Ukai, M., Moran, W. H., Jr., and Zimmermann, B.: The role of visceral afferent pathways on vasopressin secretion and urinary excretory patterns during surgical stress. Ann. Surg. *168*:16–28, 1968.

Van Winkle, W., Jr.: The tensile strength of wounds and factors that influence it. Surg. Gynec. Obstet. *129*:819–842, 1969.

VandenBerg, H. J., Jr., Chen, S. C., Blatt, C. J., and Berkas, E. M.: A comparison of wound healing between irradiated and nonirradiated patients after radical neck dissection. Amer. J. Surg. *110*:557–561, 1965.

Vaughn, D. L., Gunter, C. A., and Stookey, J. L.: Endotoxin shock in primates. Surg. Gynec. Obstet. *126*:1309–1317, 1968.

Vernon, S.: The ideal initial infusion in unexpected shock. Surg. Gynec. Obstet. *131*:748–749, 1970.

Wagner, M.: Evaluation of diverse plastic and cutis prostheses in a growing host. Surg. Gynec. Obstet. *130*:1077–1081, 1970.

Walike, J. W.: Tube feeding syndrome in head and neck surgery. Arch. Otolaryng. *89*:117–120, 1969.

Watson, T. A.: Irradiation in the management of tumors of the head and neck. Amer. J. Surg. *110*:542–548, 1965.

Weale, F. E., and Rothwell-Jackson, R. L.: The efficacy of cardiac massage. Lancet *1*:990–992, 1962.

Wilkinson, T. S., and Rybka, F. J.: Experimental study of prevention of tip necrosis in ischemic Z-plasties. Plast. Reconstr. Surg. *47*:37–38, 1971.

Wynder, E. L.: Etiological aspects of squamous cancers of the head and neck. J.A.M.A. *215*:452–453, 1971.

Zimmerman, J. E.: Respiratory failure complicating post-traumatic acute renal failure: Etiology, clinical features and management. Ann. Surg. *174*:12–18, 1971.

3. THE SINUSES AND MAXILLA

INTRANASAL ANTROSTOMY

Highpoints

    1. Site of opening must be behind anterior wall of antrum.
    2. Direction of instrument must be either horizontal or pointed slightly downward to avoid injury to floor of orbit.
    3. When irrigating, no air should be injected to avoid air embolism.
Refer to plates 5 and 6.

Anesthesia

    Local, topical 2 per cent tetracaine or 10 per cent cocaine.

A
A¹ A small hollow antral trocar (Douglas) is placed beneath the inferior turbinate. Occasionally the turbinate will hang and obstruct the approach. In such cases it is fractured medially and elevated with a blunt instrument. Its mucosa should not be injured. With steady pressure, the trocar punctures the medial wall of the antrum (the lateral wall of the inferior meatus). The antrum is then gently irrigated with sterile normal saline or other suitable alkaline solution (Alkalol). The return flow is through the natural ostium. If the bony wall is very thin, a spinal needle may be substituted for the trocar.

B
B¹ When the medial wall of the antrum is thick, a Faulkner trocar chisel is used to perform the antrostomy.

B²
B³ If an antral window is desirable for continuous drainage of the antrum, the instrument is rotated 180 degrees after the antral wall is punctured. The undercut edge of the instrument then engages the rim of the opening. As the instrument is withdrawn, the opening is thus enlarged.

    To enlarge the antrostomy further, several techniques are available.

C
C¹ A curved rasp (Wiener) is inserted and with to and fro motion the opening is enlarged. Care must be taken that the tip of the rasp is pointed downward. This avoids injury to the floor of the orbit and removes the bone at the base of the medial wall, allowing adequate drainage. No ledge of bone should remain at the base.

D A bone cutting punch is also utilized to enlarge the opening, as is a double action cutting forceps if the bone is thick. Again the important direction is downward so that the nasoantral ridge is removed at the antrostomy site. The floor of the nasal cavity usually is slightly lower than the antral floor, allowing free flow of secretions from the antrum into the nose if the nasoantral ridge is adequately removed. At times, however, the floor of the antrum may be lower than the floor of the nose.

D¹ A Kerrison forceps is used to enlarge the opening.

E The antrum may be explored using Coakley curets. Cysts and diseased mucous membrane can be removed if so indicated. Any sizable polyp, however, should be removed through a Caldwell-Luc approach.

Complications

    1. Injury to the orbit.
    2. Air embolism.
    3. Insertion of trocar anterior to anterior wall of antrum and then into soft tissue of cheek.

Plate 27   The Sinuses and Maxilla

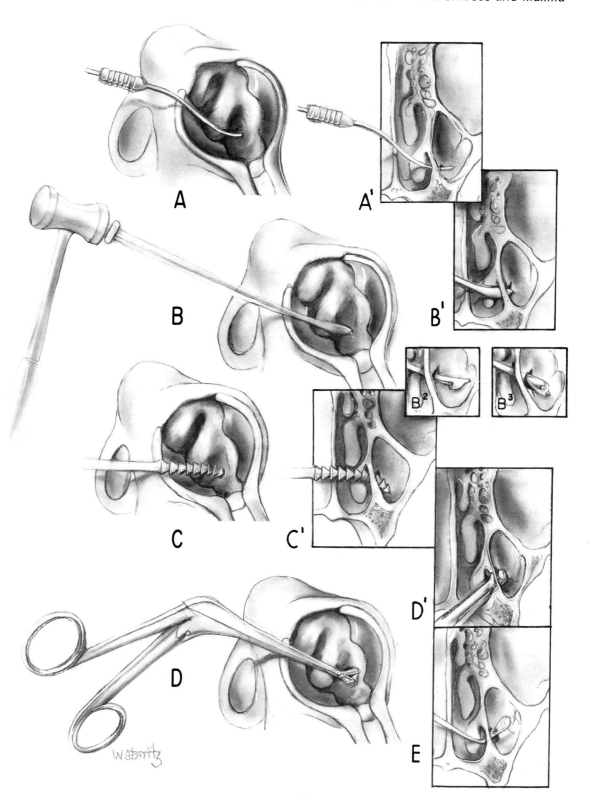

A

A'

B

B'

B²

B³

C

C'

D

D'

E

CALDWELL-LUC ANTROTOMY

Indications

1. Benign tumors.
2. Chronic empyema resistant to conservative treatment.
3. Complicated fractures of maxilla.
4. Exploration.

Refer to plates 1, 5 and 6.

A In the gingivobuccal sulcus (canine fossa), well above the tooth sockets, an incision is made through mucosa and periosteum several centimeters from the midline. Sufficient mucosa is preserved inferiorly for ease of closure.

B The periosteum is elevated. The insertion of the facial muscles may require sharp dissection to free them from the anterior wall of the antrum.

C The exposure is carried upward to a point just below the infraorbital rim where the infraorbital nerve is identified and carefully preserved. Using an osteotome, the anterior wall of the antrum is opened. This opening must be well above the tooth sockets and above the floor of the antrum. All the fractured fragments of bone are removed.

D Using a Kerrison back biting forceps, the opening is enlarged to the desired size to permit exploration.

E Removal of benign tumors and cysts is then easily accomplished by grasping forceps and scissors. Normal mucosa should not be injured; however, all diseased mucosa is removed.

Plate 28   The Sinuses and Maxilla

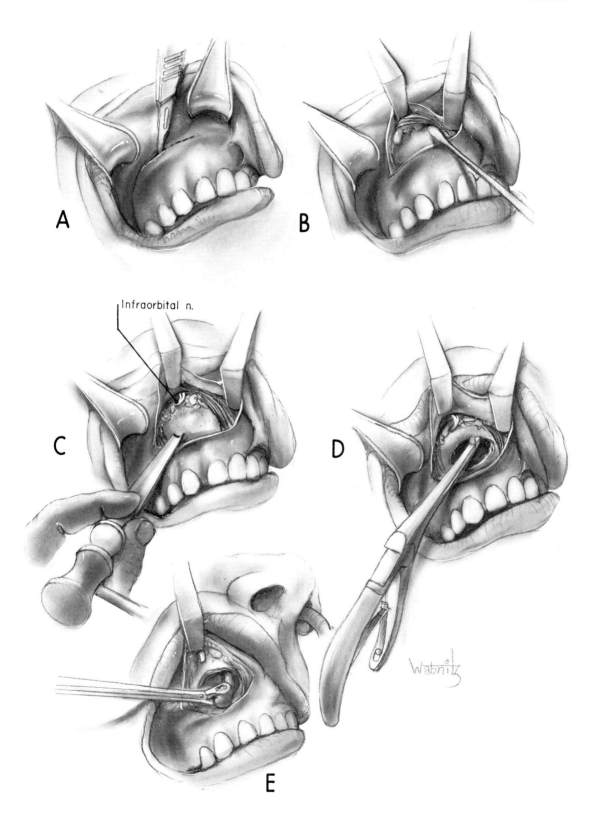

Infraorbital n.

CALDWELL-LUC ANTROTOMY (*Continued*)

F   Usually an intranasal antrostomy beneath the inferior turbinate is done to facilitate drainage (plate 27).

G   This intranasal antrostomy may be enlarged through the original operative opening using forward bone cutting forceps, depending on the purpose of the operation.

H   Close-up of step G.

I   Cross-sectional anatomy to show the dependent intranasal opening. The arrow depicts the natural ostium.

J   The mucosal flap over the anterior wall opening is approximated with interrupted 4-0 nylon.

Complications

1. Injury to infraorbital nerve.
2. Injury to roots of teeth.
3. Injury to the floor of the orbit.

This procedure should be avoided when a malignant lesion is suspected. Needle aspiration through the inferior meatus or the use of an intranasal antrostomy with curettage using Coakley curets is preferred (plate 27). If these methods fail, then do not hesitate to explore the antrum through this Caldwell-Luc antrotomy.

Plate 29   The Sinuses and Maxilla

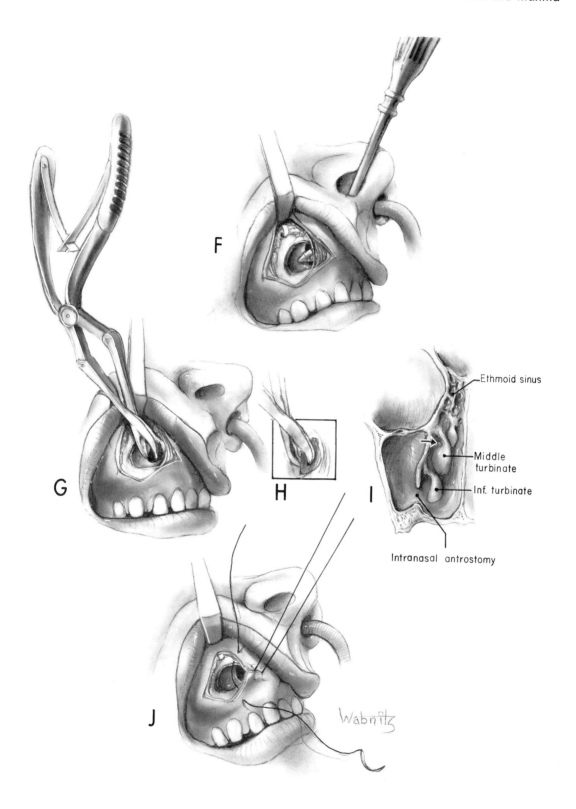

F

G

H

I

Ethmoid sinus

Middle turbinate

Inf. turbinate

Intranasal antrostomy

J

Wabnitz

INTRANASAL ETHMOID SURGERY FOR BENIGN DISEASE

Indications

1. Chronic ethmoid sinusitis.
2. Ethmoid polyposis.

Highpoints

1. Avoid injury to thin lacrimal plate laterally.
2. Avoid injury to cribriform plate superiorly.
3. Never use curet in an upward fashion; always downward and slightly medially.

Uncapping of Anterior Ethmoid Cells

A The point of entrance is just lateral to the attachment of the middle turbinate. The middle turbinate may require displacement medially. This is done with a blunt instrument to minimize damage. The turbinate is not removed. If the turbinate is cystic, it may be gently crushed.

B Using an asymmetrical, oval, thin beaked curet, the anterior ethmoidal cells are opened with a downward and inward motion. The curve of the curet is turned medially to avoid injury to the lacrimal plate.

C Further curettage is downward and backward. A 1 to 2 cm introduction often suffices for simple drainage. However, if there is evidence of extensive involvement, further exenteration becomes necessary.

Ethmoidectomy

D
E Using a Faulkner curved ring curet, the ablation of the more posterior cells is performed, always with a downward and slightly medial motion. This will avoid injury to the cribriform plate. The lacrimal plate is the lateral guide while the middle turbinate is the medial guide.

F As the operation progresses posteriorly, a smaller ring curet is employed if the space narrows.

G The exenteration continues up to the anterior wall of the sphenoid sinus.

H Ethmoidal type blunt forceps are used to remove any remaining diseased cells. The superior turbinates may be removed with scissors if additional space superiorly is required. However, the less injury and the less removal of nasal lining mucosa that is done, the better. In any case atrophic rhinitis must be avoided.

Some surgeons prefer an external ethmoidectomy for extensive disease. The approach is similar to that depicted in plate 95.

Complications

1. Hemorrhage either intranasally or into orbit usually from ethmoidal arteries arising from the ophthalmic artery.
2. Injury to the orbit and optic nerve.
3. Meningitis.

If periorbital edema occurs, extreme care and evaluation of the globe is necessary. Decompression of the orbit may be required to prevent permanent damage to the optic nerve.

Plate 30   The Sinuses and Maxilla

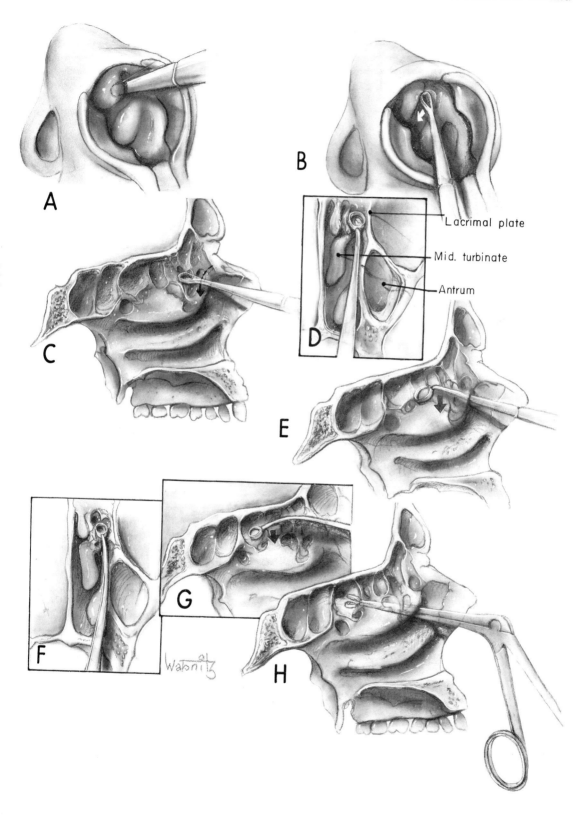

Lacrimal plate

Mid. turbinate

Antrum

RADICAL RESECTION OF MAXILLA WITH ORBITAL AND ETHMOID EXENTERATION

Malignant tumors of the maxillary sinus (antrum of Highmore) amenable to surgical treatment, unless very early and limited, are handled better by a more radical operation than by a limited one because of the intimate and complex relationship of the antrum to the ethmoid and sphenoid sinuses as well as the orbital contents. Hence the radical resection with orbital and ethmoid exenteration will be described first.

Highpoints

1. Antrum is not entered.
2. Orbital contents should be resected with roof of antrum in any extensive carcinoma of maxilla or with involvement of roof of antrum.
3. Resect as much of ethmoid en bloc as possible. Remainder will require curettage.
4. Skin graft raw surfaces with split thickness skin.
5. Leave orbital skin defect open to future inspection for early detection of recurrences.
6. Preserve soft palate.
7. Tracheostomy indicated.

Refer to plates 1 through 6 for radiographic anatomy.

A A Weber-Dieffenbach (Fergusson) incision is made with an extension into the floor of the nose. The upper lip incision is staggered to minimize postoperative contracture. The vertical line is just medial to the philtrum and the horizontal line follows the vermilion border. The eyelids are sutured together and are left attached to either the skin flaps or the eye. If an orbital prosthesis is intended, it may be advantageous to preserve the lids with the skin flaps. An incision in the floor of the naris is optional since the transection of the floor of the nose can be done without this incision. An acute angle of the skin incision is to be avoided near the medial canthus.

B The bony area resected includes the entire antrum with hard palate and floor of the orbit, lateral orbital rim, body of the zygoma (malar bone) and portion of zygomatic arch (the dotted lines on the arch indicate the portion of arch excised to facilitate the application of silver clips to the internal maxillary artery), ethmoid labyrinth, anterior wall of sphenoid sinus and complete lateral wall of the nasal cavity with all three turbinates. The nasal septum is left intact unless the septum is involved. If it is involved, the line of resection through the floor of the nose is on the contralateral side.

C Skin flaps are dissected preserving the orbicularis oris and buccinator muscle in the lateral flap. The remaining facial muscles are for the most part left attached to the anterior wall of the antrum. The incision from the lip is carried along the gingivobuccal sulcus posterolaterally to beyond the maxillary tuberosity. Attachments of the buccinator muscle to the lower edge of the maxilla extending back to the tuberosity are transected. The nasal (frontal) process of the maxilla is then sectioned with a chisel or a sagittal plane saw up to the level of the inner canthus of the eye. This area corresponds to the suture line of the maxilla with the frontal bone and serves as a marker for the level of the cribriform plate of the ethmoid—the floor of the anterior cranial fossa. This is the superior level of resection medially.

D The upper incisor tooth on the side of the resection is removed. A stab wound is made into the nasal cavity at the posterior edge of the hard palate. Through the stab wound a curved clamp is inserted into the nasal cavity grasping the end of the Gigli saw which is passed into the nares. If any tooth fragments remain on the edge of the saw cut, these should be removed.

E The hard palate is transected longitudinally through the floor of the right nasal cavity with the Gigli saw. An incision is then carried across the posterior edge of the hard palate (dotted line) separating it from the soft palate. The soft palate is left intact.

F The anterior attachment of the masseter muscle has been cleared from the anterior portion of the zygomatic arch. A 2 cm section of the zygomatic arch is excised with a Gigli saw. This opening affords access to pterygomaxillary fossa and exposure of a portion of the internal maxillary artery which is then transected between silver clips (see Plate 33, step L). *(Text continued on page 80.)*

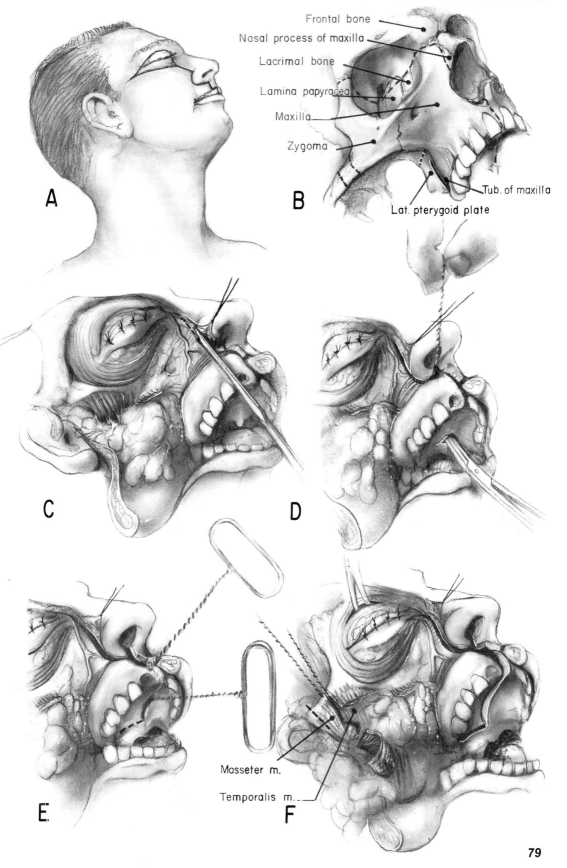

Plate 31   *The Sinuses and Maxilla*

Frontal bone

Nasal process of maxilla

Lacrimal bone

Lamina papyracea

Maxilla

Zygoma

Tub. of maxilla

Lat. pterygoid plate

A

B

C

D

E

F

Masseter m.

Temporalis m.

79

RADICAL RESECTION OF MAXILLA WITH ORBITAL
AND ETHMOID EXENTERATION (*Continued*)

G With the globe retracted downward and medially, a curved clamp is passed through the inferior orbital fissure to grasp the Gigli saw. Occasionally a fracture of some thin bone will be required in order to introduce the clamp.

H The lateral orbital rim is transsected by directing the Gigli saw upward and forward. The optic nerve is severed midway between the globe and the optic foramen (dotted line).

I A cut is made with a chisel or sagittal plane saw starting at the upper extent of the osteotomy performed in step C. This separates the maxilla from the frontal bone. The chisel is directed slightly downward and inward hugging the inner aspect of the cribriform plate. This must be performed slowly and carefully to prevent injury to the cribriform plate. The cut extends across the superior margin of the lacrimal bone and through the upper third of the lamina papyracea of the ethmoid to the anterior lateral extent of the sphenoid sinus. In this manner as much of the ethmoid labyrinth as possible is removed en bloc with the maxilla.

If gross disease has invaded the superior ethmoidal cells or frontal sinus, extension of the operation to include these areas is performed by exposing the dura and anterior cranial fossa. This may require a craniotomy in a combined approach (Ketcham, 1963). Coverage of the dura or even exposed cerebral cortex is achieved with a free split thickness graft. The use of forehead flaps to close the orbital defect completely is believed unwise since recurrence of disease would be obscured.

J The posterolateral attachment of the maxilla is freed in one of two ways. The pterygoid process is transected near its origin from the body and the great wing of the sphenoid bone (J^1). This is accomplished by first sectioning the external and internal pterygoid muscles from the lateral and medial pterygoid plates and then transecting the pterygoid process with angulated rongeurs. Overlying the pterygoid muscle is the main trunk and some branches of the internal maxillary artery. These vessels are the source of significant hemorrhage if not individually ligated or occluded with silver clips.

Plate 32   The Sinuses and Maxilla

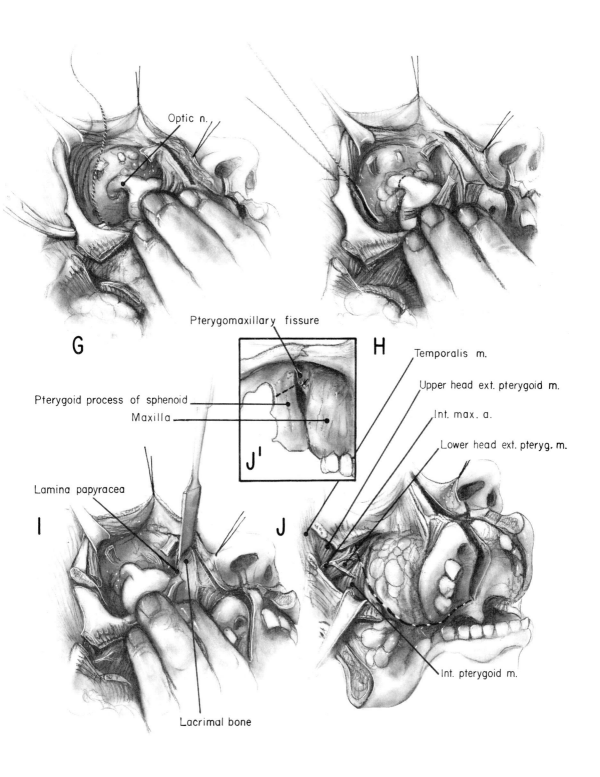

Optic n.

G

Pterygomaxillary fissure

H   Temporalis m.

Upper head ext. pterygoid m.

Pterygoid process of sphenoid

Maxilla

Int. max. a.

Lower head ext. pteryg. m.

J¹

Lamina papyracea

I

J

Int. pterygoid m.

Lacrimal bone

RADICAL RESECTION OF MAXILLA WITH ORBITAL
AND ETHMOID EXENTERATION (*Continued*)

K   An alternate method of freeing the posterolateral attachment of the maxilla is by directing a chisel between the pterygoid process and the maxilla. This cut extends into the pterygomaxillary fissure. Again branches of the internal maxillary artery require ligation. This method is not recommended if there is any suspicion of bone erosion in the posterior wall of the antrum.

L   The entire specimen is now usually free enough so that the remaining weak attachments of the maxilla deep in the medial aspect of the orbit are broken by rocking the specimen back and forth. If necessary, a chisel may be used gently to cut these attachments along the dotted line. The line of transsection extends across the posterior reaches of the posterior ethmoid air cells, usually removing the anterior wall of the sphenoid sinus.

   Proximity to the base of skull is well depicted in plate 1. The internal maxillary artery and its branches are shown in this step. Silver clips are utilized to occlude the vessel. The head is tilted backward and sideward in the drawing, thus throwing the zygomatic arch somewhat upward. Exposure of the vessels is facilitated by Langenbeck long retractors. Occasionally, this maneuver fails. This approach also affords evaluation of the extent of disease in the pterygomaxillary space. Additional exposure of this area can be obtained by transecting the base of the coronoid process of the mandible. This is rarely necessary.

M   Any remaining cells of the anterior and posterior ethmoids are removed with curettage. The curet is used in a downward motion rather than upward to avoid injury to the cribriform plate of the ethmoid. The anterior wall of the sphenoid sinus, if still intact, is removed with forward grasping forceps (Jansen-Middleton) or back biting forceps (Hajek or Kerrison) (see plates 38 and 39).

N   After bleeding has been controlled, all bare surfaces both deep in the bony defect and on the under surface of the skin flap are covered with split thickness skin. Where possible the graft is sutured with 4-0 chromic catgut. The remaining opposition is achieved with a pack of absorbent cotton saturated with liquid Furacin.

O   The orbital defect filled with this type of packing.

P   Sutures of 3-0 nylon are used across the palate defect, acting as slings to hold this pack in place. The skin flaps are approximated in two layers throughout.

   As soon as the skin graft has taken and certainly within two weeks, the first temporary impression is made for the prosthesis. If this is delayed, contractures of the anterior skin flap will occur and hamper proper fitting for the final upper denture. Some prefer the use of an immediate though temporary prosthesis for the palate defect which is made prior to the surgery. The packing is thus held in place by the prosthesis.

Complications

1. Hemorrhage.
2. Cerebrospinal fluid leak.
3. Airway obstruction unless a tracheostomy is performed.
4. Separation of wound between cheek and nose unless a two-layer closure is used.

Plate 33   *The Sinuses and Maxilla*

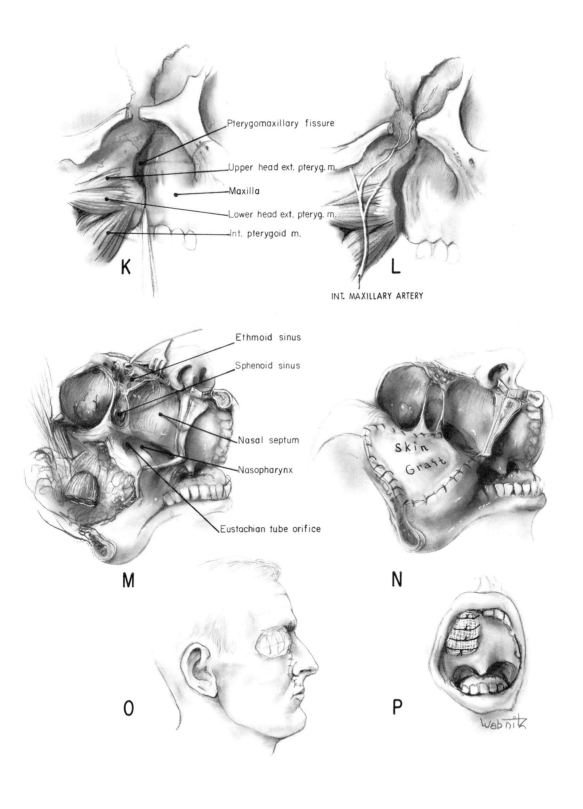

Pterygomaxillary fissure

Upper head ext. pteryg. m.

Maxilla

Lower head ext. pteryg. m.

Int. pterygoid m.

K

L

INT. MAXILLARY ARTERY

Ethmoid sinus

Sphenoid sinus

Nasal septum

Nasopharynx

Eustachian tube orifice

M

N

Skin Graft

O

P

wabnitz

RESECTION OF MAXILLA INCLUDING THE FLOOR
OF ORBIT WITH PRESERVATION OF THE GLOBE
(After Baker)

This procedure is indicated when there is no erosion of the orbital floor but the tumor involves somewhat more than half of the contents of the antrum.

The technique combines the initial steps of resection of the maxilla with orbital exenteration except that the globe is preserved. The globe is then supported by a temporal muscle flap across the inferior aspect of the globe (Wise and Baker, 1958). The orbicularis oculi muscle is preserved.

Steps are shown which modify the basic operation depicted in plates 31, 32 and 33. The globe is protected by a temporary tarsorrhaphy. The skin has been elevated superiorly to the orbicularis oculi muscle, which is preserved and carefully retracted upward with a Cushing vein retractor.

A Exploration of the floor of the orbit is performed with an incision (dotted line) along the superior aspect of the infraorbital rim. By careful elevation of the periosteum at this point, palpation of the orbital contents is possible. If there is no gross evidence of disease in the orbit, if the floor of the orbit is intact and preoperative laminograms reveal no bone erosion, the floor of the orbit (roof of the antrum) is resected, preserving the globe.

B The frontal process and arch of the zygoma are transected with a Gigli saw. The medial attachment of the infraorbital rim is transected with a sagittal plane saw just inferior to the medial canthal ligament. The dotted lines depict the extent of the osseous resection. The central incisor tooth on the involved side is extracted.

C Using a small malleable or curved retractor, the globe with the orbicularis oculi muscle and periosteum is gently retracted upward. Posteriorly and inferiorly the floor of the orbital floor is transected with a curved osteotome.

D The remaining steps in the procedure are similar to the more radical operation except that the globe is preserved. A temporal muscle flap (X) is then mobilized by separating a 1 cm strip of the muscle from its insertion and attaching this free distal end near the inner canthus of the eye. This attachment can be made to the fascia in the area or through a small hole drilled in the remaining bone on the medial aspect of the orbit. The temporal muscle flap thus forms a sling to support the globe.

Plate 34   The Sinuses and Maxilla

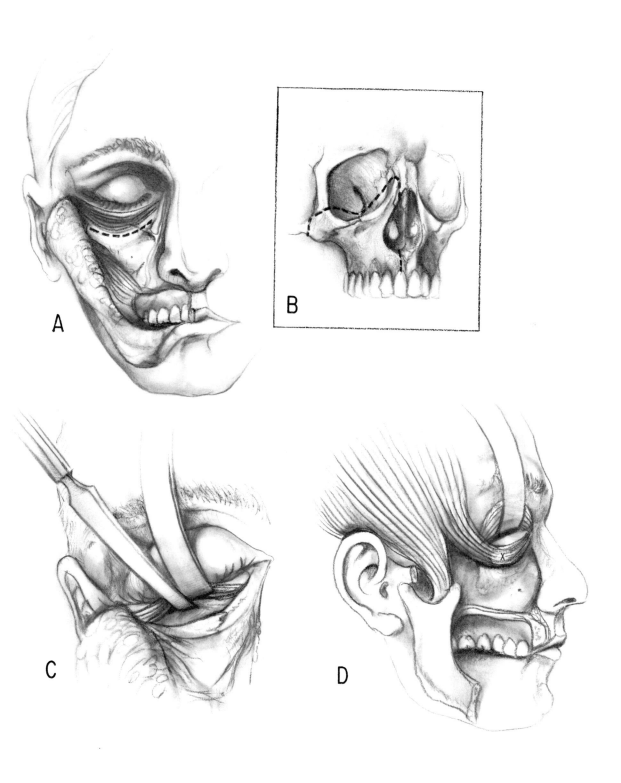

LIMITED RESECTION OF THE MAXILLA

The technique of this procedure follows the basic principles of the radical maxillary resection except that the orbit is left intact and the ethmoid labyrinth is not removed en bloc but cleared by curettage.

Highpoints

1. This procedure is indicated mainly in carcinomas involving only the floor of the antrum.
2. A portion or all of the floor of the orbit is preserved as well as all the orbital contents.
3. The skin incision is made as close as possible to lower eyelashes—otherwise troublesome edema of lower lid will result.
4. Ethmoid air cells are removed by curettage.
5. Preserve soft palate.
6. All raw areas are covered with split thickness skin.

A   After the eyelids are approximated (temporary tarsorrhaphy, plate 161), a Weber-Dieffenbach (Fergusson) skin incision is started across the midportion of the upper lip in stepladder fashion to minimize scar contracture. The incision is carried upward in the nasolabial sulcus to the level of the inner canthus and thence horizontally just beneath the eyelashes of the lower lid and beyond the outer canthus. The orbicularis oculi muscle is left intact and preserved at its orbital location.

An incision is made in the gingivobuccal fold, and the cheek flap including the buccinator muscle is reflected back to the tuberosity of the maxilla.

B   The area resected is schematically represented. This includes the lower two thirds of the maxilla including the juxtaposed hard palate. A Gigli saw is used to transect the hard palate as in steps *D* and *E* of plate 31. The nasal process of the maxilla is sectioned with a chisel for a distance of 1.0 to 1.5 cm to the level of the infraorbital rim.

The inferior turbinate (a separate bone) is thus included in the resected specimen, while the superior and middle turbinates which are part of the ethmoid are excised as separate fragments after the main specimen is removed.

If the tumor grossly involves the medial wall of the antrum, the middle turbinate and superior turbinate are removed en bloc with the main specimen. When the tumor involves the septum, the floor of the nose is transected on the contralateral side. The septum is thus removed with the main specimen. If possible, the columella is preserved; otherwise, an anterior strut graft is inserted for support.

C   The orbicularis oculi muscle is retracted upward. A Stryker saw transects the upper third of the maxilla preserving most of the infraorbital rim and floor of the orbit. This cut is extended laterally across the body of the zygoma. The posterolateral attachment of the maxilla is separated from the pterygoid process of the sphenoid bone with a chisel as depicted in step *K* of plate 33. The posterior wall of the maxilla is then usually free enough for removal of the specimen by rocking the maxilla. The branches of the internal maxillary artery, especially those in the pterygomaxillary fissure, will require ligation.

The anterior and posterior ethmoids are curetted as in step *M*, plate 33, with the same precautions as in an ethmoidectomy (plate 30). A split thickness skin graft is used to line all bare areas (*N*, plate 33).

D   Furacin-soaked cotton is used as packing (step *P*, plate 33).

The packing is removed in seven to 10 days and a temporary prosthesis inserted. In two weeks the temporary tarsorrhaphy is released.

Plate 35   The Sinuses and Maxilla

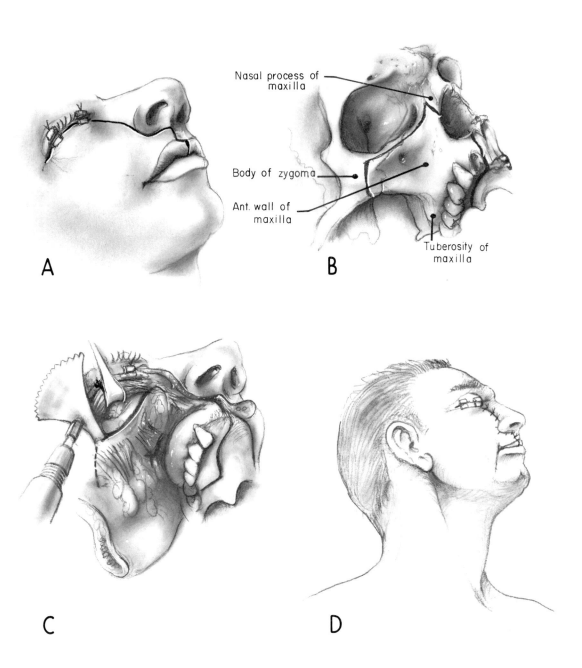

Nasal process of
maxilla

Body of zygoma

Ant. wall of
maxilla

Tuberosity of
maxilla

A

B

C

D

A more extensive resection of the maxilla can be performed in which the entire maxilla is resected as in plates 31, 32, 33 and 34, with preservation of the eye. In such procedures, a portion or slip of the temporalis muscle is detached from the coronoid process of the mandible and swung as a sling under the eye for support. The distal end of the muscle is sutured in the region of the inner canthus of the eye.

SPHENOID SINUSOSTOMY

General Highpoints

1. Check x rays for possible ossification of sphenoid sinus.
2. Asymmetry of sphenoid sinuses is the rule rather than the exception.
3. Dividing partition almost never in midline.

Refer to plates 2, 3, 4 and 7.

CANNULATION OF SPHENOID SINUS THROUGH NATURAL OSTIUM

Highpoints

1. Distance from anterior nasal spine to sphenoid ostium in adult is from 6.5 to 8 cm.
2. Using floor of nose as base line, the angle to reach sphenoid ostium is between 20 and 30 degrees.
3. Ostium is usually located just behind and slightly above posterior end of superior turbinate.

Indications

For emergency irrigation of acute empyema of the sphenoid sinus.

A With topical anesthesia and use of a vasoconstrictor, a malleable cannula is inserted into the nasal cavity closely hugging the septum. It is directed toward the posterior ends of the middle and superior turbinates at an angle of 20 to 30 degrees from the
B floor of the nose. The anterior wall of the sphenoid sinus is thus reached and by gentle manipulation the ostium is located and entered. If necessary, x-ray film may be used to confirm the location of the cannula. Gentle irrigation is then performed. Deviation of the nasal septum and other anomalies may make access to the ostium impossible.

The sphenoid cannula pictured is the Van Alyea instrument which is 10 cm in length and equipped with markers on the proximal end at 9 cm. These markers are placed at an angle of 23.5 degrees from the shaft, thus simulating the angle of insertion using the floor of the nose as the base line. The distal end of the cannula has a smooth 4 mm curve laterally.

Plate 36   *The Sinuses and Maxilla*

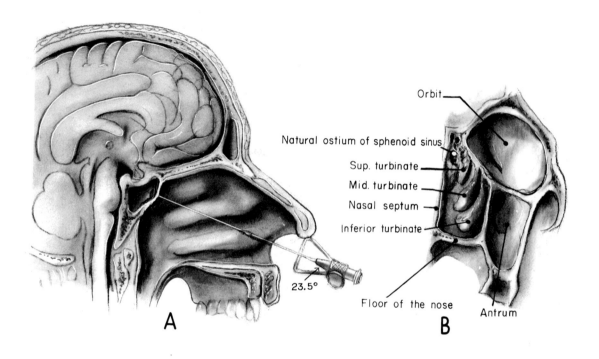

23.5°

A

Orbit
Natural ostium of sphenoid sinus
Sup. turbinate
Mid. turbinate
Nasal septum
Inferior turbinate
Floor of the nose
Antrum

B

SPHENOID SINUSOSTOMY (*Continued*)

PUNCTURE OF ANTERIOR WALL OF SPHENOID SINUS

Highpoints

1. Keep to midline — laterally are the internal carotid artery and cavernous sinus.
2. Keep low and posterior — high and anterior are the floor of the anterior cranial fossa and cribriform plate of the ethmoid. The level of the inner canthus of the eye corresponds to the level of the cribriform plate.
3. Hook on instrument must face downward.
4. Check x-ray films of patient.

Refer to plates 2, 3, 4 and 7.

Indications

Puncture of the anterior wall of the sphenoid sinus is performed if cannulation of the natural ostium is not feasible.

C A sharp pointed instrument with hook facing downward (Sluder or Hajek sphenoid hook preferably with a Tremble guard) is inserted into the nasal cavity keeping close to the nasal septum. It is directed toward the plane of the posterior end of the middle
D turbinate. The anterior wall of the sphenoid sinus is thus reached and the instrument inserted through a thin section of the wall (**X**). The point of entry is as close to the midline as possible and as low and posterior as possible. The lower and more posterior one goes, however, the thicker the anterior wall of the sinus becomes. Puncture then becomes somewhat more difficult.

ENLARGEMENT OF NATURAL SPHENOID OSTIUM OR ANTERIOR WALL PUNCTURE SITE

Highpoints

1. Avoid injury to or removal of posterior end of middle turbinate.
2. Keep angle of biting forceps facing downward.

Indications

Usually used for emergency sphenoid sinus drainage when irrigation through natural ostium or anterior wall puncture appears inadequate. It is also used for exploration and biopsy of sphenoid sinus.

E Using either the natural ostium or anterior wall puncture site as the point of entry, a Hajek or Kerrison biting forceps is employed to enlarge the opening. The enlargement is directed downward. It must be remembered that the dividing septum of the sphenoid may not be in the midline, and hence the sinus entered may not be the one corresponding to the side of the nasal approach. In such cases, careful breakdown of the dividing partition is necessary. Confirmation is obtained by x-ray examination when necessary.

Complications

Injury to sella turcica, internal carotid artery and cavernous sinus.

Plate 37   *The Sinuses and Maxilla*

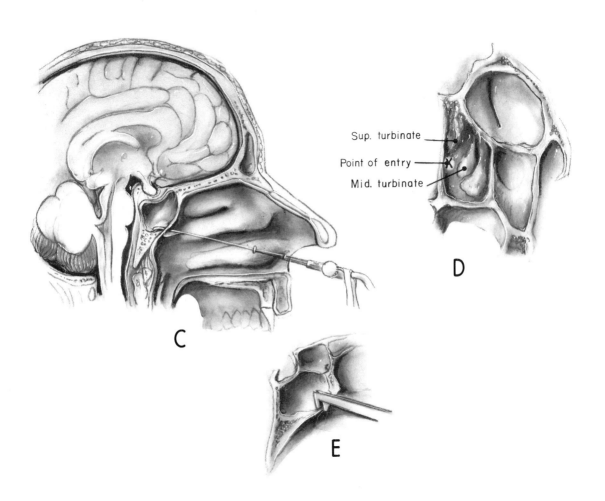

Sup. turbinate

Point of entry

Mid. turbinate

C

D

E

TRANSSEPTAL TRANSSPHENOIDAL HYPOPHYSECTOMY — CRYOSURGICAL AND SURGICAL

Basically, there are two surgical approaches for hypophysectomy:

I Transcranial — usually frontal.
II Transsphenoidal.

The transsphenoidal approach has a number of modifications or intermediate variations in the manner in which the sphenoid sinus is reached.
These include:

1. Transantral ethmoidal — through a Caldwell-Luc operation and then an ethmoidectomy (Hamberger, 1961; Tollefsen, Miller and Gerold, 1966).
2. Transethmoidal — through an external ethmoidectomy (Chiari, 1912).
3. Transnasal — through an osteoplastic approach near the glabella (Macbeth and Hall, 1962).
4. Transpalatal.
5. Transseptal — through an extended submucous resection of the nasal septum (Hirsch, 1910).

In addition, various methods aside from the surgical techniques have been and are utilized for oblation of the pituitary. These include:

1. Insertion of radioactive material into the pituitary, e.g., yttrium, using stereotactic method.
2. Crysosurgical, using either stereotactic or direct vision method.
3. Ultrasound.
4. Hormonal.

The following five plates outline the transseptal approach to the sphenoid sinus and the pituitary gland for surgical hypophysectomy and cryosurgical hypophysectomy. Steps A through D describe the septal and sphenoid portion of the operation. Steps E through O describe the exposure of the pituitary gland. Steps P and Q depict the direct vision cryoprobe technique while steps R through X depict the surgical removal of the pituitary gland.

Indications for Hypophysectomy

1. Tumors of pituitary.
2. Metastatic carcinoma of the breast and prostate.
3. Diabetic retinopathy (some difference of opinion).

Anesthesia

Topical and general endotracheal anesthesia are both suitable. Ten per cent cocaine with a vasoconstrictor is combined with general anesthesia to minimize bleeding. General anesthesia is to be avoided in the debilitated patient with poor cough reflex and pulmonary metastases. When cryosurgery is utilized, topical anesthesia should be utilized in order to evaluate vision and to avoid permanent damage to the optic nerves.

Highpoints

1. Careful preoperative evaluation:
   a. By ophthalmologist and endocrinologist depending on purpose of operation.
   b. X-ray films of sphenoid sinus and sella turcica for their relationship and whether or not the sphenoid sinus is small or nonpneumatized. This latter finding is a contraindication to this approach.
   c. Be sure there is no active nasal or sinus infection — nose and throat cultures are routine.

TRANSSEPTAL TRANSSPHENOIDAL, HYPOPHYSECTOMY — CRYOSURGICAL AND SURGICAL (Continued)

2. Removal of posterior nasal septum gives access to sphenoid sinus.
3. There should be complete elevation of nasal septal mucosa posteriorly and mucosa on anterior and inferior walls of sphenoid sinuses.
4. Preserve this elevated mucosa intact since most of the blood vessels lie within this mucosal layer and bleeding will be much less if mucosa is not torn.
5. Be certain opening is made in midline vertical plane of sella turcica to avoid cavernous sinuses and internal carotid arteries laterally. This incidentally is an advantage of the transseptal approach.
6. Incise both layers of dura of sella turcica.
7. X-ray facilities in operating room for lateral films to ascertain proper angle of approach and depth of sella turcica.
8. Corticosteroids preoperatively, operatively and postoperatively.

Complications

1. Cerebrospinal fluid rhinorrhea.
2. Meningitis.
3. Hemorrhage.
4. Intracranial damage if diaphragma sella is penetrated.
5. Aspiration with respiratory embarrassment.

G. H. Bateman has described a technique of hypophysectomy utilizing a dual simultaneous approach through the septum and right ethmoid. After the sphenoid sinus is entered (see plate 38), the wound is packed and an external right ethmoidectomy is performed. The incision is similar to that described in step *B*, plate 95; however, the nasal cavity is not entered. The lateral wall of the nose is fractured medially. The anterior ethmoid vessels are coagulated and packing inserted to hold the orbital contents laterally. The ethmoid wound is utilized for suction and visualization using a Zeiss operating microscope while the septal wound is used for instrumentation. The midline is carefully checked through the septal exposure. An opening is then made in the anterior wall of the pituitary fossa (steps *F* and *G*, plate 39). The remaining technique is similar to that described.

A
A¹ If an anterior deviation of the nasal septum is present, the routine submucous resection of the nasal septum is performed (see plates 64 and 65); otherwise, the mucoperichondrial incision may be made farther posteriorly. The approach may be from either the left or right as desired. In any event the posterior bony nasal septum is removed up to its attachment on the anterior wall of the sphenoid sinus. After the posterior bony nasal septum has been removed, further elevation of mucosa is necessary over the anterior and inferior walls of both sphenoid sinuses as depicted.

B
B¹ The crest and rostrum (triangular spine on inferior surface) of the sphenoid sinus are thus well exposed. The crest is the anterior ridge on the sphenoid sinus which articulates with the perpendicular plate of the ethmoid forming the most posterior superior portion of the nasal septum. The crest is continuous inferiorly with the rostrum of the sphenoid to which the vomer bone is articulated. Sometimes by removing the sphenoidal crest and rostrum with forward grasping forceps (Jansen-Middleton or vomer), one or both sphenoidal sinuses can be entered. Otherwise, an anterior wall puncture is made close to the midline (see plate 37, steps *C* and *D*). If there is any question regarding location, a lateral x-ray film is taken.

Plate 38   The Sinuses and Maxilla

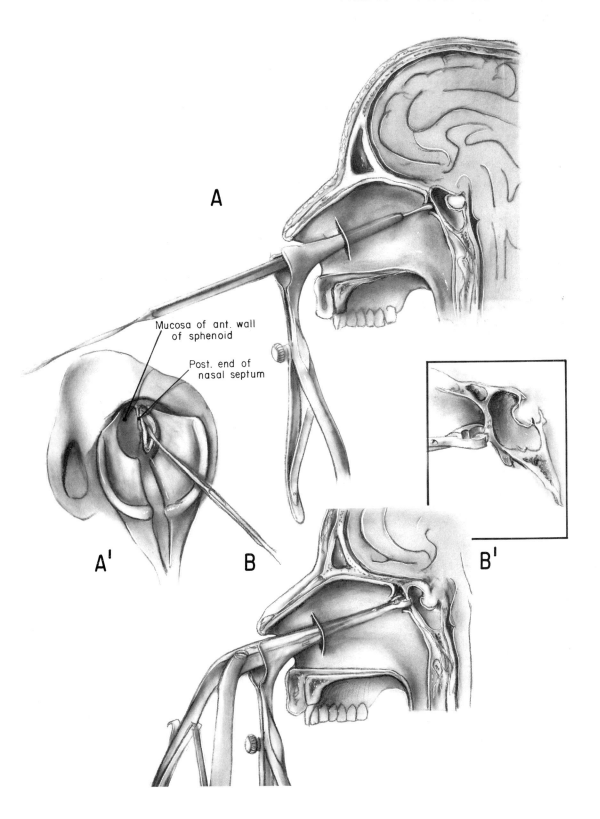

A

Mucosa of ant. wall
of sphenoid

Post. end of
nasal septum

A'

B

B'

TRANSSEPTAL TRANSSPHENOIDAL HYPOPHYSECTOMY — CRYOSURGICAL AND SURGICAL (*Continued*)

C Using Hajek or Kerrison forceps, the opening in the anterior and inferior wall of the sphenoid sinus is enlarged to 2 cm in diameter.

D The anterior portion of the intersinus septum is removed with forward biting forceps. If this intersinus septum is far from the midline and the sella turcica is well visualized, the septum need not be removed.

E The removal of the intersinus septum is completed.

F The bulge of sella turcica on the posterior wall of the sphenoid sinus is exposed. Position is checked by lateral x-ray film with a probe against the sella turcica. If feasible, the mucous membrane overlying the sella turcica is incised to form inferiorly based flaps as outlined along the dotted lines.

One of two techniques can now be utilized to expose the dura.

G Depicted is a small dental-type bur with a long shank used to expose the dura. This is especially useful if the presenting bone of the sella turcica is exceptionally thick.

H Lateral view of the bur technique.

I The opening made with the bur is enlarged with Hajek or fine Kerrison forceps.

Plate 39   The Sinuses and Maxilla

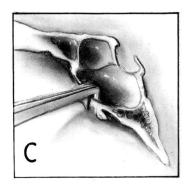

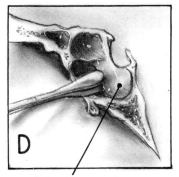

Intersinus septum

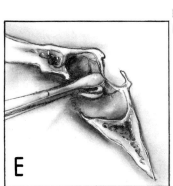

Base of intersinus septum

Mucous membrane of
post. wall of sinus

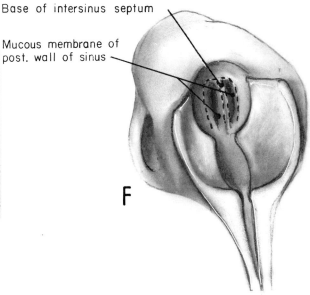

Posterior sinus wall

Dura overlying pituitary

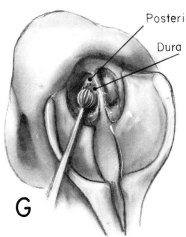

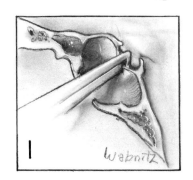

Wabnitz

TRANSSEPTAL TRANSSPHENOIDAL HYPOPHYSECTOMY—
CRYOSURGICAL AND SURGICAL (*Continued*)

J   The other technique for exposure of the dura when the bone is thin is the use of a specially designed right angle osteotome. This method affords better visualization than with the bur. The presenting bulge of the sella turcica is gently fractured in cruciate fashion.

K   Lateral view of osteotome against the sella turcica.

L   A blunt angulated hook is then placed under the fractured fragments of the sella turcica, pulling the fragments outward, thus exposing the outer layer of dura. Depicted are the two layers of dura surrounding the pituitary gland. At this stage, the operation microscope with six to 10 times magnification is utilized. The microscope is not as necessary when the cryosurgical probe is to be used as when surgical ablation of the gland is planned.

M   The opening in the sella turcica is enlarged with fine Kerrison forceps.

Plate 40   The Sinuses and Maxilla

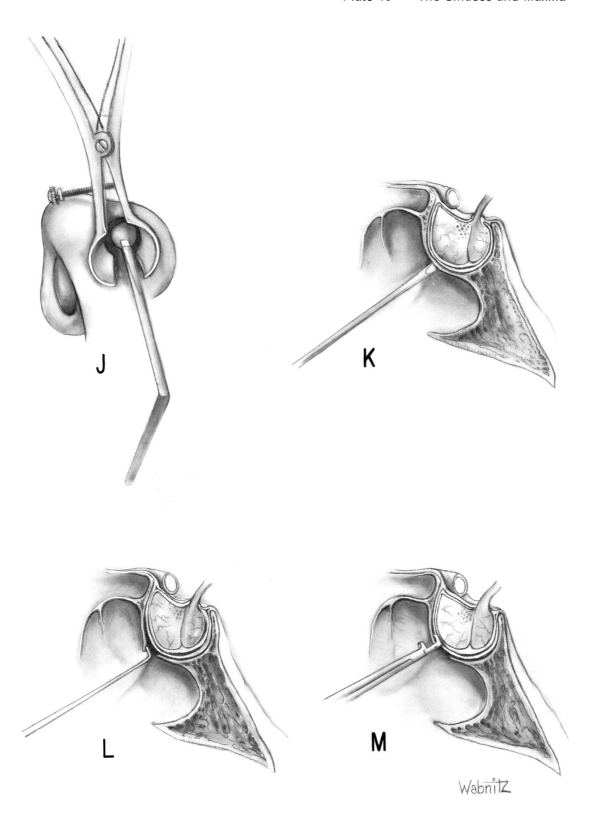

J

K

L

M

Wabnitz

TRANSSEPTAL TRANSSPHENOIDAL HYPOPHYSECTOMY — CRYOSURGICAL AND SURGICAL (*Continued*)

CRYOSURGICAL HYPOPHYSECTOMY

The size of this opening in the sella turcica depends on the procedure contemplated. When cryosurgical hypophysectomy is the choice, a 5 to 7 mm opening suffices for exposure of the dura.

Cryosurgical technique is preferred in extremely poor risk patients, or when excessive hemorrhage accompanies an attempted surgical hypophysectomy or in secondary procedures.

N   With an angulated myringotome, the two layers of dura are incised in cruciate fashion (*O'*). It is most important to incise both layers of dura since a venous sinus exists between the two layers of dura. The yellow-colored pituitary gland is now exposed.

O   Cerebrospinal fluid will be seen dripping through the incised dura. Usually there will be no significant bleeding at this stage.

P   A 4.9 mm cryosurgical probe (Rand-Linde) is inserted several millimeters through the dural opening and the position checked by x-ray film. The probe is then advanced to within several millimeters of the posterior clinoid process.

Q   Lateral roentgenogram demonstrating the cryoprobe within the pituitary gland. The probe is low, and refreezing at a higher level is indicated.

The cryotherapy consists in lowering the temperature from −160 to −180°C for a period of 15 to 20 minutes. This necessitates topical rather than general anesthesia since the visual fields should be checked every few minutes during the period of refrigeration. If visual disturbance occurs, refrigeration is terminated. Any impairment is usually reversible since the venous sinuses act as excellent buffers. The probe is removed after a defrosting period of seven to eight minutes. If a special heating attachment is available, the defrosting time is markedly shortened.

Another technique of cryotherapy is the freezing, defrosting and refreezing and defrosting method. The temperature need not be lowered as much as above, e.g., from −40 to −80°C. This technique is based on the theory that freezing and defrosting several times is the actual process which destroys living tissue.

In any event, this direct vision method of cryotherapy has distinct advantages over the stereotactic method which is cumbersome and time-consuming.

SURGICAL HYPOPHYSECTOMY

The opening in the sella turcica has been enlarged with fine Kerrison forceps to a diameter of 15 to 18 mm as described by Heck (1957). The cruciate incision (*O'*) in the two layers of dura has also been enlarged. This must be performed with extreme care to avoid nicking the anterior transverse communicating sinus.

R   With a Tumarkin double-headed mastoid dissector, the inner layer of dura is separated from the pituitary gland. Inner and upper dissection is performed cautiously,

S   keeping in mind the cavernous sinuses laterally and the communicating sinuses superiorly and inferiorly.

Plate 41   The Sinuses and Maxilla

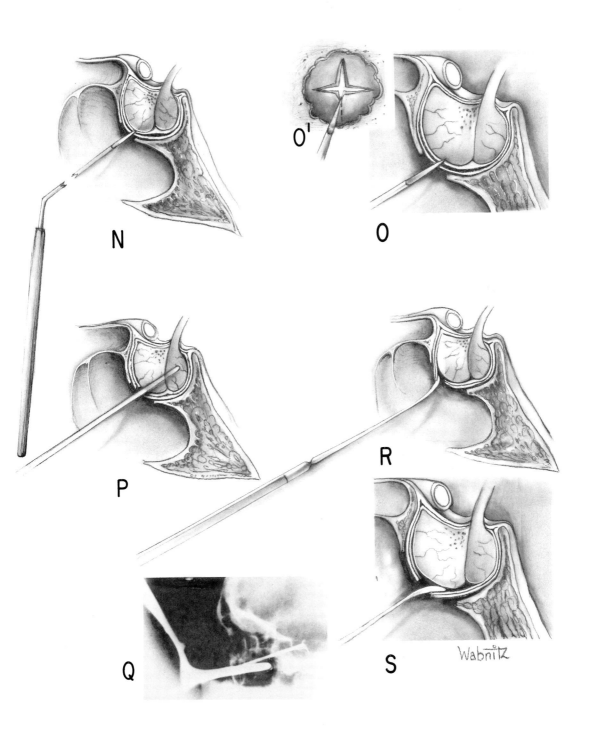

N

O'

O

P

Q

R

S

Wabnitz

SURGICAL HYPOPHYSECTOMY (*Continued*)

T   The inner layer of dura is further separated from the gland using Angell-James modified Olivekrona pituitary dissectors. At this stage, troublesome bleeding may occur

U   and can be controlled by temporary packing. If severe bleeding continues, it is best to stage the procedure or use cryotherapy.

V   A small ring curette can also be used to separate the gland from the dura. For improved visualization, especially through the microscope, the handles on all these dissectors are angulated to suit the surgeon.

W   The stalk of the pituitary gland is transected with fine forceps and ideally the entire gland is removed intact. If the gland fragments, this is no worry; the forceps and curet are utilized to complete the removal. Zenker's solution can be applied to the empty fossa to destroy any remaining cells of the gland.

In the removal of an adenoma, simple suction has achieved it completely.

X   A section measuring 2.5 × 1.5 cm of the vastus intermedius muscle is inserted into the sella turcica and the sphenoid sinus. Both cavities should be obliterated to prevent cerebrospinal fluid leak. The muscle plug is dipped in bacitracin solution (20,000 units in 100 cc) before insertion.

The septal incision anteriorly is closed with two sutures of 4-0 nylon.

Half inch plain strip gauze soaked in the same bacitracin solution is inserted in each naris and left in place for three to seven days. The bacitracin solution is applied to this packing every four hours. Prophylactic antibiotics are utilized during this time, the choice depending on preoperative nose and throat cultures.

Corticosteroids are administered before, during and after the operation as follows. One day prior to the operation, 25 mg of cortisone acetate is administered orally four times that day; the morning of the operation, 100 mg of Solu-Cortef intramuscularly; during the operation, 100 to 200 mg of Solu-Cortef intravenously. Postoperatively, 100 to 200 mg of Solu-Cortef daily is administered intramuscularly or intravenously in divided doses until the patient is able to tolerate 25 mg of cortisone acetate by mouth four times a day. This dose is gradually reduced over a period of one week to a permanent maintenance dose of 12.5 mg of cortisone acetate three times a day.

The only other maintenance medication necessary is 2 to 3 gm of thyroid extract in divided doses. Polyuria and polydipsia are always present postoperatively and continue for some time. They gradually decrease and cause little concern. However, if they are troublesome, 3 to 5 units intramuscularly of Pitressin tannate in oil every two to five days or posterior pituitary powder insufflated in the nose three to four times a day may be administered.

Postoperative leakage of cerebrospinal fluid is rare; if it persists to any extent, reinsertion of a larger muscle graft into the pituitary fossa and sphenoid sinus may be required. Cerebrospinal rhinorrhea has a high content of reducing sugar.

Plate 42   The Sinuses and Maxilla

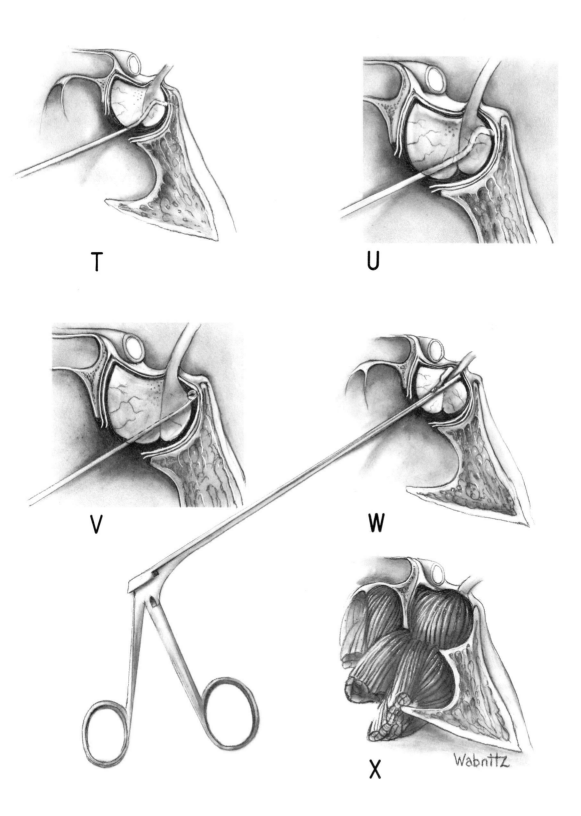

T

U

V

W

X

Wabnitz

FRONTAL SINUSOTOMY (Trephination)

1. Purulent acute frontal sinusitis refractory to conservative management; e.g., nasal decongestants and 10 per cent cocaine applied on cotton tampon plus antibiotics in large doses.
2. Persistent pain and tenderness with or without local edema.
3. Exploration for chronic frontal sinusitis.
4. Biopsy.

Refer to plates 2 through 7 for radiographic anatomy.

Highpoints

1. Keep incision well above medial canthal ligament.
2. Continue conservative management.
3. Careful x-ray evaluation pre- and postoperatively, especially for any evidence of dehiscence of the inner wall, thus exposing dura. Remember x-ray films of the frontal sinus can be deceptive.
4. Avoid injury to the globe.
5. Trephine is made in the floor, not the anterior wall, thus avoiding cancellous bone containing marrow which could be an excellent avenue for osteomyelitis.

A   A slightly curved incision is made just below the eyebrow. It is carried through the periosteum exposing the bone.

B   A small periosteal elevator exposes the underlining bone just below the prominence of the frontal sinus. The exact point of entrance is checked on the x-ray films. Using a small bur or curet, the sinus is entered. Cultures of any purulent material should be taken followed by gentle irrigation with normal saline. Potency of the nasofrontal duct can be checked with methylene blue inserted through the tubes. The duct usually should not be probed since it may result in stenosis.

   A nasopharyngoscope can be inserted through the trephine to inspect the inner lining of the sinus. One must be certain that the inner bony wall is intact, otherwise a more radical operation is indicated.

C   Two small plastic tubes are inserted and held in place with 4-0 Tevdek sutures. One tube can be used for daily irrigations with a suitable antibiotic solution (e.g., neomycin, 1 per cent) for a period of 24 to 48 hours. The other tube acts as the release for the irrigation fluid.

Plate 43   *The Sinuses and Maxilla*

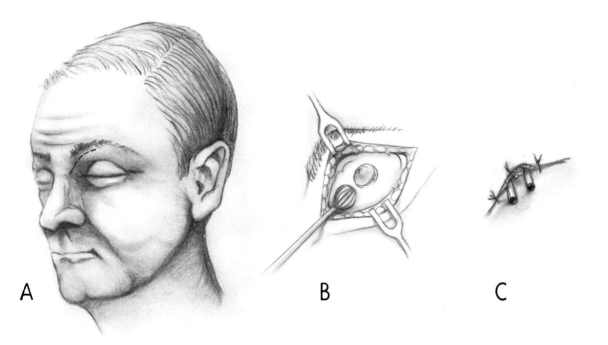

A

B

C

EXTERNAL FRONTOETHMOIDECTOMY (After Lynch, 1921)

Indications

Severe recurrent frontoethmoid sinusitis refractory to conservative management, including intranasal ethmoidectomy, submucous resection of the nasal septum and frontal sinusotomy. In this day and age, this operation is seldom indicated for chronic sinusitis. It is not suitable for malignant lesions. Another consideration for use of this procedure is severe polyposis and inverted papillomatosis. This approach is also used by some surgeons (Bateman, 1961) for hypophysectomy (page 93). Refer to plates 2 through 7 for radiographic anatomy.

Highpoints

1. Meticulous hemostasis.
2. Avoid injury to the eye and associated structures:
   a. Medial palpebral ligament.
   b. Lacrimal sac and duct.
3. Do not perforate cribiform plate.
4. Preserve as much normal mucous membrane as compatible with a good drainage operation.
5. Problems with adequate and safe removal of frontal sinus disease:
   a. Incomplete removal.
   b. Entrance into anterior cranial fossa through a bony dehiscence in long-standing disease.
6. Remove entire floor of frontal sinus and establish a wide new frontonasal communication. This is one of the main objectives of the operation.

D   Outline of incision which is 2.5 to 3.5 cm long, extending about 1 cm below the level of the medial palpebral (canthal) ligament. It lies midway between the attachment of this ligament (see plates 143 and 157.) and the dorsum of the nose. A temporary tarsorrhaphy is performed to protect the globe.

The incision exposes the orbicularis oculi (orbicularis palpebrum) and the superior portion of the quadratus labii superioris muscles as well as the superior palpebral vessels (branches of angular vessels) which are ligated. The medial palpebral ligament is exposed and preserved.

The periosteum is incised, elevated and retracted laterally, carefully freeing the superior portion of the lacrimal sac. The periosteal dissection is continued posteriorly exposing the entire lamina papyracea and the floor of the frontal sinus. Avoid tearing the periosteum and periorbita fascia especially along the frontoethmoidal suture where the former is quite adherent. Otherwise, periorbital fat will herniate through obstructing vision. Two smooth retractors or a Loungo self-retaining retractor is inserted. The anterior and posterior ethmoidal arteries are occluded as per plate 52.

E   At a point just posterior to the lacrimal fossa, the medial orbital wall is entered with a sharp perforator. Using bone Kerrison forceps and curet, the bone posteriorly (dotted line) is now removed including the posterior edge of the nasal process of the maxilla (preserve the nasal mucous membrane) and thence the lacrimal bone and lamina papyracea. The preserved mucoperiosteum will be used as a superior-based flap to line the new nasofrontal communication. The anterior ethmoidal cells are then removed.

The upper medial orbital bone is then removed, thus entering the frontal sinus and removing the entire floor of this sinus. As much as possible of the lining mucous membrane is removed from the frontal sinus. Loculations and septa can make this step difficult and frustrating. Care must be exercised that if dehiscence in the posterior or roof of the frontal sinus exists perforation of dura lining the anterior cranial fossa does not occur. If incomplete removal occurs, this could lead to recurrent frontal sinus problems especially with marked polyposis—a failure for this procedure. An

Plate 43 Continued   *The Sinuses and Maxilla*

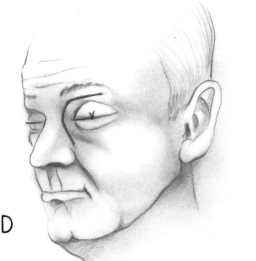

D

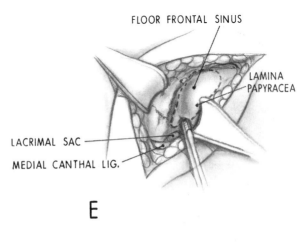

FLOOR FRONTAL SINUS

LAMINA PAPYRACEA

LACRIMAL SAC

MEDIAL CANTHAL LIG.

E

osteoplastic frontal sinus operation may then be necessary at a later stage (see plate 44).

As much of the middle turbinate is removed (by punch, not tearing) as is necessary to provide a suitable communication into the nasal cavity. This is accomplished both through the operation wound and through the naris.

EXTERNAL FRONTOETHMOIDECTOMY (*Continued*)

F   The posterior cells are removed with punch forceps both through the wound and naris, taking care not to perforate the cribriform plate. This is most important.

The complete operation with removal of the floor of the frontal sinus, portion of lacrimal bone, lamina papyracea, ethmoid cells and portion of middle turbinate.

If the sphenoid is to be entered, this is accomplished by either making an opening with a sharp curet or enlarging the natural opening. Kerrison or Hajek forceps are used to enlarge the opening. Inferiorly and anteriorly the sphenopalatine vessels may be encountered which then will require occlusion with silver clips or electrocoagulation.

If the purpose of the operation is a hypophysectomy, the frontal sinus portion of the operation is deleted. From here on the reader is referred to the section dealing with hypophysectomy (pages 93–103).

G   The preserved superior-based mucoperiosteal nasal flap is now used as lining for the new frontonasal communication. Gauze impregnated with antibiotic ointment or a soft tube is utilized to coapt this flap and extend into the nasal cavity. The tubing or gauze is removed in one week.

Complications

1. Orbital injuries.
2. Hemorrhage.
3. Stenosis of frontonasal communication.
4. Recurrent sinusitis, polyposis or mucocele.
5. Perforation of cribriform plate or inner wall of frontal sinus to dura.

Plate 43 Continued   The Sinuses and Maxilla

F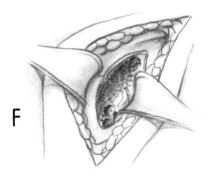

G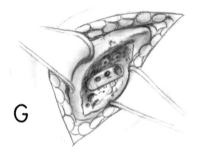

OSTEOPLASTIC APPROACH TO THE FRONTAL SINUS
(After Goodale and Montgomery, 1964; Alford, 1964)

Highpoints

1. Use template of frontal sinus cut from x-rays.
2. Cosmetic incision — choice at eyebrows or coronal hairline.
3. Leave periosteum attached to bone forming anterior wall of frontal sinus. The periosteum acts as a hinge attaching the bone fragment inferiorly.
4. Bevel bone incision inward toward sinus and slightly smaller than x-ray template.
5. If mucous membrane is hopelessly diseased, it should be removed completely and meticulously using a power driven bur and the nasofrontal duct, likewise stripped and obliterated.
6. If the major portion of the mucous membrane is normal, e.g., in an osteoma, the mucous membrane of the sinus and nasofrontal duct should be carefully preserved.
7. Do not shave the eyebrows since they may not be regenerate.
8. Do not enter the anterior cranial fossa.

A   The incision may be just above or below the eyebrows as shown. The upper incision is slightly curved.

B   A superior based skin flap is developed consisting of all layers down to periosteum. The periosteum is left attached to the underlying bone. A template of the left frontal sinus containing an osteoma has previously been cut, slightly smaller, from the Caldwell view and gas sterilized. The template is placed over the frontal sinus and an incision is made through the periosteum along the superior and lateral edges. The inferior edge is left intact forming the hinge for the anterior frontal sinus bone window.

C   The line of incision through the periosteum is slightly widened with a narrow elevator to allow free access for the saw blade. Using a Stryker sagittal plane saw, a cut is made, beveled slightly inward and downward. This protects the edges forming the boundaries of the sinus and later on supports the bone flap when it is returned. The dotted line indicates the hinge of intact periosteum and the line of fracture of the bone-periosteum flap. Additional bone may be transected on the edges of the dotted line for a distance of a few millimeters inferiorly.

D   Using an osteotome along the cut edges, the bone periosteum flap is elevated and fractured along its inferior margin.

E   The flap of bone and periosteum is reflected downward, exposing the pathologic change in the frontal sinus which in this case is an osteoma. The osteoma is removed revealing the major portion of mucous membrane to be intact and normal. The mucous membrane is left undisturbed; the nasofrontal duct is left inviolate. If the pathologic change consists of chronic sinusitis with diseased mucous membrane, all mucous membrane is meticulously removed. Small spurs of bone are leveled off with a bur destroying any minute infolding of mucous membrane. The operation microscope can be of help. Too much time at this stage cannot be criticized. The nasofrontal duct will likewise be stripped of mucous membrane and obliterated. Any remaining mucous membrane in the sinus will be the nidus for future problems. At this point, some surgeons place an autogenous adipose tissue graft into the sinus cavity and duct remnant to aid in their obliteration; others perform a transfrontal ethmoidectomy.

F   The flap of bone and periosteum is returned and the periosteum approximated with 4-0 catgut sutures. The skin flap is closed in two layers. A cutaneous drain is used only in those patients with active infection.

G   An outline of the extension of the brow incision in bilateral frontal sinus disease. Occasionally the opposite sinus may be approached through the original exposure by removing the sinus septum. This depends on the extent of disease and size of the sinus. It is usually more opportune to perform a bilateral approach.

Plate 44   *The Sinuses and Maxilla*

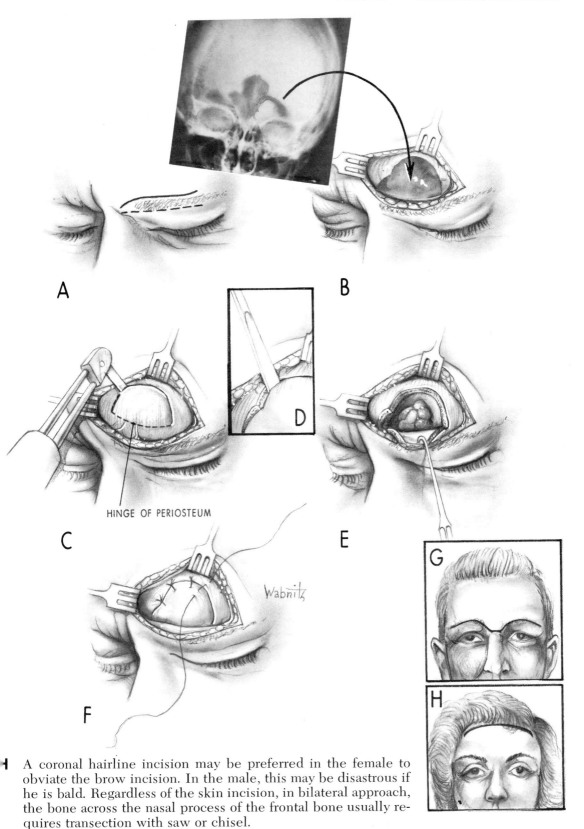

A

B

D

HINGE OF PERIOSTEUM

C

E

Wabnitz

F

G

H

A coronal hairline incision may be preferred in the female to obviate the brow incision. In the male, this may be disastrous if he is bald. Regardless of the skin incision, in bilateral approach, the bone across the nasal process of the frontal bone usually requires transection with saw or chisel.

CYSTS OF MAXILLA

    I Odontogenic cysts
        Radicular—dental root or dentoperiosteal.
        Follicular—dentigerous (contains a tooth).
    II Developmental fissural or inclusion cysts
        Nasoalveolar.
        Nasopalatine.
        Globulomaxillary.

Highpoints for Resection of All Maxillary Cysts

1. Preoperative x-ray films should be taken to evaluate extent of bone encroachment.
2. Entire cyst wall must be removed including juxtaposed portion of nasal or antral mucous membrane if necessary.
3. Teeth to be retained if compatible with adequate cyst wall removal. Devitalized teeth require root canal treatment.
4. Frozen section should be performed if there is any question regarding neoplasm.

Resection of odontogenic cysts follows much of the same technique and approach as with the basic Caldwell-Luc operation (plates 28 and 29). When possible, the juxtaposed normally located teeth are preserved by dental care. The oroantral communication is closed and drainage is obtained with an intranasal antrostomy.

Plate 45   The Sinuses and Maxilla

ODONTOGENIC

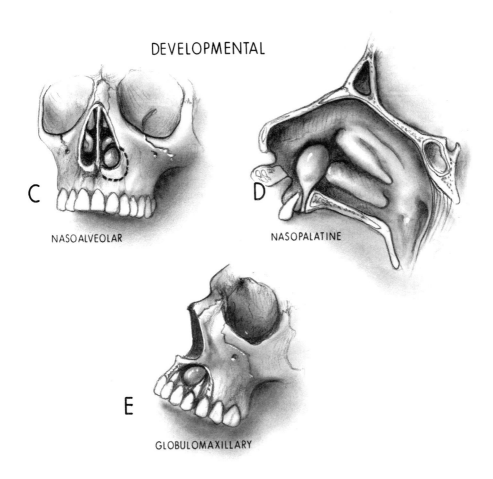

A

RADICULAR

B

FOLLICULAR (DENTIGEROUS)

DEVELOPMENTAL

C

NASOALVEOLAR

D

NASOPALATINE

E

GLOBULOMAXILLARY

EXCISION OF NASOALVEOLAR CYST

A   Cystic swelling at lateral base of right ala nasi and vestibule with partial obstruction of anterior naris. Cavitation of the bone is not present and rarely occurs in these cysts.

B   An incision is made along a portion of the nasolabial fold forming the lateral base of the ala nasi. If the presenting portion of the cyst were lower, an approach in alveolar labial gutter could be utilized.

C   Using blunt and sharp dissection, the presenting wall of the cyst is exposed. If the cyst is extremely large, aspiration will facilitate easier enucleation without extension of the incision.

D   Using a small, curved, blunt-nosed scissors, the cyst is then enucleated with intact wall. In this patient there was a line of cleavage between the cyst wall and the nasal mucous membrane. The nasal cavity was not entered. If there were no line of cleavage, the adherent nasal mucosa would require excision.

    The wound is closed with 5-0 nylon sutures without drainage. Nasal packing impregnated with an antibiotic ointment may be placed in the vestibule to coapt the elevated nasal mucous membrane to the concavity of the defect.

Plate 46   The Sinuses and Maxilla

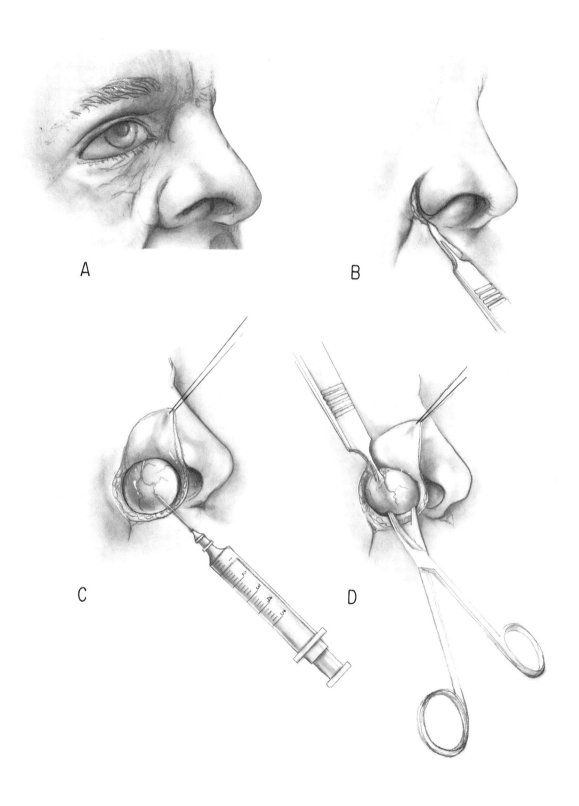

A

B

C

D

EXCISION OF NASOPALATINE DUCT CYST

A   Depicted is a form of nasopalatine duct cyst presenting with a sinus tract through the hard palate just behind the right medial incisor tooth. This would correspond to the right incisive canal. The cyst presents in the right nasal cavity displacing the inferior turbinate superiorly, reaching the nasal septum and causing severe nasal destruction.

A¹   An incision is made in the gingivolabial sulcus slightly across the midline transecting the superior labial frenulum. The incision is so placed that sufficient mucous membrane remains on the gingival side to facilitate placement of sutures for closure. The dotted line around the sinus tract indicates the incision in order to remove the lining of the sinus tract.

B   Using blunt and sharp dissection, the labial flap is elevated exposing the anterior wall of the cyst. A small probe can be passed through the sinus tract to demonstrate the communication with the cystic cavity.

C   Cross section showing the location of the sinus tract and cyst with a small blunt curet attempting to separate the mucous membrane of the floor of the nose from the cyst wall. This is not possible posteriorly and hence juxtaposed nasal mucous membrane and cyst wall are removed together. It is most important that all portions of the cyst wall be excised; otherwise, recurrence will most likely occur. Any bone projecting into the nasal cavity is removed with rongeur forceps.

D   The entire lining of the sinus tract must likewise be removed. This requires an elliptical incision around sinus tract in the hard palate with careful curettage along the walls of the defect in the bone. Considerable bleeding may occur from terminal branches of the greater palatine artery or the nasopalatine artery in the tract. Electrocautery is used to control this bleeding. Cautery is also utilized to destroy any possible remaining epithelial elements of cyst and duct. A single suture of 4-0 nylon is placed through the mucous membrane of the hard palate to close the defect while a continuous 4-0 nylon suture closes the gingivolabial incision. Packing of ½ inch strip gauze impregnated with antibiotic ointment or Furacin is inserted in the defect in the floor of the nose and brought out through this defect. Additional nasal packing may be required to control any oozing blood.

E   Another type of nasopalatine cyst which presents in the roof of the mouth rather than in the nasal cavity.

F   A palatal flap based posteriorly is elevated with an incision just behind the gingiva, thus preserving the greater palatine vessels. The cyst and wall are resected using much the same technique as for the previous nasopalatine cyst. Closure is with 4-0 nylon and a drain brought out anteriorly if necessary.

Plate 47   The Sinuses and Maxilla

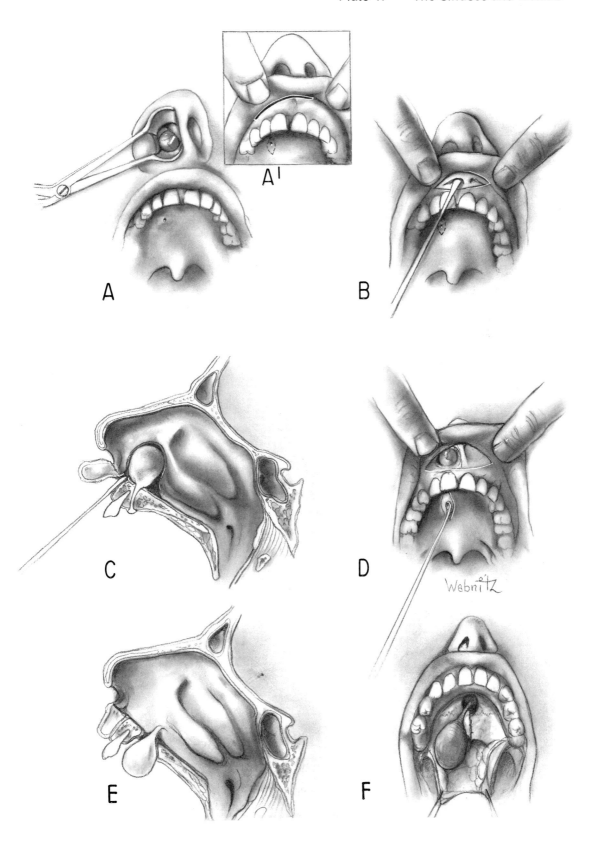

A

A¹

B

C

D

Wabnitz

E

F

CLOSURE OF OROANTRAL FISTULA

Highpoints

1. Small oroantral fistulae, 1 to 2 mm in size, usually close spontaneously. Those from 3 to 4 mm in size are usually successfully closed with a buccal flap (step *F*).
2. Fistulae 5 mm and larger as well as those of longstanding duration associated with severe sinus disease require a more extensive surgical procedure using a large palatal flap.
3. Adequate sinus surgery with antrostomy is necessary in this latter group.
4. Flaps must be rotated and sutured without tension.
5. The suture line must be well away from the bony defect.
6. All diseased bone must be removed. In large fistulae, the tooth on either side of the fistula is extracted.
7. If an active purulent sinusitis exists, antral washings through an antrostomy with systemic antibiotics are indicated preoperatively.
8. Any projecting bone should be leveled off so that no undue pressure is exerted on the flap.

A The dotted line depicts the diseased edematous mucous membrane to be excised. Since the anterior located tooth is close to the fistula, it will be extracted. The solid line on the palate outlines the mucoperiosteal palatal flap based on the greater palatine artery (dotted line). A broad based buccal flap is also elevated to expose the canine fossa through which a Caldwell-Luc operation (see plates 28 and 29) can be performed as indicated. Large fistulae over 5 mm usually require this antral surgery, depending, of course, on the antral pathologic change.

B Frontal section through the fistula shows the diseased mucous membrane extending into the fistula. All this diseased tissue, as well as surrounding osteomyelitis in adjacent bone, is excised. If the bone disease is extensive, adjacent teeth or alveolar ridge is to be removed.

 Arrow indicates position of Caldwell-Luc approach to the antrum through which diseased mucous membrane is removed. If the oroantral defect is extremely large, a Caldwell-Luc exposure may not be necessary since access to the antrum may be through the fistula defect. An intranasal antrostomy (see plate 27) is performed into the inferior meatus. This is enlarged if considerable sinus disease is present.

C The palatal flap is elevated, preserving the greater palatine artery. The buccal flap is turned upward to expose the canine fossa when Caldwell-Luc procedure is deemed necessary. The tooth anterior to the fistula has been extracted and diseased bone and mucous membrane have been excised.

C¹ Following the technique of Proctor (1969), a bone plug may be fitted into the bony defect when it is large (0.5 to 2.5 cm). The bone plug is taken from the iliac crest and consists only of cancellous bone, the hard cortical bone having been discarded. The bone plug is tapered and shaped to fit the defect. It is tapped into the fistula. Any protruding portion of the bone plug is removed so that it is flush with the surrounding bone.

Plate 48   The Sinuses and Maxilla

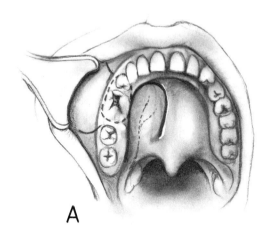

A

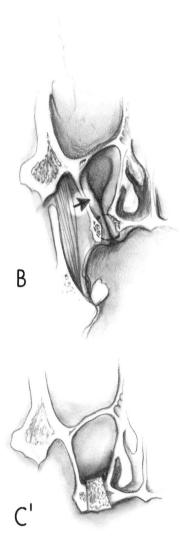

B

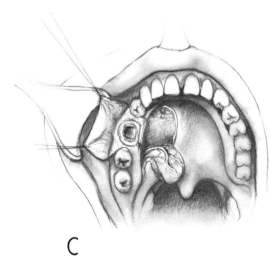

C

C'

CLOSURE OF OROANTRAL FISTULA (*Continued*)

D   The palatal flap is rotated across the defect without tension. The suture line must rest on sound bone and not cross the fistula. If tension occurs posteriorly at the second molar tooth, this unfortunately is removed. The donor site on the palate may be allowed to granulate, or, if objectionably large, grafted with free dermis or epidermis.

E   The frontal section depicts the palatal flap closure with suture lines well away from fistula. The locations of the Caldwell-Luc operation and the intranasal antrostomy are shown on the lateral wall and medial wall of the antrum, respectively. A rubber drain is through the intranasal antrostomy.

F   With smaller fistulae (under 5 mm in diameter), buccal flap is advanced to cover the fistula. Care must be taken not to injure Stenson's duct in the mobilization of the flap.

G   The frontal section showing the buccal flap in position. An intranasal antrostomy has been performed. A disadvantage of the buccal flap is that it crosses the buccogingival gutter and partially obliterates it—a possible source of trouble with denture-wearing patients. However, this will stretch in time. In the immediate postoperative period, the patient must not wear his denture since this would place undue tension and pressure on the flap. Another disadvantage is the possible tension placed on this flap with motion of the lips and cheek.

Usually no dressing is used in either procedure; however, with large palatal flaps, cotton soaked with Furacin and secured to surrounding teeth may be used if the flap appears to buckle or separate from the underlying bone. The intranasal antrostomy drain is likewise optional. Antibiotics are used.

Plate 49   The Sinuses and Maxilla

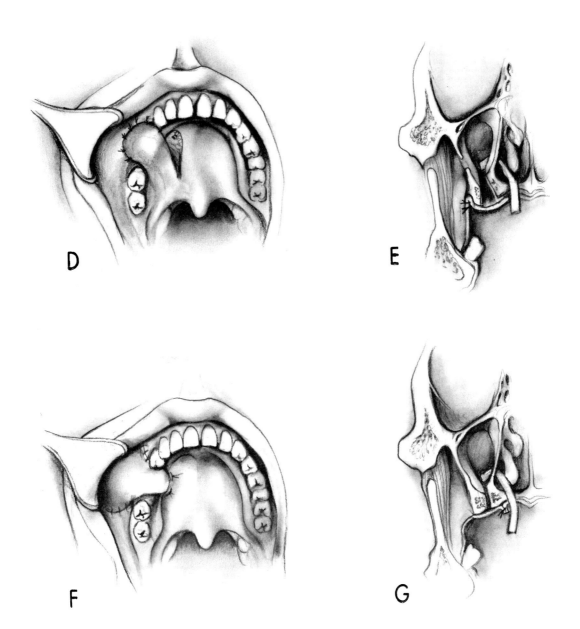

D

E

F

G

BIBLIOGRAPHY

Alford, B. R.: Osteoplastic approach to the frontal sinus for osteoma. Arch. Otolaryng. *80*:16–21, 1964.

Arlen, M., Tollefsen, H. R., Huvos, A. G., and Marcove, R. C.: Chondrosarcoma of the head and neck. Amer. J. Surg. *120*: 456–460, 1970.

Bateman, G. H.: Personal communication, 1960.

Bateman, G. H.: Technique of hypophysectomy. Presented at Trans. Amer. Acad. Ophthal. Otolaryng., Chicago, 1961.

Bateman, G. H.: Trans-sphenoidal hypophysectomy. Otolaryng. Clin. N. Amer. *4*:205–215, 1971.

Bordley, J. E., and Bischofberger, W.: Osteomyelitis of the frontal bone. Laryngoscope 77:1234–1244, 1967.

Bosley, W. R.: Osteoplastic obliteration of the frontal sinuses. A review of 100 cases. Laryngoscope 82:1463–1475, 1972.

Briant, T. D. R.: Trans-sphenoidal hypophysectomy. Amer. Acad. Ophthal. October, 1967.

Brownson, R. J., and Ogura, J. H.: Primary carcinoma of the frontal sinus. Laryngoscope *81*:71–89, 1971.

Catlin, F. I., Cluff, L. E., and Reynolds, R. C.: The bacteriology of acute and chronic sinusitis. Southern Med. J. *58*:1497–1502, 1965.

Chandler, J. R.: Iatrogenic cerebrospinal rhinorrhea. Trans. Amer Acad. Ophthal. Otolaryng. 74:576–584, 1970.

Chandler, J. R., Langenbrunne, D. J., and Stevens, E. R.: *The pathogenesis* of orbital complications in acute sinusitis. Laryngoscope 80:1414–1428, 1970.

Chiari, O.: Zur Kasuistik der Erkrankungen der Unterkieferspeicheldrüse. Wien Klin. Wschr. 25:1562–1567, 1912.

Cocke, E. W.: Use of Gigli saw in resection of the superior maxilla. Presented at James Ewing Society Meeting, New York, April, 1956.

Cocke, E. W., Jr., and Braund, R. R.: Superior maxillary resection. *In* Cooper, P.: The Craft of Surgery. 2nd ed. Boston Little, Brown and Company, 1971.

Fracchia, A. A., Farrow, J. H., Miller, T. R., Tollefsen, R. H., Greenberg, E. J., and Knapper, W. H.: Hypophysectomy as compared with adrenalectomy in the treatment of advanced carcinoma of the breast. Surg. Gynec. Obstet. *133*: 241–246, 1971.

Gallagher, T. M., and Boles, R.: Symposium: Treatment of malignancies of paranasal sinuses. I. Carcinoma of the maxillary antrum. Laryngoscope *80*: 924–932, 1970.

Gass, H. H., and Klein, S.: Transethmoidal drainage and arrest of craniopharyngioma by Zenker's solution. Acta Neurochir. (Wien) *17*:196–203, 1967.

Gatti, W. M., Mason, J. H., and Kosmala, R. L.: Fibrocementoma of the maxilla. Arch. Otolaryng. *84*:114, 1966.

Goodale, R. L., and Montgomery, W. W.: Technical advances in osteoplastic frontal sinusectomy. Arch. Otolaryng. *79*:522–529, 1964.

Grayhack, J. T.: Adrenalectomy and hypophysectomy for carcinoma of the prostate. J.A.M.A. *210*:1075–1076, 1969.

Hamberger, C. A., Hammer, G., Norlen, G., and Sjogren, B.: Transantrosphenoidal hypophysectomy. Arch. Otolaryng. *74*:2–8, 1961.

Harner, S. G., and Newell, R. C.: Treatment of frontal osteomyelitis. Laryngoscope *79*:1281–1294, 1969.

Heck, W., McNaught, R. C., Greenspan, F. S., and Kaplan, H. S.: Trans-septal-sphenoid pituitary surgery. Laryngoscope 67:906–943, 1957.

Hiranandani, L. H., and Kamdar, H. H.: Treatment of chronic oro-antral fistula by complete palatal flap. J. Laryng. *75*:744–752, 1961.

Hiranandani, L. H., Chandra, O., Melgiri, R. D., and Hiranandani, N. L.: Aberrant salivary tumours. J. Laryng. *80*:564–570, 1966.

Hirsch, O.: Eine neue Methode der endonasalen Operation von Hypophysentumoren. Wien. Med. Wschr. 636, 1939.

Hirsch, O.: Über Methoden der operativen Behändlung von Hypophysentumoren auf endonasalen Wege. Arch. Laryng. Rhin. (Berl.) *24*:129, 1910.

Jesse, R. H.: Preoperative versus postoperative radiation in the treatment of squamous carcinoma of the paranasal sinuses. Amer. J. Surg. *110*:552–556, 1965.

Kenan, P. D., and Hudson, W. R.: Chromophobe adenoma: Evaluation and management. Trans. Amer. Acad. Ophthal. Otolaryng. 73:52–59, 1969.

Ketcham, A. S., Wilkins, R. H., Van Buren, J. M., and Smith, R.: A combined intracranial facial approach to the paranasal sinuses. Amer. J. Surg. *106*:698, 1963.

Ketcham, A. S., Hoye, R. C., Van Buren, J. M., Johnson, R. H., and Smith, R. R.: Complications of intracranial facial resection for tumors of the paranasal sinuses. Amer. J. Surg. *112*:591–596, 1966.

Kimmich, H. M.: Radical palliative surgery about the orbit. Arch. Otolaryng. *94*:338–346, 1971.

Kirchner, F. R., Toledo, P. S., and Robison, J. T.: Modified osteoplastic approach to the frontal bone, sinuses, and/or the orbit. Laryngoscope 77:1706–1713, 1967.

Kurohara, S. S., Webster, J. H., Ellis, F., Fitzgerald, J. P., Shedd, D. P., and Badib, A. O.: Role of radiation therapy and of surgery in the management of localized epidermoid carcinoma of the maxillary sinus. Amer. J. Roentgen. *114*:35–42, 1972.

Lewis, J. S.: Sarcoma of the nasal cavity and paranasal sinuses. Ann. Otol. *78*:778, 1969.

Loeb, H. W.: Operative Surgery of the Nose, Throat and Ear. Vol. II. St. Louis, C. V. Mosby Company, 1917.

Loré, J. M.: Diseases of the maxillary sinus and their relationship to the oral cavity. Laryngoscope, *48*:724–737, 1938.

Loré, J. M., Jr.: Cryosurgical aspects of hypophysectomy. J. Cryosurg. *1*:216–219, 1968.

Loré, J. M., Jr.: Transseptal transsphenoidal hypophysectomy. Amer. J. Surg. *112*:577–582, 1966.

Lynch, R. C.: The technique of a radical frontal sinus operation which has given me the best results. Laryngoscope *31*:1–5, 1921.

Macbeth, R.: Caldwell-Luc operation 1952–1966. Arch. Otolaryng. 87:630–636, 1968.

Macbeth, R., and Hall, M.: Hypophysectomy as a rhinological procedure. Arch. Otolaryng. 75:440–450, 1962.

Manace, E. D., and Goldman, J. L.: Acinic cell carcinoma of the paranasal sinuses. Presented at Meeting of Eastern Section of Amer. Laryng. Rhinol. Otol.

Soc., Paradise Island, Nassau, January, 1971.

Marchetta, F. C., Sako, K., Mattick, W. L., and Stinziano, G. D.: Squamous cell carcinoma of the maxillary antrum. Amer. J. Surg. *118*:805–807, 1969.

Martinson, F. D., Alli, A. F., and Clark, B. M.: Aspergilloma of the ethmoid. J. Laryng. *84*:857–861, 1970.

Miglets, A. W., and Saunders, W. H.: Dural replacement with split thickness skin. Long term experimental and clinical results. Laryngoscope *81*:8–17, 1971.

Montgomery, W. W.: Transethmoidosphenoidal hypophysectomy with septal mucosal flap. Arch. Otolaryng. 78:68–77, 1963.

Montgomery, W. W.: Symposium on surgery of the nasal sinuses. Otolaryng. Clin. N. Amer. *4*:97–126, 1971.

Newsome, J. F., Timmons, R. L., Van Wyk, J., and Dugger, G. S.: Pituitary stalk section for metastatic carcinoma of the breast. Ann. Surg. *174*:769–773, 1971.

Niho, S., Niho, M., and Niho, K.: Decompression of the optic canal by the transethmoidal route and decompression of the superior orbital fissure. Canad. J. Ophthal. 5:22–40, 1970.

Norrell, H., Alves, A. M., Winternitz, W. W., and Maddy, J.: A clinicopathologic analysis of cryohypophysectomy in patients with advanced cancer. Cancer 25:1050–1060, 1970.

Otty, J. H.: Exploration of the sphenoid sinus. *In* Rob, C., and Smith, R. (eds.): Operative Surgery: Eye, Ear, Nose and Throat. Philadelphia, F. A. Davis Company, 1958.

Pastore, P. N.: Mucormycosis of the maxillary sinus and diabetes mellitus. Southern Med. J. *60*:1164–1167, 1967.

Pearson, B. W., MacKenzie, R. G., and Goodman, W. S.: The anatomical basis of transantral ligation of the maxillary artery in severe epistaxis. Laryngoscope 79:969–984, 1969.

Proctor, B.: Bone graft closure of large or persistent oromaxillary fistula. Laryngoscope 79:822–826, 1969.

Rafla, S.: Mucous gland tumors of paranasal sinuses. Cancer 24:683–691, 1969.

Reed, P. I., and Pizey, N. C. D.: Transsphenoidal hypophysectomy in the treatment of advanced breast cancer. Brit. J. Surg. 54:369–374, 1967.

Ritter, F. N.: Surgical anatomy of the paranasal sinuses. Instruction Section, Trans. Amer. Acad. Ophthal. Otolaryng., 1970.

Roca, A. N., Smith, J., and Jing, B.: Osteosarcoma and parosteal osteogenic sarcoma of the maxilla and mandible: Study of 20 cases. Amer. J. Clin. Path. 54:625–636, 1970.

Ross, D. E.: Radical en bloc ethmoidectomy for cancer. Surg. Gynec. Obstet. 108: 109–114, 1959.

Saunders, W. H., and Miglets, A.: Surgical techniques for eradicating far advanced carcinoma of the orbital-ethmoid and maxillary areas. Trans. Amer. Acad. Ophthal. Otolaryng. 71:426–431, 1967.

Schmitz, G. L., Peters, R., and Lehman, R. H.: Thorium induced carcinoma of the maxillary sinus. Presented before the Wisconsin Otolaryng. Soc., February, 1969.

Schuknecht, H. F.: The surgical management of carcinoma of the paranasal sinuses. Laryngoscope 61:874–890, 1951.

Sisson, G. A.: Modern management of malignancies of the maxilla. Proceedings of Ninth International Oto-Rhino-Laryngology Congress, Mexico, D. F., 1969.

Sisson, G. A.: Symposium – Paranasal sinuses. III. Discussion and summary. Laryngoscope 80:945–953, 1970.

Sisson, G. A., Johnson, N. E., and Amiri, C. S.: Cancer of the maxillary sinus. Ann. Otol. 72:1050, 1963.

Smith, A. T.: Acute and chronic sphenoid and ethmoid sinus disease. Maloney, W. H. (ed.): Otolaryngology. Volume III. Hagerstown, Maryland, Harper & Row, 1969.

Smith, H. W.: Cystic lesions of the maxilla. Arch. Otolaryng. 88:426–435, 1968.

Smith, R. R., Klopp, C. T., and Williams, J. M.: Surgical treatment of cancer of the frontal sinus and adjacent areas. Cancer 7:991, 1954.

Sofferman, R. A., Smith, R. O., and English, G. M.: Albers-Schönberg's disease (osteopetrosis). A case with osteomyelitis of the maxilla. Laryngoscope 81: 36–46, 1971.

Tabb, H. G.: Carcinoma of the antrum: An analysis of 60 cases with special reference to primary surgical extirpation. Laryngoscope 67:269, 1957.

Tabb, H. G., and Barranco, S. J.: Cancer of the maxillary sinus. An analysis of 108 cases. Laryngoscope 81:818–827, 1971.

Terz, J. J., Alksne, J. F., and Lawrence, W., Jr.: Craniofacial resection for tumors invading the pterygoid fossa. Amer. J. Surg. 118:732–740, 1969.

Tollefsen, H. R., Miller, T. R., and Gerold, F. P.: Transantral sphenoidal hypophysectomy. Amer. J. Surg. 112:569–576, 1966.

Van Alyea, O. E.: Maxillary sinus. In Jackson, C., and Jackson, C. L. (eds.): Diseases of the Nose, Throat and Ear. 2d ed. Philadelphia, W. B. Saunders Company, 1959.

Ward, P. H., Alley, C., and Owen, R.: Monostotic fibrous dysplasia of the maxilla. Laryngoscope 79:1295–1306, 1969.

Wilder, L. W., Beyer, C. K., Smith, B., and Conley, J. J.: Ocular findings following radical maxillectomy. Trans. Amer. Acad. Ophthal. Otolaryng. 75:797–801, 1971.

Wise, R. A., and Baker, H. W.: Surgery of the Head and Neck. 1st Ed. Chicago, Year Book Medical Publishers, Inc., 1958.

Wise, R. A., and Baker, H. W.: Surgery of the Head and Neck. 3rd ed. Year Book Medical Publishers, 1968.

Worsoe-Petersen, J.: Colloid carcinoma of the nasal cavity and sinuses. Arch. Otolaryng. 82:181–185, 1965.

4. THE NOSE AND THE NASOPHARYNX

ANATOMY OF EPISTAXIS
(After Hollinshead, 1954; Montgomery, 1971)

Epistaxis can be either a very minor or a very major problem. The most common area in children and young adults is anteriorly on the septum (Kiesselbach or Little area) and is the easiest controlled (plate 51, steps *E* and *F*). The more complicated areas are posterior and superior both on the lateral wall of the nose and septum in older adults (plate 51, steps *A*, *B*, *C*, *D* and *F*).

The important factors in the control of epistaxis are etiology, location and management.

Etiology

A. Local disease
   1. Crusting and ulceration
   2. Nose picking
   3. Infection
   4. Neoplasms
      a. Malignant neoplasms
      b. Juvenile nasopharyngeal fibromas
      c. Angiomas
   5. Trauma
   6. Foreign body
B. Generalized disorders and disease
   1. Arteriosclerosis — hypertension
   2. Rheumatic heart disease
   3. Blood dyscrasia and associated diseases
      a. Anemia
      b. Polycythemia vera
      c. Thrombocytopenia purpura
      d. Hemophilia
   4. Leukemia
   5. Familial telangiectasia (Rendu-Osler-Weber disease)
   6. Hepatic diseases
   7. Chronic nephritis
   8. Vicarious menstruation
   9. Atmospheric pressure changes, e. g., scuba divers; caisson disease.
   10. Generalized infectious diseases
   11. "Stigmata"?

ANATOMY OF EPISTAXIS (*Continued*)

Location

Exact determination of the bleeding site must be made, if at all possible, to facilitate direct attack. Occasionally a submucous resection (plates 64 and 65) or septoplasty (plates 66, 67 and 68) is necessary to visualize the site. Often under such circumstances these procedures will achieve control of the hemorrhage. Lateral rhinotomy may be necessary especially in familial telangiectasia to insert a dermal graft for septal dermoplasty (plate 53) (Saunders, 1960).

Technique of Management

1. Cauterization
2. Nasal packing—anterior, posterior or both
3. Ligation of vessels—ligation should be as close as possible to the feeding vessel.
   a. Ethmoid vessels
   b. Internal maxillary and sphenopalatine vessels
   c. External carotid vessel
4. Septal dermoplasty—removal of offending mucosa and application of a dermal graft rather than split thickness epidermis.
5. Basic care of severe hemorrhage—frequency and selection depends on degree of severity of blood loss.
   a. Vital signs—every one to two hours
   b. Hemaglobin and hematocrit determination, one to three times per day
   c. Blood transfusion
   d. Central venous pressure (James and Myers, 1972)
   e. Blood volume
   f. Venous cutdown or intracatheter in vein
   g. Blood urea nitrogen determination—elevation result of swallowing and absorbing blood

ANATOMY OF EPISTAXIS (*Continued*)

Angiography

Seldom necessary but of distinct use in persistent and refraction epistaxis to determine feeding vessels.

Complications

1. Shock
2. Aspiration of blood with airway obstruction causing respiratory arrest and then cardiac arrest. Never have patient keep head back. If bleeding is to occur, let it run out of the nose rather than down the pharynx and into the larynx. Oversedation can be the cause of this complication.

Axiom

Treat all patients with severe epistaxis as a serious problem.

A Anatomy of septal vessels.

B Anatomy of vessels on lateral wall of nose.

Plate 50   *The Nose and the Nasopharynx*

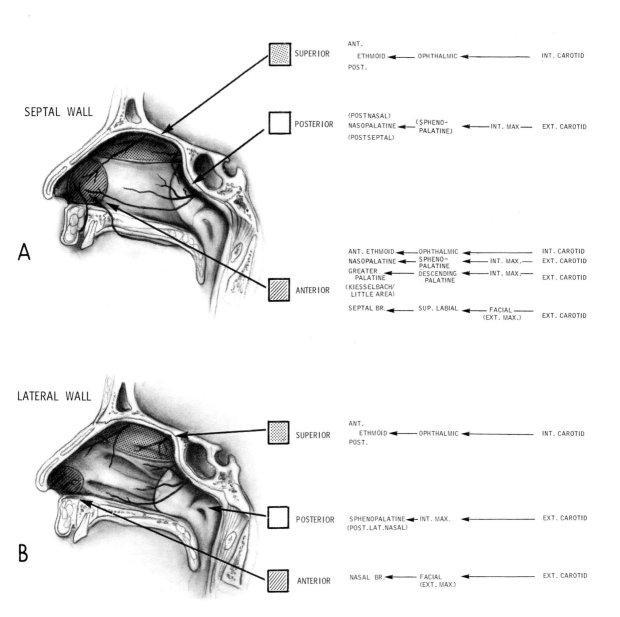

SEPTAL WALL

SUPERIOR

ANT.
ETHMOID ← OPHTHALMIC ← INT. CAROTID
POST.

POSTERIOR

(POSTNASAL)
NASOPALATINE ← (SPHENO-PALATINE) ← INT. MAX ← EXT. CAROTID
(POSTSEPTAL)

ANTERIOR

ANT. ETHMOID ← OPHTHALMIC ← INT. CAROTID
NASOPALATINE ← SPHENO-PALATINE ← INT. MAX. ← EXT. CAROTID
GREATER PALATINE ← DESCENDING PALATINE ← INT. MAX. ← EXT. CAROTID
(KIESSELBACH/LITTLE AREA)

SEPTAL BR. ← SUP. LABIAL ← FACIAL (EXT. MAX.) ← EXT. CAROTID

A

LATERAL WALL

SUPERIOR

ANT.
ETHMOID ← OPHTHALMIC ← INT. CAROTID
POST.

POSTERIOR

SPHENOPALATINE ← INT. MAX. ← EXT. CAROTID
(POST.LAT.NASAL)

ANTERIOR

NASAL BR. ← FACIAL (EXT. MAX.) ← EXT. CAROTID

B

ANTERIOR AND POSTERIOR PACKING FOR EPISTAXIS

Highpoints

1. Attempt to locate bleeding site by cleansing nasal passages with cotton-tipped applicator dipped in solution of cocaine, 10 per cent, or tetracaine, 2 per cent, and a vasoconstrictor.
2. Anterior septal vessels (Kiesselbach's plexus) most common site.
3. In the absence of hypertension, bleeding at this common site is usually controlled with a pledget of cotton gauze soaked with cocaine or tetracaine and a vasoconstrictor. If bleeding persists from this location, cauterization with either a silver nitrate stick or electrocautery is performed (*E*). Anterior packing (*F*) may also be necessary.
4. Fatal hemorrhage is very rare, especially in hypertension, if meticulous care is given.
5. Epistaxis in hypertension is looked upon as a fortunate safety valve mechanism.
6. Aspiration and swallowing of blood should be avoided. If oozing persists, allow blood to run from anterior nares with head flexed forward.
7. Ligation of one or both external carotid arteries is occasionally necessary (see plate 374).
8. Occlusion of anterior ethmoidal, posterior ethmoidal (plates 52 and 53) or internal maxillary arteries (plates 54 and 55) with silver clips may be necessary.
9. Ligation of common carotid or internal carotid is neither necessary nor justified.
10. Nasal packing of any type should be accompanied by systemic antibiotics. Strip gauze one-half inch, impregnated with an antibiotic ointment, is ideal.
11. Occasionally in persistent epistaxis, e.g., in familial telangiectasia, an arteriogram may be helpful. Collateral blood supply has been demonstrated via the vertebral artery and the occipital artery into the internal maxillary artery in a patient with external carotid artery ligation.
12. A nasal mucous membrane dermoplasty (excision of diseased mucous membrane and coverage with dermal graft) may be required in familial telangiectasia (plate 53).

Posterior Packing

A Topical anesthesia may be applied to the nasal mucosa. A small rubber catheter (#10 French), to which an 18 inch length of soft-bodied string is tied, is inserted into one naris. The forward end is grasped with a small sponge stick and pulled out through the mouth leaving the string in the nasal cavity and mouth. This maneuver is repeated through the other naris.

B The oral ends of the string are then secured to a prearranged roll of gauze impregnated with antibiotic ointment to which is tied a third section of string.

Plate 51   The Nose and the Nasopharynx

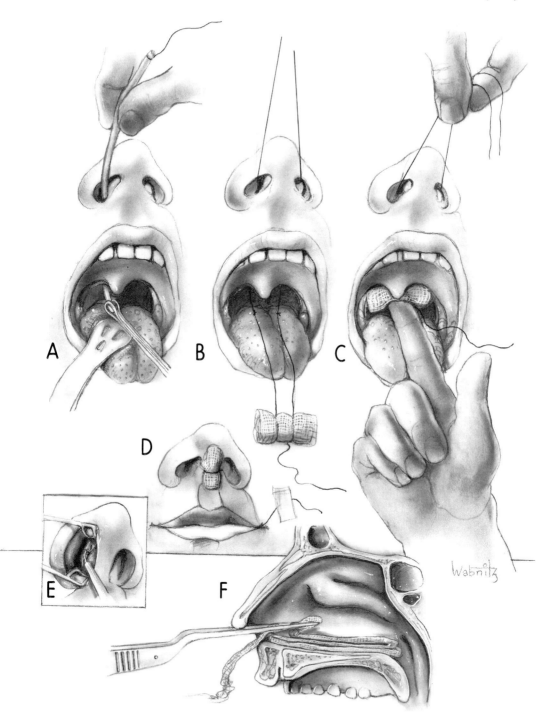

A

B

C

D

E

F

Wabnitz

C   Steady traction is then applied to the nasal ends of the strings and, with the index finger of the opposite hand, the roll of gauze is firmly directed into the nasopharynx. The third string protrudes from the corner of the mouth.

D   The two nasal ends of the string are tied securely over a small cushion of gauze or dental roll across the columella. The oral string is loosely taped to the cheek. This latter string facilitates easy removal of the posterior pack.

    When the above equipment is not available, a Foley catheter is inserted through one naris. When the tip has passed the nasopharynx the bag is inflated and pulled forward into the posterior naris. The catheter is secured with folded gauze tied at the anterior naris.

    The Stevens nasal balloon with or without a built-in breathing tube can also be used. Its use is similar to that of the Foley catheter.

Control of Anterior Hemorrhage

E   Cauterization of the anterior septal vessels is done after initial control with topical application of cocaine, 10 per cent, or tetracaine, 2 per cent, and a vasoconstrictor. Either silver nitrate (stick or 50 to 100 per cent solution) or electrocautery is used as the agent.

F   When anterior nasal packing is necessary, one-half inch gauze impregnated with Furacin or antibiotic ointment is placed in horizontal layers. In this manner more complete and uniform pressure is obtained or selective pressure at one level is obtained by simply raising or lowering the packing. This latter technique leaves a small air passage for respiration. Systemic antibiotics are used with any type of nasal packing.

Complications

1. Persistent hemorrhage leading to hypovolemic shock and death.
2. Aspiration of blood passing down through nasopharynx. Oversedation may well be a contributing cause to this avoidable complication which has caused death.
3. Elevation of BUN from absorption of ingested blood.
4. Any other complication resulting from hypovolemic shock, e.g., myocardial infarction, kidney shutdown.

Plate 51 Repeated   The Nose and the Nasopharynx

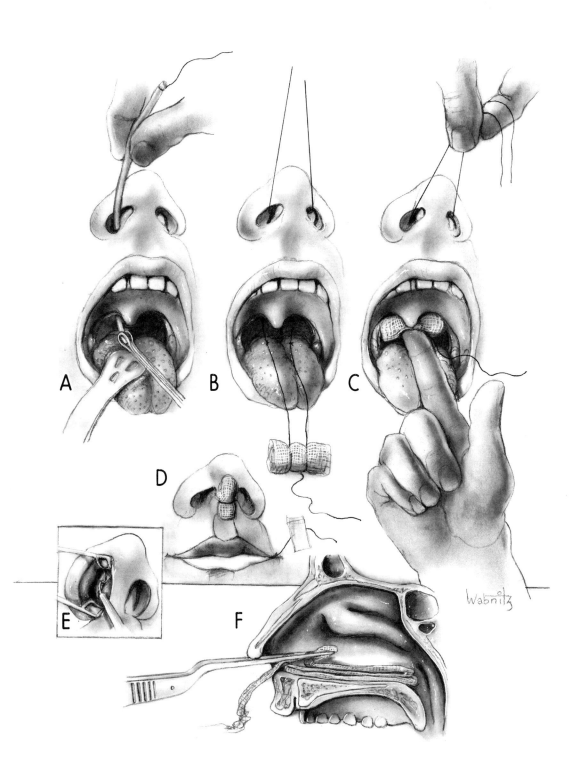

A

B

C

D

E

F

Wabnitz

LIGATION OF ETHMOIDAL ARTERIES

Indication

Epistaxis superiorly (above the middle turbinate) (see plate 50).

A Depicted is the anatomy of the origin and relationships of the anterior and posterior ethmoidal arteries as they arise from the ophthalmic artery which is the first branch of the internal carotid artery (refer to plates 1 through 6 for bony relationships). A number of excellent articles by Weddell, Macbeth, Sharp and Calvert (1946) and Kirchner, Yanagisawa and Crelin (1961) refer to the details of the surgical anatomy of these vessels. An important relationship is the proximity of the posterior ethmoid artery to the optic nerve which "entering at a small angle with the medial orbital wall, lies only 1 or 2 mm from the point where the posterior ethmoid artery leaves the orbital soft tissue to enter the foramen" (Kirchner, 1961). The posterior ethmoidal foramen is between 4 to 7 mm in 84 per cent of the skulls from the optic foramen. Hence the admonition of caution if electrocautery is used to obliterate this vessel. It must be applied meticulously to the bony foramen with retraction of the orbital contents. Silver clips are preferred. The distance relationships depicted on the illustration are from Kirchner but he hastens to emphasize that there are such variations that these distances may be of little help to the surgeon. The anterior ethmoid artery is usually the larger but the reverse can be true. One or the other vessel may be absent.

B An anterior view of the anatomy of the medial bony wall of the orbit showing the more typical location of the foramena of the anterior and posterior ethmoid arteries in the region of the frontoethmoidal suture line.

The relationship of the medial canthal ligament and the lacrimal sac to the region of the surgical approach is depicted in plate 157, step *B*.

The reference point is the frontomaxillolacrimal suture junction in both steps *A* and *B*.

Highpoints

1. Avoid injury to the medial canthal ligament and the lacrimal sac below and the trochlear of the superior oblique muscle above.
2. Subperiosteal dissection.
3. Avoid injury to the globe and optic nerve.
4. Do not fracture the thin lamina papyracea of the ethmoid bone.
5. Control all bleeding meticulously—postoperative intraorbital hemorrhage could damage the optic nerve by pressure.

Plate 52   The Nose and the Nasopharynx

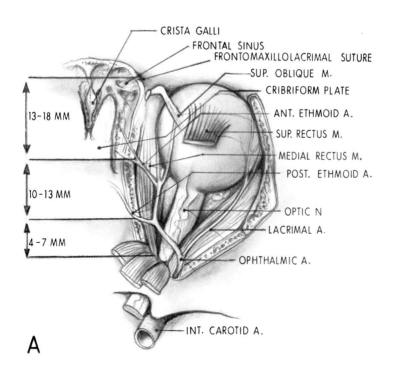

CRISTA GALLI
FRONTAL SINUS
FRONTOMAXILLOLACRIMAL SUTURE
SUP. OBLIQUE M.
CRIBRIFORM PLATE
ANT. ETHMOID A.
SUP. RECTUS M.
MEDIAL RECTUS M.
POST. ETHMOID A.
OPTIC N
LACRIMAL A.
OPHTHALMIC A.
INT. CAROTID A.

13-18 MM
10-13 MM
4-7 MM

A

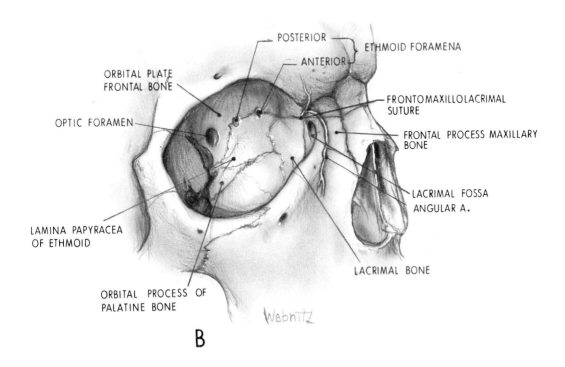

POSTERIOR
ETHMOID FORAMENA
ANTERIOR
ORBITAL PLATE
FRONTAL BONE
FRONTOMAXILLOLACRIMAL
SUTURE
OPTIC FORAMEN
FRONTAL PROCESS MAXILLARY
BONE
LACRIMAL FOSSA
ANGULAR A.
LAMINA PAPYRACEA
OF ETHMOID
LACRIMAL BONE
ORBITAL PROCESS OF
PALATINE BONE

Wabnitz

B

LIGATION OF ETHMOIDAL ARTERIES (*Continued*)

C   A temporary tarsorrhaphy may be performed. A slightly curved incision about 3 cm in length is made as depicted extending more above the medial canthal ligament than below it. Branches of the angular vessel will require ligation. This artery anastomoses with the dorsal nasal branch of the ophthalmic artery.

D   The periosteum is incised and elevated above the medial canthal ligament avoiding the lacrimal sac below and the trochlear above. This exposes the suture line (vertical) between the frontal (nasal) process of the maxilla and the lacrimal bone and the suture line (horizontal) between the orbital plate of the frontal bone and the lamina papyracea of the ethmoid bone. A suitable self-retaining retractor with interchangeable slatted and solid blades (Loungo) is inserted. If necessary, a small malleable retractor can also be used to retract the periosteum and the globe laterally. Following the frontoethmoid suture line, the anterior ethmoid artery is identified. Silver clips are placed proximally and distally—if possible, two on each side—and the vessel transected. This is necessary to facilitate deeper exposure of the posterior ethmoidal artery, which is then simply occluded with one or two silver clips. Care is taken not to dislodge the silver clips on the ends of the transected anterior ethmoid artery during the maneuver.

At this point extreme care is exercised to avoid injury to the optic nerve (see step A).

When hemostasis is incomplete, electrocautery can be used for small vessels if extreme care is taken not to injure the optic nerve nor any other contents of the orbit; the wound is closed without drain.

Complications

1. Hematoma.
2. Optic nerve damage.

Plate 52 Continued   The Nose and the Nasopharynx

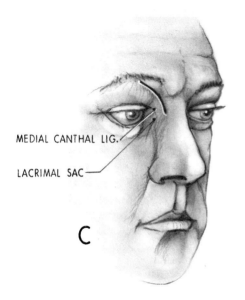

MEDIAL CANTHAL LIG.

LACRIMAL SAC

C

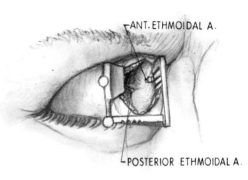

ANT. ETHMOIDAL A.

POSTERIOR ETHMOIDAL A.

D

SEPTAL DERMOPLASTY (After Saunders, 1960)

Indications

Repeated epistaxis secondary to familial telangiectasia (Rendu-Osler-Weber disease). This disease is systemic with possible bleeding from any epithelial or mucosal surface including the gastrointestinal tract. Cardiac failure secondary to anemia must be carefully evaluated and managed prior to any surgical intervention.

Highpoints

1. Remove entire mucous membrane in area to be treated, leaving intact the underlying perichondrium.
2. If there is any question regarding the viability of the septal cartilage from use of electrocautery, it may be wiser to stage a procedure on the opposite side to avoid perforation.
3. Remove as much of diseased area as possible from one side—this usually includes mucous membrane not only on the septum but also on the lateral wall of the nose, including turbinates.
4. Give adequate exposure.
5. Avoid aspiration of blood; if performed under general anesthesia, pack hypopharynx in addition to using a cuffed endotracheal tube since the bleeding may be profuse.

A Depicted is a lateral rhinotomy (see plate 93) which affords adequate exposure of the nasal septum and a portion of lateral wall of the nasal cavity. The dotted line outlines area of mucous membrane excised. All the mucous membrane must be excised so that no islands remain under the skin graft. The perichondrium is preserved. Bleeding is usually copious and is controlled with electrocautery. Care must be taken not to perforate the nasal septum.

A¹ Since it is quite impractical to place sutures completely around the edges of the mucosal defects on the skin graft, the grafts are merely sutured anteriorly using 5-0 continuous nylon. The grafts are then folded in over the defects on the septum and lateral wall of the nose, leaving excess graft posteriorly. This will slough off in due time. One half inch gauze packing impregnated with antibiotic ointment is carefully and loosely placed within the nasal cavity separating the two grafts, medially and laterally.

B Frontal section through the nasal cavity showing the location of the skin graft. Both split thickness epidermal and dermal grafts have been utilized, more recently the latter. Although not proven, it is believed that the dermal grafts may possibly assume some of the morphologic characteristics of mucosa in the nose as they do in the oral cavity and pharynx. One caution would be the possible adherence of the dermal grafts on the septum and the turbinate to one another. Hence, packing or splint (see plate 67, step I) should be maintained until epithelialization of the dermis occurs. Another possible criticism would be the increased thickness of the dermal graft over the epidermal graft thus compromising the nasal airway.

The nasolabial incision for the lateral rhinotomy is closed in layers. There must be no bleeding at the close of the operation. Antibiotic ointment is used freely during the postoperative period.

Complications

1. Recurrent epistaxis.
2. Cardiac failure.
3. Graft failure.
4. Septal perforation.
5. Atrophic rhinitis with varying degrees of crusting.

Plate 53   The Nose and the Nasopharynx

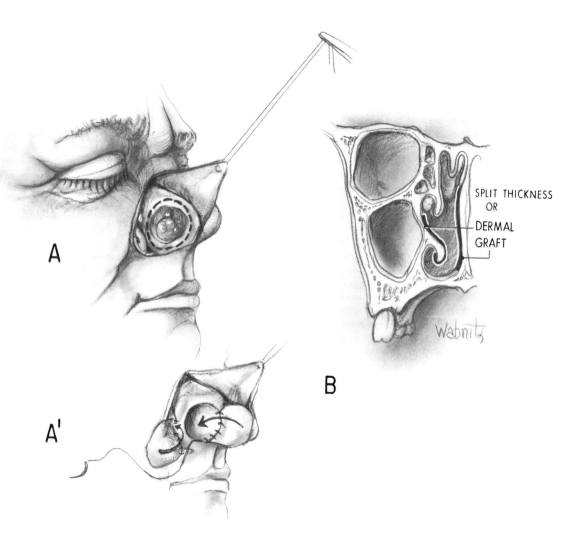

A

A'

B

SPLIT THICKNESS
OR
DERMAL
GRAFT

Wabnitz

LIGATION OF (INTERNAL) MAXILLARY ARTERY

Indications

Epistaxis posteriorly (from the sphenopalatine artery and its nasopalatine branch) (see plate 50).

A   Depicted is the basic anatomy of the internal maxillary artery (now known as simply the maxillary artery while the external maxillary artery is known as the facial artery) (see plates 1 through 7 for bony relationships). This main terminal branch of the external carotid artery (along with the superficial temporal artery) is of prime concern to the surgeon. It is divided into three parts. There may be some confusion regarding terminology, and alternate names are in brackets. The following classification is after Pearson, MacKenzie, and Goodman (1969); Hollinshead (1954); Anson and McVay, (1971); and Sobotta (1936).

Part I

(Medial to mandible)
1. Deep auricular
2. Anterior tympanic
3. Middle meningeal (and accessory meningeal)
4. Inferior alveolar

Part II

(Relationship deep or superficial to external pterygoid muscle — all muscular branches)
1. Masseteric
2. Deep temporal (2)
3. Buccinator
4. External and internal pterygoid

Part III

Pterygopalatine part lies against posterolateral aspect of maxilla and passes in a plane lying between two heads of external pterygoid muscle to enter pterygopalatine fossa (lateral portion).

Lateral	Posterior superior alveolar
Anterior	Infraorbital
	Descending palatine (somewhat medial and inferior)
	Greater palatine
	Lesser palatine
Posterior	Pharyngeal
	Branch to foramen rotundum and to the pterygoid canal
Medial and	Sphenopalatine (posterior lateral nasal)
Superior	Posterior nasal (nasopalatine; posterior septal)

The branches of the third part are those involved in the transantral ligation for the control of epistaxis, specifically the terminal medial branch forming the sphenopalatine and the posterior nasal arteries and the descending palatine. There are anastomoses with the internal carotid (via ethmoids and ophthalmic), other external carotid branches (via facial), other branches of the maxillary artery (via buccinator) and crossed anastomoses with vessels of contralateral side (via sphenopalatine). Hence there is the obvious difficulty of controlling persistent epistaxis and often the necessity of performing bilateral multiple ligations of not only the maxillary artery branches but also the bilateral ethmoid arteries. In one patient (familial telangiectasia) who previously had bilateral external carotid artery ligations as well as ethmoid and sphenopalatine artery ligations, an angiogram performed via the superficial temporal artery revealed anastomoses of a branch of the maxillary artery with the vertebral artery via the occipital artery. It is in such situations that an angiogram is of help. A common carotid arteriogram would also demonstrate any significant variant of the internal carotid, which is extremely rare, as shown by Quain (1844) in which the branch to the foramen rotundum and the accessory meningeal arteries substituted for the internal carotid artery.

(Text continued on opposite page.)

Plate 54   *The Nose and the Nasopharynx*

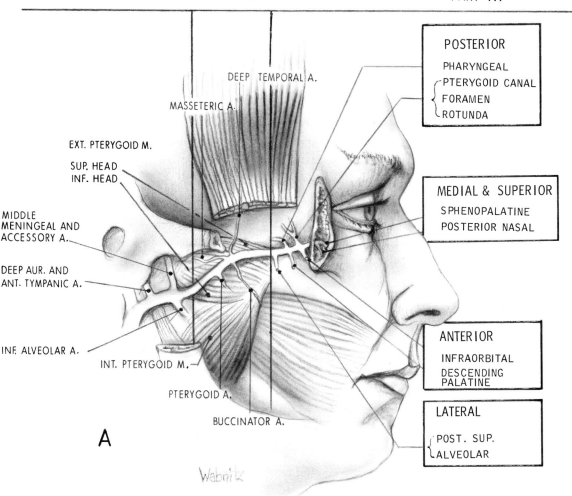

PART I   PART II   PART III

POSTERIOR

PHARYNGEAL
PTERYGOID CANAL
FORAMEN
ROTUNDA

DEEP TEMPORAL A.

MASSETERIC A.

EXT. PTERYGOID M.

SUP. HEAD
INF. HEAD

MIDDLE
MENINGEAL AND
ACCESSORY A.

DEEP AUR. AND
ANT. TYMPANIC A.

INF. ALVEOLAR A.

INT. PTERYGOID M.

PTERYGOID A.

BUCCINATOR A.

MEDIAL & SUPERIOR

SPHENOPALATINE
POSTERIOR NASAL

ANTERIOR

INFRAORBITAL
DESCENDING
PALATINE

LATERAL

POST. SUP.
ALVEOLAR

A

Highpoints

1. Check anatomy and size of antrum with x-ray. A markedly small antrum may make the procedure extremely difficult, if not impossible. The average size of an antrum is 23 mm wide × 33 mm high × 34 mm deep (Schaeffer, 1920).
2. Be cognizant of proximity of internal carotid artery.
3. Related nerves lie in a deeper plane and should easily be avoided.
4. Care not to dissect too high and enter the orbit—this may occur with the smaller antrum.
5. At least occlude the terminal medial branch forming the sphenopalatine and posterior nasal arteries and the anterior branch forming the descending palatine. Ideally at least three sites should be occluded as depicted in step *C.*
6. A portion of the orbital process of the palatine bone should be removed for access to the terminal branch of the maxillary artery forming the sphenopalatine and posterior nasal arteries.
7. Use locking clips or multiple clips and transect vessels when possible.

The approach to the antrum is a Caldwell-Luc operation (plates 28 and 29) with a large opening.

Cocaine, 10 per cent, or neosynephrine (check with the anesthesiologist regarding side effects with any general anesthetic agent, e.g., Halothane) is applied to antral mucosa to decrease bleeding.

B   An inferiorly or laterally based mucoperiosteal flap is then elevated and reflected from the posterior wall of the antrum. Using the operation microscope (300 mm lens), the thin inferior posterior wall of the antrum is removed with a burr or curet. This opening is then enlarged superiorly with fine back-biting Kerrison forceps and hooks. The bone removal is continued upward to resect a portion of the orbital process of the palatine bone (Pearson, 1969). This may require additional use of a bur, and this exposes the region of the sphenopalatine foramen.

C   The posterior layer of periosteum is then opened using a fine instrument or electro-scalpel. This exposes adipose tissue which is teased forward exposing some of the branches of the third part of the maxillary artery. A small Mixter forceps is of aid in this dissection as well as a nerve hook. Small forward grasping forceps are advantageous for removing adipose tissue. Depicted is a rather typical configuration (after Pearson, 1969). Minimally three sites are occluded with clips and, if possible, the intervening vessels are transected. It is important to occlude the maxillary artery proximally (*1*) as well as distally (*2*) where the vessel continues on to divide into the sphenopalatine and posterior nasal branches and the descending palatine artery (*3*) to prevent retrograde flow. If additional small vessels are apparent, these, too, should be occluded because of the crossed anastomoses. In other variants of the maxillary artery, multiple clips are utilized again. It may not be possible to identify each branch by name. It is adequate to occlude them all.

    If bleeding occurs during the procedure, the antrum is packed and then re-explored. All related nerve structures are usually deep to the vessels and easily avoided.

D   If the antrum is small, a somewhat different dissection of the antrum is performed:
1. Remove lateral inferior wall of antrum, and if necessary, communicating this exposure with the Caldwell-Luc opening, the upper and lower heads of the external pterygoid muscle will be exposed. The maxillary artery may lie over the lower head or pass between the two heads. All branches of the vessel are then occluded with clips.
2. Ligation of the maxillary artery will then be lateral and posterior to the antrum.
3. Be careful not to enter the orbit.

   After hemostasis is assured, the posterior mucoperiosteal flap is replaced. A piece of Gelfoam can be placed against the flap. An antral window is usually not required unless antral packing is necessary. The Caldwell-Luc incision is closed with continuous 4-0 nylon without drainage.

Plate 55   The Nose and the Nasopharynx

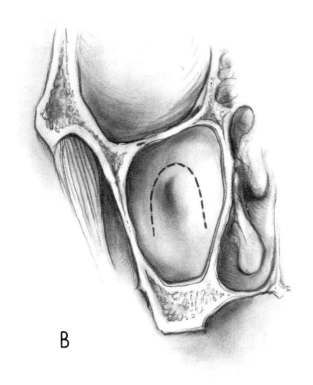

B

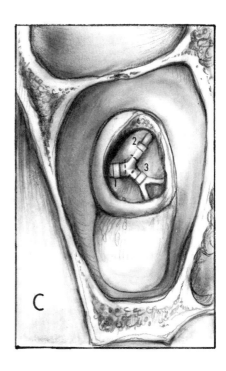

C

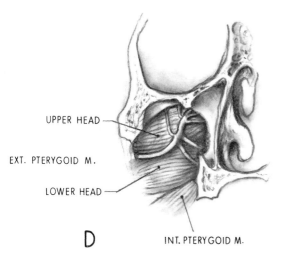

UPPER HEAD

EXT. PTERYGOID M.

LOWER HEAD

INT. PTERYGOID M.

D

NASOPHARYNGOSCOPY

Indications

1. Every head and neck examination.
2. Specifically:
   a. Nasal obstruction.
   b. Following epistaxis.
   c. Enlarged spinal accessory lymph nodes (posterior cervical triangle), e.g., undifferentiated squamous cell carcinoma or lymphoma of the nasopharynx (previously known as Schminke tumor or lymphoepithelioma).
   d. Paralysis of any cranial nerves.

Highpoints

1. Simplest technique is mirror.
2. Topical anesthesia often necessary.
3. Frequent use and practice of mirror technique.

A
B The tongue is depressed and the patient asked to breathe through his nose. This usually throws the soft palate forward. A suitable-sized warmed mirror is then inserted, using a head mirror or headlight for illumination. The angle of the mirror may require adjustment depending on the configuration of the vault of the nasopharynx. Occasionally grasping the tongue as is done in mirror laryngoscopy (see plate 289) is of aid.

C The area so visualized is depicted. To obtain complete visualization, the mirror is simply rotated a few degrees. The posterior wall of the vault is first examined for any tumefaction, benign or malignant. The ostia of the sphenoid sinus may be seen. The roof of the vault is likewise scrutinized and then the posterior end of the nasal septum. The posterior tips of all six turbinates should be visualized lying in the posterior nares. Laterally, the eustachian tube orifices in Waldeyer's ring are evaluated. The posterior-superior aspect of the soft palate is checked.

D Another technique of nasopharyngoscopy is the use of a nasopharyngoscope. Following topical anesthesia to the nasal cavity, the instrument is inserted through the anterior nares. Rotation of the scope at various depths is necessary to cover the nasopharynx. Since only smaller visual fields are available at each degree point, a composite picture is more difficult. This technique is best reserved for occasions when the mirror method fails or when a specific area noted on mirror examination requires more scrutiny.

An oral nasopharyngoscope is preferred by others. The advantage over the nasal introduced type is that it has a larger field of vision. A number of models are available: Beck, Proud-Beck and Wolf.

Digital examination is also performed to evaluate the consistency of any abnormality visualized. The index finger is inserted through the mouth and behind the soft palate. The operator may find that standing to the side of the patient facilitates this.

Retraction of Soft Palate

When the soft palate obstructs visualization of the vault either during examination or biopsy or in minor operations, it may be retracted in several ways.

E A specific soft palate retractor is available which has its fixed point on the upper lip and alveolar ridge. The drawbacks of the instrument are its size and the fact that it tends to slip.

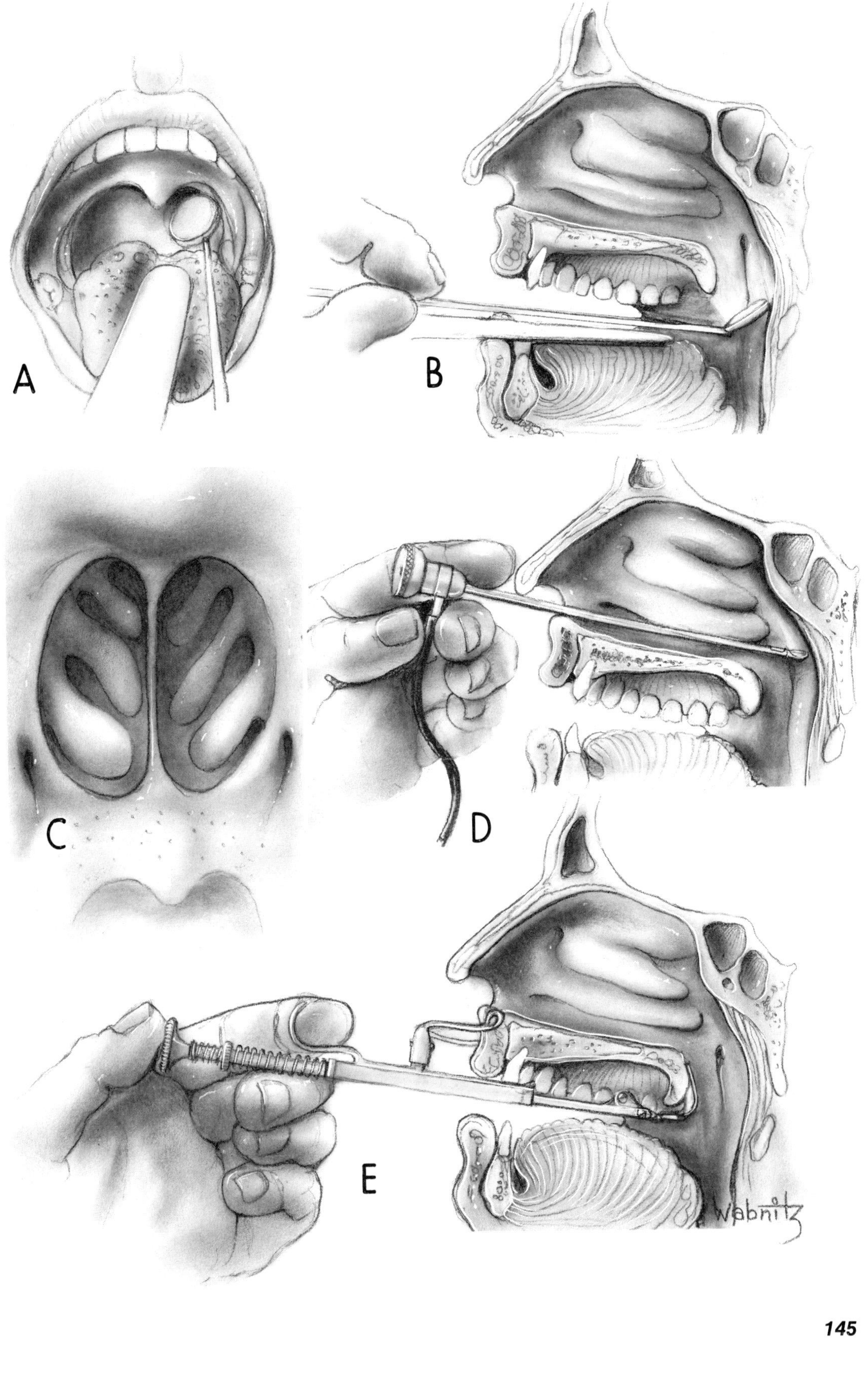

Plate 56   The Nose and the Nasopharynx

A

B

C

D

E

wabnitz

RETRACTION OF SOFT PALATE (*Continued*)

F A small curved retractor of the Cushing venous type may be used. Usually the tongue must also be depressed, in which case an assistant is necessary.

G A small catheter may be inserted through one naris and out through the mouth. Traction with a clamp retracts the soft palate.

Biopsy of Nasopharynx

H Using the mirror method for visualization, a very slender cup forceps is inserted through one naris. The tip of the forceps and the tumor are visualized in the mirror and the biposy is performed.

I A transoral biopsy requires a specially curved forceps (a Lawton instrument). Visualization is in either a mirror or a nasopharyngoscope or through the nasal cavity. Visualization through the nasal cavity is seldom possible and requires complete shrinkage of the nasal mucosa. Only lesions in the visual range of the posterior nares can be seen.

   "Blind" biopsies are also resorted to in the search for an unknown primary tumor in the head and neck.

   A word of caution—Do *not* perform a biopsy if any mass is suspected to be an angiofibroma. If biopsy is necessary this should be performed in the operating room with blood replacement available.

Plate 57   The Nose and the Nasopharynx

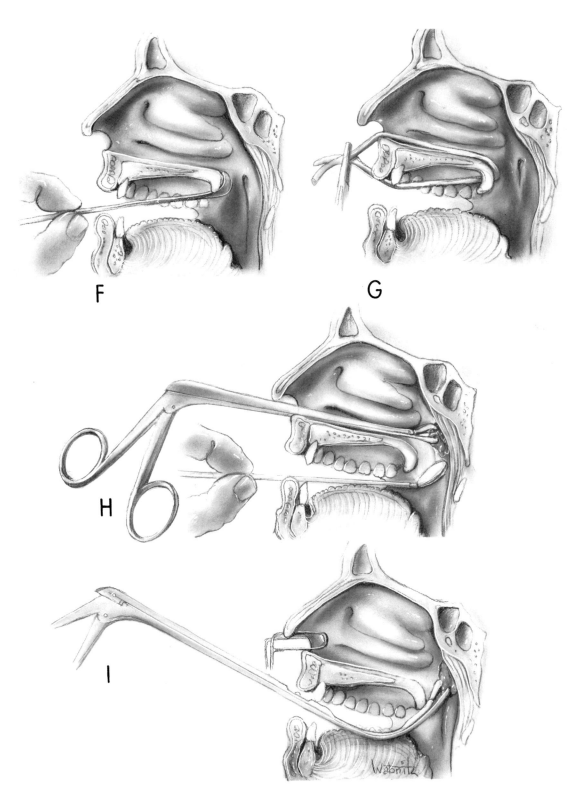

F

G

H

I

REMOVAL OF NASAL AND NASOPHARYNGEAL POLYPS

Highpoints

1. Anesthesia: Topical tetracaine, 2 per cent, or cocaine, 10 per cent, with or without a vasoconstrictor.
2. Usually more polyps will become visualized after removal of initial polyps.
3. Suspect polypoid disease in sinuses and some type of allergic background.
4. Most polyps tend to recur.
5. Do not confuse a polypoid turbinate with a true polyp.
6. In infants a nasal glioma may simulate an innocent polyp (see plates 95 and 96).
7. Do not confuse an angiofibroma with a nasopharyngeal polyp.

A A nasal polyp snare is slipped around the polyp under direct vision through a nasal speculum.

B The snare is tightened only after it is worked up to the base of the pedicle. If possible, the snare is not completely closed, thus not completely transecting the pedicle. At this point, the snare has a firm grip on the pedicle; snare and polyp are removed together. If the pedicle is completely transected, a bayonet forceps or duckbill forceps is used to remove the free polyp. If it is inaccessible, the patient is asked to blow his nose gently and this will expel the polyp.

C Some large posterior polyps presenting in the nasopharynx cannot be encircled with a snare alone.

D A grasping forceps through the mouth is used to introduce the dependent portion of the polyp into the loop of the snare. Gentle traction on both instruments works the snare upward to the pedicle.

E When the snare meets resistance, it is at the base of the pedicle; it is then completely closed. This severs the pedicle completely and the polyp is removed orally using the grasping forceps.

Smaller polyps and remnants are removed with punch forceps. Extension of polypoid disease into the sinuses may require sinus surgery. Refer to uncapping of ethmoids, ethmoidectomy, antral window and Caldwell-Luc operations.

All polyps and, for that matter, all tissue should be submitted for histological examination at all times.

Complications

1. Hemorrhage.
2. Aspiration of blood or, conceivably, polyps, causing respiratory embarrassment.

Plate 58   The Nose and the Nasopharynx

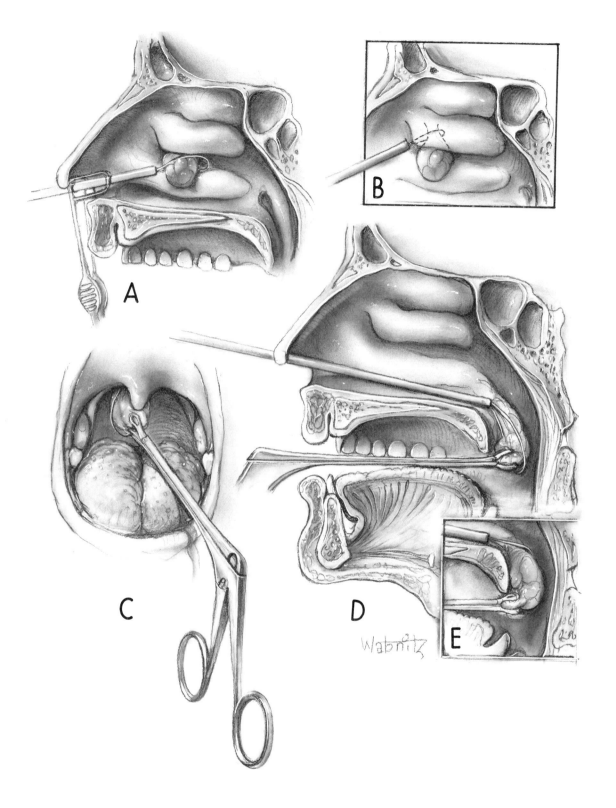

A

B

C

D

E

Wabnitz

TRANSPALATINE EXPOSURE OF THE NASOPHARYNX

Indications

1. Removal of large benign and locally invasive lesions (juvenile angiofibroma).
2. Exposure for surgical correction of posterior choanal atresia.
3. Diagnostic exploration when other methods have failed.
4. If lesion extends beyond confine of nasopharynx, another approach or combination of approaches is necessary.

Alternate Techniques

1. Most benign pedunculated lesions in the nasopharynx can be removed with nasal snare (see plate 58).
2. Posterior choanal atresia also can be surgically treated via the nasal cavity with or without the operation microscope.

Highpoints

1. Mucoperiosteal hard palate flap.
2. Remove and discard major portion of hard palate.
3. Preserve greater palatine arteries bilaterally. Elevate vessels and nerves with mucoperiosteal hard palate flap.
4. Safeguard as much mucous membrane as possible, e.g., along floor of nose, septum, vomer and palatal crest. If lesion is malignant, mucous membrane is removed with lesion.
5. Additional exposure can be achieved by mobilization of the greater palatine vessels by removing surrounding bone.

Additional Criteria and Characteristics of Juvenile Angiofibroma

1. Carotid arteriogram is helpful in delineating feeder vessels which are usually the internal maxillary and ascending pharyngeal arteries.
2. Tumor can extend into orbit, any paranasal sinus, pterygomaxillary space, nasal cavity and temporal fossa and involve foramen of skull and extend intracranially.
3. Bleeding is usually profuse—have up to 12 units of blood available.
4. Preoperative estrogens (2 to 2.5 mg stilbestrol three times a day for two to four weeks) may reduce the degree of hemorrhage during the operation. The use of hormones alone as definitive treatment has not been proved to be of value.
5. A planogram is of help in the evaluation of the extent of tumor.
6. Temporary occlusion of the external carotid artery. The vessel should not be permanently ligated since subsequent arteriograms for recurrence will then be quite difficult. Yet such an arteriogram can be performed with permanent ligation via a catheter in the superficial temporal artery.
7. Transpalatine approach is usually preferred. The pterygomaxillary space can be reached via this approach. The combination of a transmaxillary and lateral rhinotomy approaches may be necessary depending on the extent of the tumor (Pressman, 1962).
8. Cryosurgery has been utilized in conjunction with the surgical procedure to reduce the size of the tumor and to reduce the hemorrhage but late hemorrhage has occurred.
9. Radiation therapy is achieved contraindicated because of the subsequent danger of malignant change. Hypotensive anesthesia, although used by some surgeons, carries too great a risk.

TRANSPALATINE EXPOSURE OF THE NASOPHARYNX (*Continued*)

A Anatomy of the palate and outline of the palatal flap. The incision is made parallel to the gingival margin, leaving enough mucous membrane on the gingival side for placement of closure sutures. The important greater palatine arteries are depicted.

B The palatal flap, including the periosteum, is mobilized with the aid of an elevator. The vessels and nerves are within the flap. The crucial point is at the site of emergence from the greater palatine foramen which is juxtaposed to the third molar region. To facilitate further retraction of the palatal flap, the posteromedial wall of the greater palatine foramen and canal can be removed to give more length to the greater palatine artery. In addition, the tensor veli palatine muscle can be sectioned or the hamulus of the pterygoid bone fractured. The incision, extended behind the third molar and along the anterior tonsillar pillar, is necessary.

C The palatal flap is retracted and the hard palate removed with rongeur forceps. The hard palate found directly under the incision should be left intact so that the closure has underlying intact bone. The mucous membrane along the floor of the nasal cavity is left intact, if possible. In angiofibroma, the hard palate and mucous membrane may be eroded. Occasionally, the greater palatine artery can be sacrificed on one side if the integrity of all the vessels on the contralateral side is preserved. These include the lesser palatine artery and branches of the ascending palatine artery (A). In these instances, on the contralateral side, extension of the incision is not made nor the flap developed.

D A transverse incision through the mucous membrane of the floor of the nose is made as far anterior as the lesion extends. Laterally, this incision may be lengthened to reach the anterior angle of the eustachian tube. If the lesion is an angiofibroma, care should be taken to avoid trauma to the tumor and its feeding vessels.

If the angiofibroma extends into the pterygomaxillary space with a presenting mass in the cheek, exposure can be gained through an incision in the buccal sulcus (after Sardana, 1965). Profuse hemorrhage will likely occur from the internal maxillary artery which will require occlusion either with ties or clips.

Plate 59   The Nose and the Nasopharynx

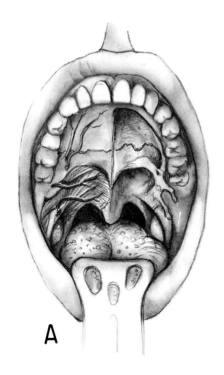

A

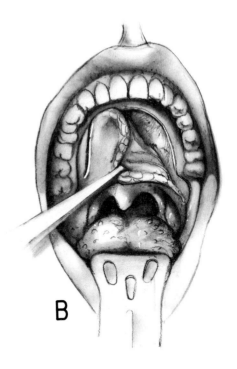

B

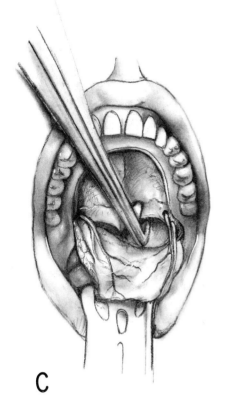

C

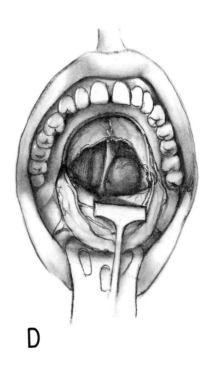

D

TRANSPALATINE EXPOSURE OF THE NASOPHARYNX
(*Continued*)

E   Depicted is a tumor arising from the left posterior nasal cavity and the left side of the nasopharynx. The septum is displaced to the right and the turbinate to the left.

F   The lesion is resected by sharp and blunt dissection. Depending on the histology, there may be profuse bleeding. If this is the case, pressure with gauze, suction or cauterization may be necessary. Complete hemostasis is achieved after total removal of the tumor. If necessary, the septum or the posterior portion of the inferior turbinate can be excised.

G   The completed resection.

Plate 60   *The Nose and the Nasopharynx*

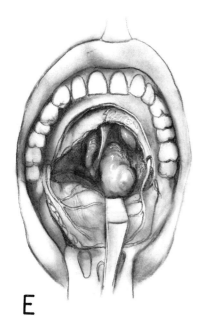

E

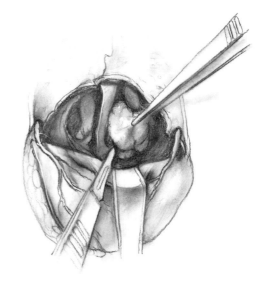

F

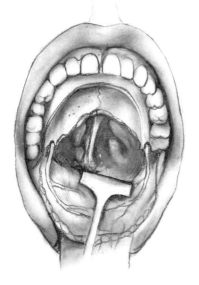

G

TRANSPALATINE EXPOSURE OF THE
NASOPHARYNX (*Continued*)

H   Anterior and posterior packing has been inserted depending on the hemostasis necessary. Closure consists of the best possible approximation of the mucous membrane

I   of the floor of the nose. The palatal flap is sutured with 4-0 nylon to the gingival mucous membrane. Care in closure is important to avoid oronasal fistula formation.

J   If pressure is required to maintain the palatal flap in position, this is achieved by securing gauze or cotton soaked in liquid Furacin with cross sutures of 3-0 nylon passed around the teeth. When this is bulky and there is any question of postoperative bleeding, an elective tracheostomy is indicated.

Complications

1. Naso-oral fistula.
2. Related specifically to angiofibroma:
   a. Profuse hemorrhage during and following surgery.
   b. Incomplete removal.
   c. Neurological sequelae from vertebral arteriogram — possibly due to blood flow stasis from catheter in vertebral artery or bolus of the radiopaque material.
3. Rhinism.
4. Oro-nasal fistula at anterior portion of palatal flap, especially if this flap is too long.

Plate 61   The Nose and the Nasopharynx

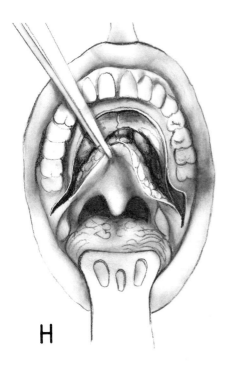

H

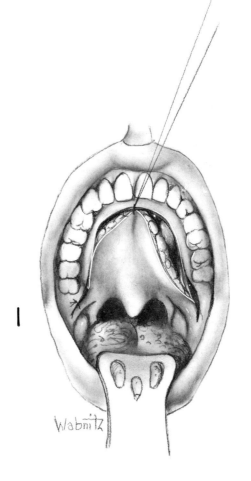

I

Wabnitz

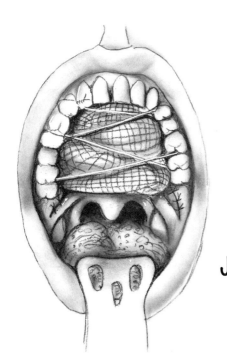

J

POSTERIOR CHOANAL ATRESIA
(After Beinfield, 1961 and 1965)

NEWBORN AND YOUNG CHILDREN

Highpoints

1. Bilateral choanal atresia is usually an airway emergency (the newborn usually breathes through the nose). Use an oropharyngeal airway until the infant is brought to the operating room.
2. Extreme care is needed not to injure the spinal cord between the axis and the atlas.
3. Extreme care is needed not to injure the base of the skull.
4. Mark instrument—curette and sound—from tip along shank to a distance of 4.4 cm. This will indicate distance of posterior pharyngeal wall to edge of anterior nares along the *floor* of the nose. A safe distance more superiorly is reduced to 3.2 cm.
5. The atresia can be unilateral or bilateral; it can be bony or simply membranous.
6. General oral endotracheal anesthesia is preferred, supplemented with topical cocaine, 10 per cent, and a vasoconstrictor.
7. Postoperative care is important to keep indwelling tubes patent.
8. Other congenital anomalies may be present.

Described is the technique for bony atresia. Membranous atresia is treated in basically the same fashion, eliminating the steps for removal of the bony portion. Yet with membranous atresia, a certain degree of bony stenosis can be present and this requires the steps referable to bony atresia.

Diagnosis is made by the inability to pass a nasopharyngeal catheter. Dye instilled in the nasal cavity as well as oily Dionosil with roentgenograms can be used to confirm the diagnosis. This is especially useful in older children and adults in whom the differential diagnosis may involve benign and malignant neoplasms.

A   Using either a #8 urethral sound or a #2 Lempert type mastoid curette, an initial opening is made through the nasal mucous membrane overlying the bony wall itself. The shank of the instrument is marked 3.2 cm and 4.4 cm from the tip to avoid injury to the posterior pharyngeal wall, spinal cord or base of the skull. Keep the instrument along the floor of the nose. Depicted is the use of the urethral sound. This is performed with the sense of touch. Direct vision is virtually impossible during this maneuver.

A¹   Technique of utilization of the mastoid curette. It must only be made in a downward direction.

B   If the posterior mucous membrane flap cannot be safely perforated as depicted with the urethral sound, a cruciate incision with #11 or suitable ear knife is made (*B¹*).

B¹   Using an ear speculum and the operation microscope, visualization can be obtained and the incision made with a suitable microsurgery ear knife.

After the opening is established, its diameter is increased by gradually using large diameter urethral sounds up to size #16F, #18F or #20F.

Plate 62   The Nose and the Nasopharynx

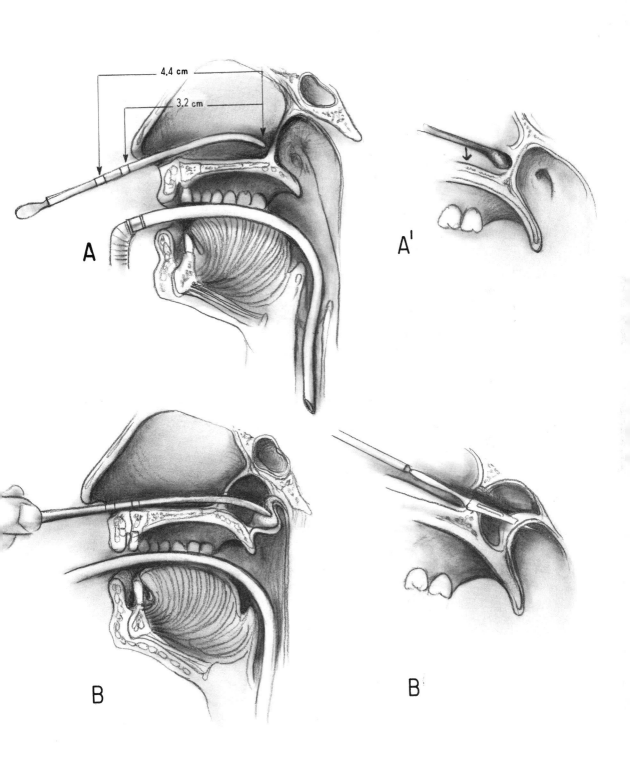

POSTERIOR CHOANAL ATRESIA (*Continued*)

C   A rubber catheter is then passed through the nose and retrieved through the mouth. A section of silicone rubber tube #16F, measuring 4.0 to 4.5 cm in length, is then sutured to the distal end of the catheter. The *inferior* aspect of the distal end (posterior end) of the silicone rubber tube is transected obliquely to increase the size of the lumen and also to prevent the end of the tube from being obstructed by the posterior nasopharyngeal wall. Then the tube is pulled into place by withdrawing the catheter. Ideally, this maneuver pulls the posterior mucous membrane edges into the newly formed posterior nares.

D   If bilateral, the same procedure is performed on the opposite side. Both tubes are sutured together with 4-0 nylon across the anterior portion of the columella with suitable padding of the columella to prevent pressure necrosis. Neosporin or aureomycin ointment is used liberally at this juncture and continued postoperatively. The presenting end (anterior) of the tube is lodged just within the alar rim to minimize necrosis of the rim. This end of the tube must be carefully observed so that it is not obstructed by the alar rim.

Postoperatively, ultrasonic mist and meticulous nursing care with suctioning of the tubes are mandatory. Gavage feeding may be necessary for days or weeks. The tubes are left in place from three to eight weeks, depending on the healing progress.

OLDER CHILDREN AND ADULTS

The technique utilized at the older ages usually is that of a transpalatine approach (see plates 59, 60 and 61). In addition to the diagnostic measures described under infants, nasopharyngoscopy is routine.

Following exposure of the posterior choanal region via the transpalatine approach, the bony wall forming the atresia is excised. The posterior end of the nasal septum may require resection.

Depicted in this plate is the midline incision; in plate 59 is the palatal flap incision.

Highpoints

1. Avoid injury to the pterygopalatine and posterior palatine canals.
2. Preserve as much nasal and juxtaposed mucous membrane as possible, using this retained tissue to line the raw edges of the resulting bone.

E   After the posterior portion of the hard palate has been exposed and the soft palate mucosa incised and a cleavage plane developed between the mucosa and palatal muscles (see plate 59), the bony portion of the hard palate is removed, as depicted by the dotted lines. The underlying mucoperiosteum should be preserved to form flaps.

F   The bony atresia has been excised and the mucoperiosteal flaps formed. A silastic tube is shown on one side with the flap on its inferior aspect. These flaps are so placed to aid in lining the new choana which helps in the prevention of subsequent stenosis.

G   The palatine incision is then closed. The tubes can be secured anteriorly as in the infant or with through-and-through sutures of nylon at the columella end of the septum (step G). The postoperative care of the tubes should be meticulous. They are left in place for about one month's time.

Plate 63   *The Nose and the Nasopharynx*

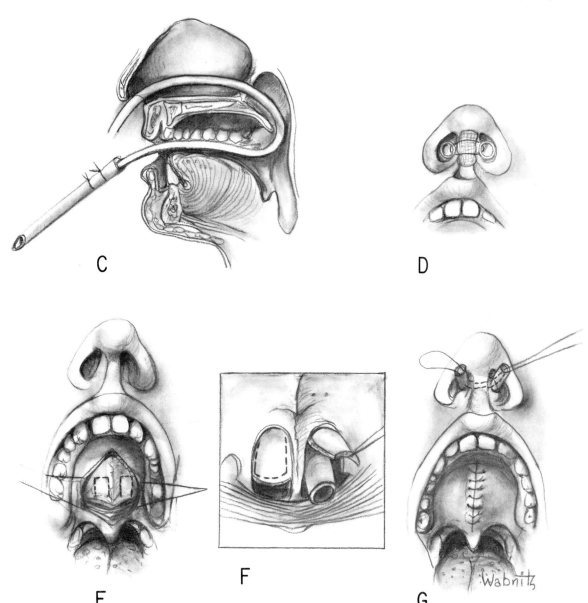

C

D

E

F

G

Wabnitz

Complications

1. Cerebral spinal fluid leak.
2. Meningitis.
3. Hydrocephalus.
4. Pressure necrosis of anterior nares rim or columella.
5. Postoperative plug of indwelling tubes.
6. Extrusion of tubes.
7. Late stenosis.
8. Regurgitation of feedings into nasopharynx—usually transient.
9. Aspiration of feedings. If this persists, an associated neuromuscular deficiency may exist—cricopharyngus myotomy has been tried in one patient without success.

SUBMUCOUS RESECTION OF NASAL SEPTUM

Highpoints

1. Subperichondrial plane of separation.
2. Leave adequate support dorsally and distally.
3. Avoid fracture of cribriform plate of ethmoid.
4. Secondary procedures on septum are difficult; hence, perform a complete operation at the first sitting.

Comment

Some surgeons are of the belief that this standard submucous resection of the nasal septum should be replaced by the septoplasty (plates 66 through 70). At this point in time, it appears that each procedure has its merits and indications and that more often than not an operation combining both techniques is ideal.

A
A¹ An incision is made 12 to 16 mm from the distal end of the septum using the index finger in the opposite naris as support. The incision extends through mucosa and perichondrium but not through cartilage.

B
B¹ With a small curet or curved elevator with the concavity facing medially, the white glistening cartilage is exposed. This marks the correct subperichondrial plane of separation of the mucoperichondrium. Again the index finger in the opposite naris lends support to initiate this step.

C
C¹ Elevation of the mucoperichondrium and mucoperiosteum is then completed by carefully hugging the cartilage and bone. At times this blunt separation fails at an old fracture site or ridge. Sharp dissection may be necessary. Care must be taken not to puncture or tear the mucoperichondrium and mucoperiosteum. If a tear does occur, satisfactory healing usually takes place if the mucosa on the opposite side is intact.

D
D¹ The cartilage is then incised through the original incision. Extreme caution is necessary to avoid a counter incision in the opposite perichondrium. The index finger is an excellent guard, for as soon as the knife blade reaches the perichondrium it may be felt. If the mucoperichondrium is cut, the defect should be sutured, along with the main incision on the opposite side; otherwise, a perforation may persist.

E
E¹ Using the small curet or curved elevator with the concavity facing the midline, the perichondrium and periosteum are elevated in the same way as on the left side. Elevation of the mucoperichondrium and mucoperiosteum should extend beyond the deviated area to be resected.

Plate 64   *The Nose and the Nasopharynx*

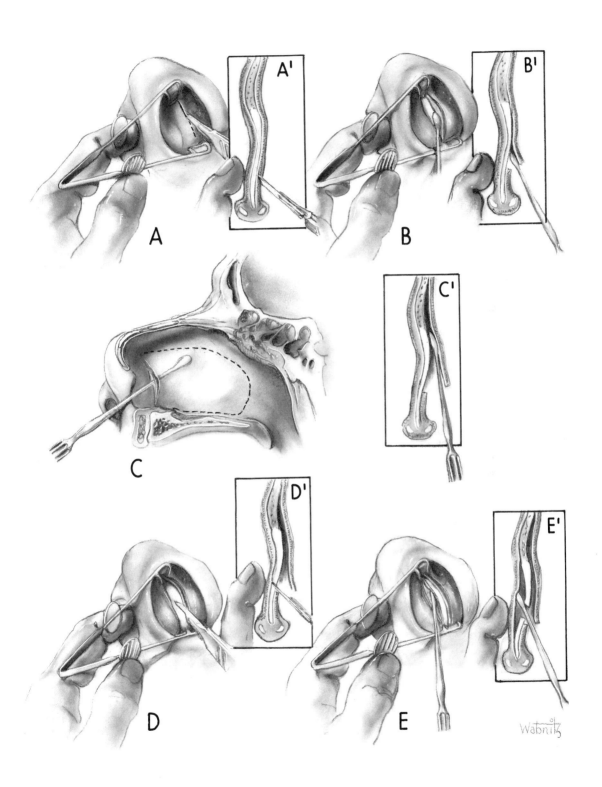

SUBMUCOUS RESECTION OF NASAL SEPTUM (*Continued*)

F   In preparation for the Ballenger swivel knife, a small cut is made with scissors at the superior edge of the incised cartilage.

G
G¹   The swivel knife is placed at this cut straddling the cartilage. Before the knife is pushed backward and upward, make certain that no portion of mucoperichondrium or mucoperiosteum is caught on the edge of the knife. The knife is then advanced to the bony septum and follows this junction downward to the vomer bone and then anteriorly. The freed cartilage is removed with forceps.

H   Cartilage cutting forceps (McCoy) remove any remaining cartilage as well as portions of the perpendicular plate of the ethmoid and vomer. A portion of septum 12 to 16 mm wide must be left dorsally to support the bridge of the nose. When removing the deviated portion of the perpendicular plate of the ethmoid, the cribriform plate of the ethmoid must not be injured. Proper use of the bone forceps is necessary. Fragments are not avulsed; small complete bits are taken carefully. When rotation of the forceps is utilized, it is done gently around a single axis. It is often best to remove such mobilized fragments with bayonet forceps since the mucoperiosteum may be adherent in several areas and require sharp separation. A Jansen-Middleton spoon-shaped biting double-action forceps is also excellent for this stage.

I   Inferiorly, portions of a broadened vomer or ridge are difficult to remove with forceps. Decussation of the periosteum and perichondrium at this point is best separated by sharp dissection (see plate 66, step A'). An open, sharp, ring curet placed posteriorly and drawn forward often removes this bone and cartilage. Again, it must be certain that no mucoperiosteum is adherent.

J   Occasionally an osteotome is necessary to remove a thick bony ridge along the base of the septum. The septal flaps are coapted and the incision approximated with 4-0 nylon. Two techniques are available:

K   A specially designed septal hollow needle with suture material already threaded is inserted as depicted. The free posterior end is grasped with forceps and the needle withdrawn.

L   The knot is tied anteriorly.

M   If such a needle is not available, the incision and anterior portion of the septum are approximated with one or two through and through sutures. In each case, a portion of the anterior cartilage strut is included in the suture. These sutures are removed in three to seven days.

   One half inch gauze impregnated with Furacin or antibiotic ointment is inserted in both nares to add support to approximate the flaps. This packing is removed the following day. If the flaps appear to separate—this will not occur if the septal needle has been used—the packing may be reinserted. Johnson reports the use of small suction catheters inserted under the septal flaps. These are connected to suction, thus removing serum and approximating the flaps.

Complications

   1. Saddleback deformity. This may occur many years later.
   2. Septal hematoma.
   3. Collapse of nasal tip and columella.
   4. Nasal obstruction—incomplete resection.

Plate 65   The Nose and the Nasopharynx

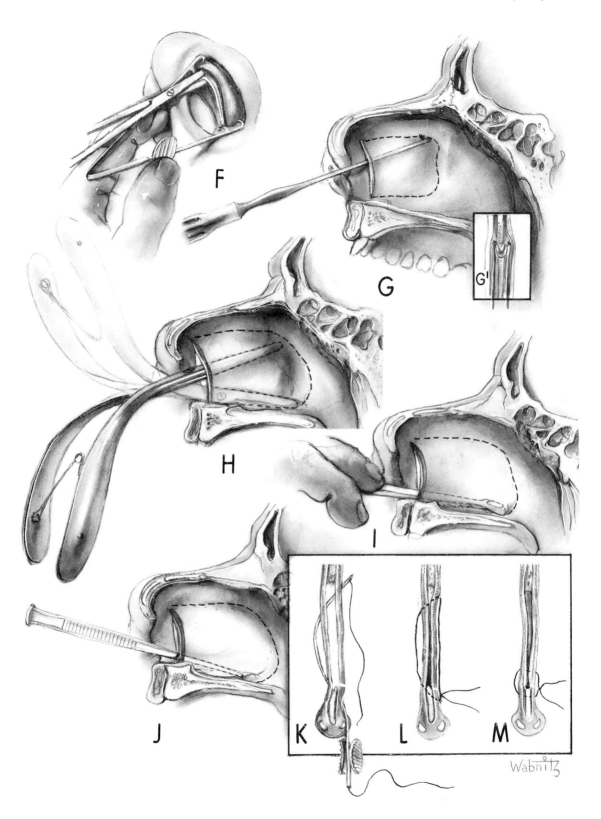

F

G

G¹

H

I

J

K

L

M

Wabnitz

SEPTOPLASTY TYPE I (After Johnson, 1964; Gorney, 1962)
(See plates 68, 69, and 70 for an alternate procedure.)

Highpoints

1. Prime indications are external nasal deformity due to deviated septum and dislocated columella. Some surgeons have substituted septoplasty for the classical submucous resection.
2. Complete mobilization of all deformed cartilage—do not depend on stents and sutures to correct deformity.
3. Precise realignment of mobilized cartilage.
4. Provide adequate cartilaginous support for tip and bridge of nose.
5. Wherever possible, leave a portion of mucoperichondrium attached to mobilized cartilage to assure complete viability of cartilage. Free cartilage grafts may absorb.
6. A rhinoplasty is necessary if part of the deformity is due to displacement of the bony framework.

A An incision is made along the dotted line at the caudal end of the deviated septum.

A¹ If an inferior obstructing septal ridge is present, it will often consist of both cartilage and bone. The perichondrium and periosteum decussate at the point where cartilage meets bone. This prevents the elevation of the mucoperichondrium and mucoperiosteum by blunt dissection with the elevator (nasal freer). Hence sharp dissection is necessary as depicted along the dotted lines. The deviated bone is removed with the osteotome at the site of the solid horizontal line.

B The deviated septum is shown causing the external nasal deformity. The dotted line depicts a portion of the alar cartilage which may require excision depending on an associated tip deformity. In similar fashion a portion of the upper lateral nasal cartilage may require excision (refer to steps *M* and *N* of plate 65).

C The caudal end of the septum is exposed.

C¹ The incision as it commences on the left side of the septum. This may be made on the right side when the deviation is to the right.

D The dotted lines depict the extent of the elevation of the mucoperichondrium. It will be noted that the mucoperichondrium is not elevated from the right side of the most caudal portion (*1*) of the septum in order to ensure viability of this most important section of the nasal septum. The next section of cartilage (*2*) may be swung into alignment with complete mobilization or be excised or be used as a free graft. If it is swung into alignment, a vertical strip of cartilage between section 1 and section 2 must be excised to prevent overriding of the two sections of cartilage. If section 3 is deviated, this portion is removed as in a standard submucous resection of the nasal septum.

E Lateral view depicting the comparable sections of cartilage corresponding to step *D*. The inferior and superior incisions mobilizing the septal cartilage depend on the type and extent of deviation. The solid line on the superior portion of cartilage (section 1) refers to the incisions between the lateral nasal cartilages and the septum. Details of this are in steps *G* and *H*. These incisions extend posteriorly only as far as is necessary to free the caudal section 1 so that it will realign in the midline. These incisions may be made with scissors as depicted or with a #11 blade knife. If made with scissors, the mucosa is elevated and preserved. If there is any question of stability, a suture is placed as in step *H* with repositioning of the relationship of the septal cartilage to the lateral nasal cartilage as depicted. It is at this stage that a portion of the alar cartilage may require excision as outlined in step *B*. All sections of cartilage must be freely mobile for realignment. Adequate support along the most caudal end (section 1) and the bridge of the nose must be assured. If a simultaneous or second stage rhinoplasty is performed, these dictums are most important.

F At the close of the operation, realignment of the nasal septum must be independent of any packing or splints or sutures. These supports are used mainly for immobilization and prevention of hematomas much as a plaster cast is used in the treatment of

(Text continued on opposite page.)

Plate 66 *The Nose and the Nasopharynx*

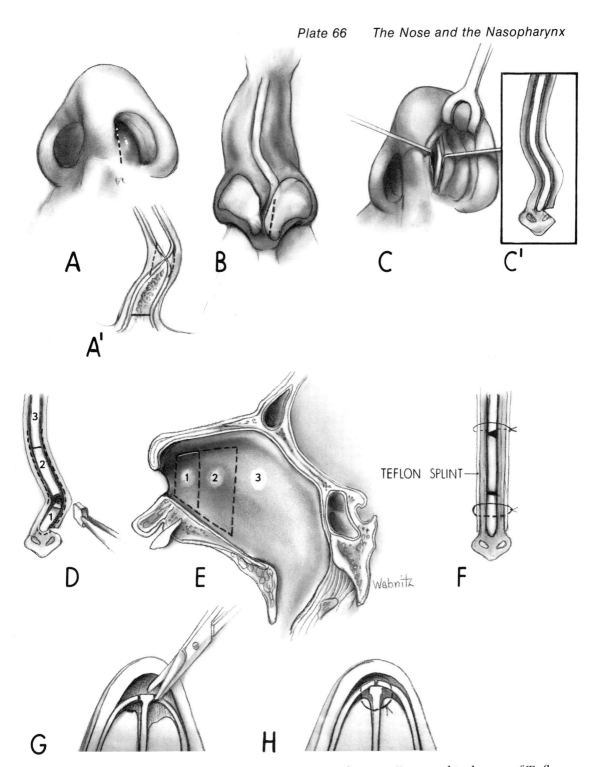

TEFLON SPLINT

Wabnitz

a Colles' fracture, i.e., immobilization but not reduction. Depicted is the use of Teflon splints to achieve this immobilization. They are secured in position with through and through 4-0 nylon sutures. Details of the use of these splints are in plate 67, steps *I, J, K and L.*

G Incision between lateral nasal cartilage and septum.

H Suture supporting repositioned cartilages.

167

SEPTOPLASTY TYPE I (Continued)

Teflon Splint

I   Outline of a typical Teflon splint cut to size of patient's nasal cavity after the technique of Johnson. The Teflon is from 0.022 (less than 1 mm) to 0.034 inch (about 1 mm) in thickness; the holes are made with an ordinary leather or paper punch. Pink dental wax as well as silastic may also be used.

J   To prevent overriding of the sections of cartilage, especially when no splint is used, a 4-0 nylon suture can be placed as depicted following the technique of Wright.

K
L   Details of placement of the Teflon splint. Also shown is another variety of cartilaginous sutures which aid in the prevention of overriding of the sections of cartilage.

A ring curet can be used to set the knot when the suture is placed deep in the nasal cavity (Johnson, 1971). Another one of Johnson's techniques is to insert the tip of the needle into the turbinate after it passes through the septum as a means of localizing the needle. The needle tip is then removed from the turbinate.

Since there is usually no bleeding with the use of splints, intranasal packing is not necessary. The splints may be left in place for up to two weeks. Care must be exercised to avoid any pressure points along the edges of the splint. A suitable surgical ointment is applied to the splints at the time of insertion and postoperatively along the free presenting edges, especially at the inferior (base) aspect of the columella.

Correction of Septal Cartilage and Anterior Nasal Spine Deformity

M   When the inferior portion of the caudal end of the septum is overriding the anterior nasal spine or maxillary crest, fixation of the realigned septal cartilage is usually necessary. This is achieved by drilling a hole using a sturdy Keith needle through the spine or crest. Exposure is either through existing incision or through sublabial incision (plate 79).

N   Fixation of the cartilage to the spine or crest is then secured with a buried 4-0 nylon suture.

O   When the septum is arched in its superior-inferior axis at the caudal end, the mucoperichondrium being elevated, a section of cartilage is removed. The septal nasal spine relationship is corrected. If the normal **V**-shaped approximation is absent and this becomes necessary to maintain the position of the cartilage, the spine is reconstructed in **V** fashion.

P   A 4-0 nylon suture is buried beneath the mucosa for fixation. A Teflon splint is usually necessary to maintain the superior and inferior sections of the nasal septum.

Composite Lateral View of Reconstructed Septum

Q   Occasionally, the deviated caudal end of the septum resists all the previously described techniques. In such circumstances, an incision through the cartilage bridge at point **x** is made to straighten the caudal end of the septum. This incision may be made through only the cartilage or, if the mucoperichondrium is not elevated in this area, the incision may be made through the mucoperichondrium on one side. If the cartilage edges are very loose, a suture of buried 4-0 nylon is used to prevent overriding as shown in the illustration. Shown also is the suture through the inferior edge of the caudal strut and the anterior nasal spine. To lend additional support, a cartilage graft from the removed or mobilized septum is placed as depicted. Teflon splints are utilized to maintain the position during the healing period.

Very rarely another incision at point **y** may be necessary to further realign a deformed nasal septum. Suture is usually not feasible nor necessary here.

With such cartilage incisions, a simultaneous rhinoplasty may not be advisable.

A septal crushing mold can also be utilized to reform severely deviated cartilage before the cartilage is reinserted as a free graft.

Plate 67   The Nose and the Nasopharynx

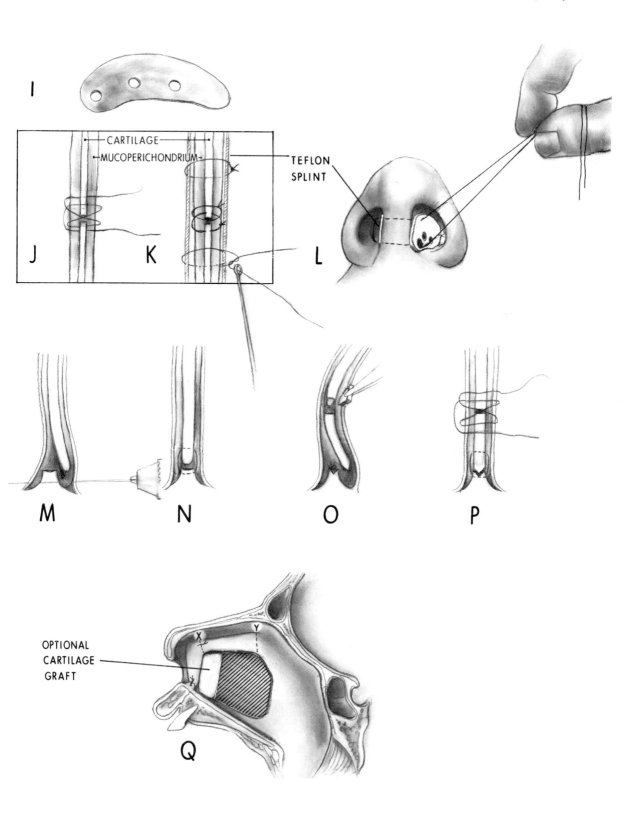

I

CARTILAGE
MUCOPERICHONDRIUM

TEFLON
SPLINT

J   K   L

M   N   O   P

OPTIONAL
CARTILAGE
GRAFT

Q

SEPTOPLASTY TYPE II

Occasionally external nasal deformity is due solely or primarily to a severely deviated septum. Correction depends on realignment of the septum. If there is associated bony deformity in the adult, it is corrected by the usual rhinoplasty (see plates 72 through 76).

Highpoints

1. Complete mobilization of the deviated septum.
2. Preservation of as much cartilage as possible.
3. If possible, leave mucoperichondrium at least partially attached to one side of the mobilized septal cartilage.

A   The external nasal deformity due to a deviated septum.

B   The usual incision for a submucous resection is made followed by elevation of muco-
C   perichondrium on the left side. (see plate 64)

D   A small right angle knife is inserted under the elevated mucoperichondrium to the point of angulation of the septum. The cartilage is then transected along the dotted line leaving a narrow bridge of cartilage intact along the upper border (**X**). Partial incision of the narrow ridge of cartilage may be required at a later stage to permit the anterior portion of the septal cartilage to be swung and maintained in the midline.

E   Through the incision in the cartilage, the mucoperichondrium is elevated posteriorly on the opposite side if there is a posterior deviation which is causing obstruction.

Plate 68   The Nose and the Nasopharynx

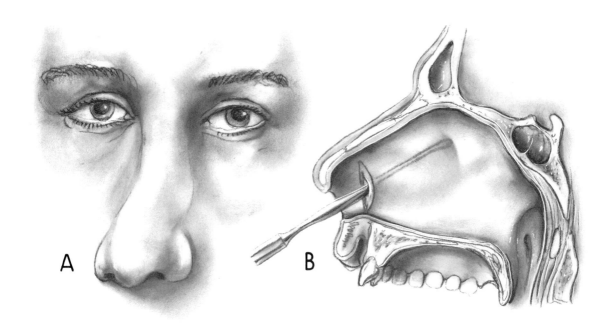

A

B

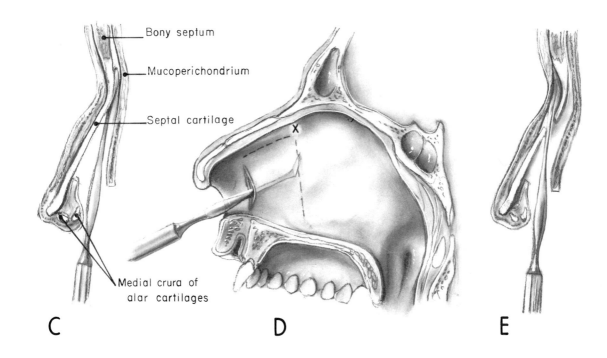

Bony septum

Mucoperichondrium

Septal cartilage

Medial crura of
alar cartilages

C   D   E

SEPTOPLASTY TYPE II (*Continued*)

F   For a posterior deviation, a Ballenger swivel knife is used to remove the cartilaginous
G   obstruction while a McCoy forceps is used to remove the thin bony obstruction. Thicker bone requires the use of Jansen-Middleton spoon-shaped forceps.

H   Using sharp and blunt dissection, the anterior portion of the septum and columella
I   are mobilized at the base down to the anterior nasal spine.

J   This anterior section of cartilage is then transected along its base. If a prominent bony ridge is present, this may require mobilization with a small curved chisel.

    The hinged anterior (lower) septal cartilage is then swung into the midline. If sufficient mobilization at the base has been done, the cartilage will stay in position. More than likely, however, the mucoperichondrium on the right side of the septum at the columella will pull the hinged cartilage out of line.

Plate 69   The Nose and the Nasopharynx

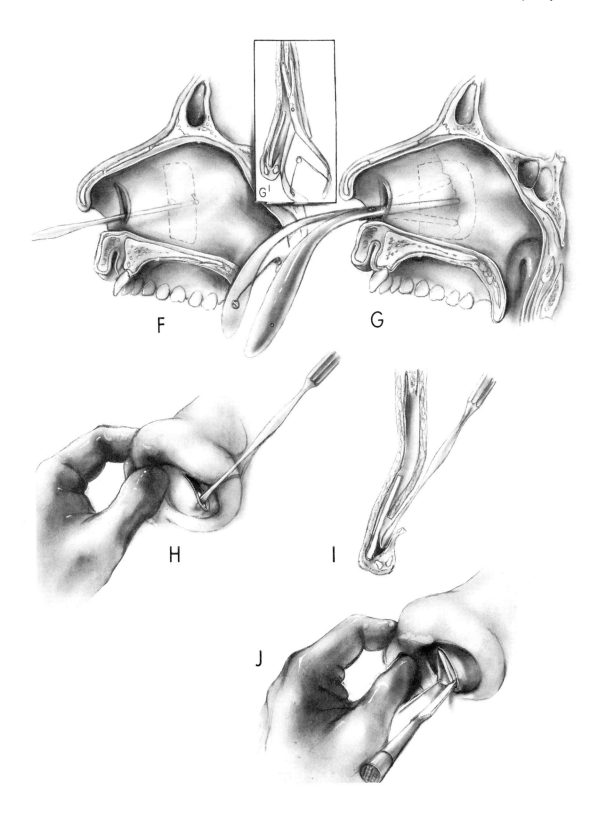

F

G

G¹

H

I

J

SEPTOPLASTY TYPE II (*Continued*)

K   If this is the case, this mucoperichondrium will require partial elevation through a separate incision on the right side. This incision is made slightly more distally than its counter incision on the opposite side.

An alternate step which is preferred if the deviation of the anterior portion of septal cartilage is very severe is the transfixion incision depicted in steps *E* and *F* of the standard rhinoplasty (plate 73). If the transfixion incision is used, elevation of the mucoperichondrium on the right side of the anterior deviated portion of septum is performed through this incision. Hence, the additional incision depicted in step *K* is not necessary. With such severe deviation, additional elevation of the mucous membrane along the floor of the nose on the right side will be advantageous.

L   The anterior septal cartilage is now swung into position. If the deviation is severe, the attachments of the lateral cartilages to the septum will require transection (L^1) with the use of a #11 blade knife (see plate 66, steps *G* and *H*).

M
N   A triangular section along the medial edge of the left lateral nasal cartilage may require removal if it overlaps the newly aligned septum.

O   Transfixion sutures are placed anteriorly. The incisions in the septum if gaping are approximated with nylon. Packing of Furacin-soaked or antibiotic-soaked one half inch gauze is inserted and an external molded aluminum splint with sponge rubber or dental compound mold is used for support.

Plate 70   The Nose and the Nasopharynx

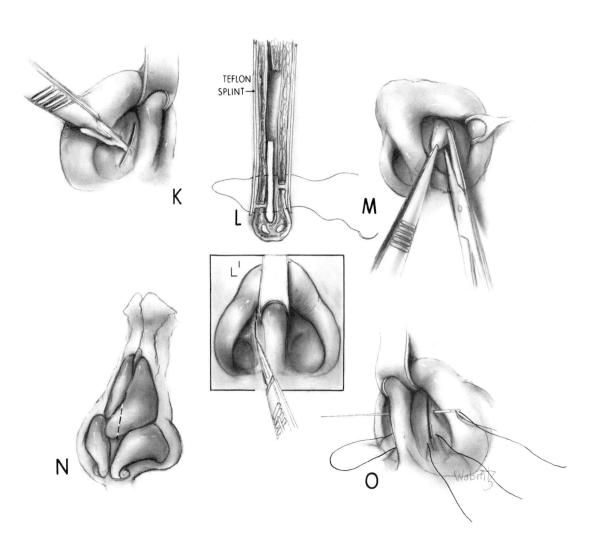

TEFLON
SPLINT

K

L

L¹

M

N

O

RHINOPLASTY

Highpoints

1. Subperichondrial and subperiosteal dissection in which the cartilage and bone are to be either modified or excised.
2. Excise the osteocartilaginous hump. Plan a nasal profile angle between 25 and 36 degrees (30 degrees is ideal).
3. When shortening the septum, if this is necessary, be certain that a careful estimate is made regarding the amount of septum excised.
4. When changing the nasolabial angle, be certain that the exact configuration of cartilage excised matches the correction desired (usually 90 degrees but can be up to 120 degrees).
5. Bilateral osteotomy of the nasal processes of the maxillae as close as possible to their bases or origins.
6. "Outfracture" the lateral bony walls before final shaping.
7. Be conservative in excision of any cartilage forming or supporting the nasal tip.
8. Preoperative photographs must be in the operating room with a careful analysis of deformity and a planned method of correction.

A   A schematic drawing showing the deformity of the hump along the bridge of the nose with the anatomic features of the osteocartilaginous framework superimposed. The dotted lines represent the lines of the saw cuts through bone and the incisions through cartilage.

A¹   Depicted are the relationships of the cartilages forming the columella.

B   An incision is made intranasally between the lateral and alar cartilage bilaterally using a #11 blade knife. The incision is carried upward to start the separation of the lateral cartilage from its perichondrium.

C   This separation of cartilage and perichondrium is continued, using a Joseph knife up to the nasal bone. At this level the tip of the knife raises the periosteum from the nasal bone.

D   A periosteal elevator (McKenty) is then inserted in the same plane and the periosteum is elevated to the upper suture line of the nasal bone and to the midline. The only exception here might be in the case of an exceptionally large hump in which the overlying periosteum is removed with the hump to prevent regeneration of excess bone.

Plate 71   The Nose and the Nasopharynx

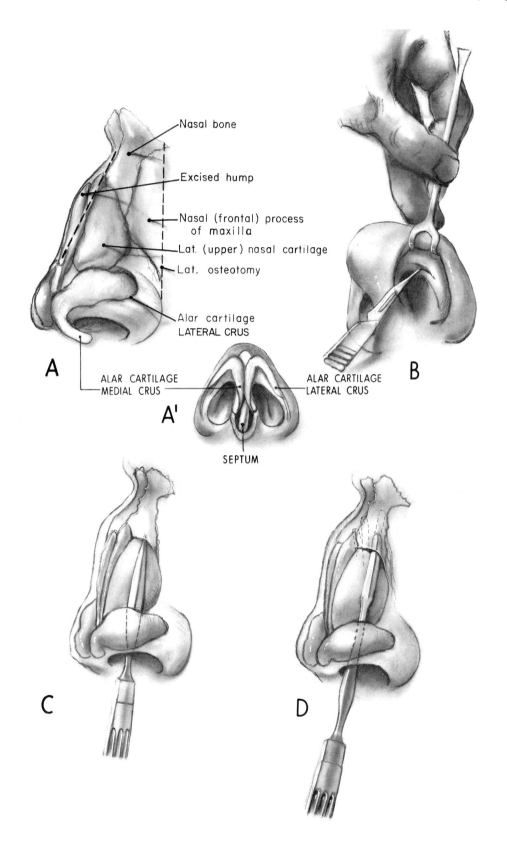

Nasal bone

Excised hump

Nasal (frontal) process of maxilla

Lat. (upper) nasal cartilage

Lat. osteotomy

Alar cartilage
LATERAL CRUS

A

A'

ALAR CARTILAGE
MEDIAL CRUS

ALAR CARTILAGE
LATERAL CRUS

SEPTUM

B

C

D

RHINOPLASTY (*Continued*)

E After the above steps are repeated on the opposite side, a button end knife initiates the so-called transfixion incision which runs along the dorsal and distal borders of the septum. To commence this incision, a curved button end knife may be more adaptable. In either case, the knife is inserted in the original intercartilaginous incision on one side reaching and lying in the subperiosteal plane over the bony hump. The knife is then brought downward over the dorsum of the septum, thus transecting the attachment of the septum along its dorsal margin. When the knife reaches the level of the opposite intercartilaginous incision, the instrument is advanced through this incision and extended to the septal tip or angle. At this point the direction changes almost at a right angle, hugging the lower or distal margin of the septum. The apices of both nares are now retracted upward as in step *F* so that the membranous distal end of the septum is placed on the stretch. In this manner the knife can follow the plane between the membranous and cartilaginous portions of the septum leaving the membranous septum with the columella.

F The lower portion of this transfixion incision is completed with a #11 blade knife or scissors down to the anterior nasal spine.

G A long narrow retractor exposes the subperiosteal plane for the bayonet saw which will be inserted through the intercartilaginous incision. Care must be taken not to injure or dull the teeth on the saw, at the same time avoiding entanglement with soft tissue.

H The bony hump is then sawed through from one side to the other. This may require a saw cut from the opposite side. Both nasal bones and the dorsum of the septum are cut in this manner. The hump usually still has lower attachments of the lateral and septal cartilages which are not cut with the saw. A small curved button end knife is used to sever these attachments in a manner similar to its use in step *F*. An osteotome may also be used to separate higher attachments The hump is then removed with a clamp.

I A rasp is used to smooth any rough areas along the bony edges as well as rounding the outer (dotted) edges of the cut surfaces of the nasal bones (*I¹*). The rasp must be used in single downward strokes and after each stroke the rasp should be cleaned of all bony fragments.

J The small curved button end knife is used to correct any irregularities of the lower portion of the incision which involves the septal and lateral cartilages. It is important that following the use of the rasp and the button end knife all fragments of bone and cartilage be removed; otherwise, they may serve as a nidus for regeneration of bone and cartilage.

Plate 72   The Nose and the Nasopharynx

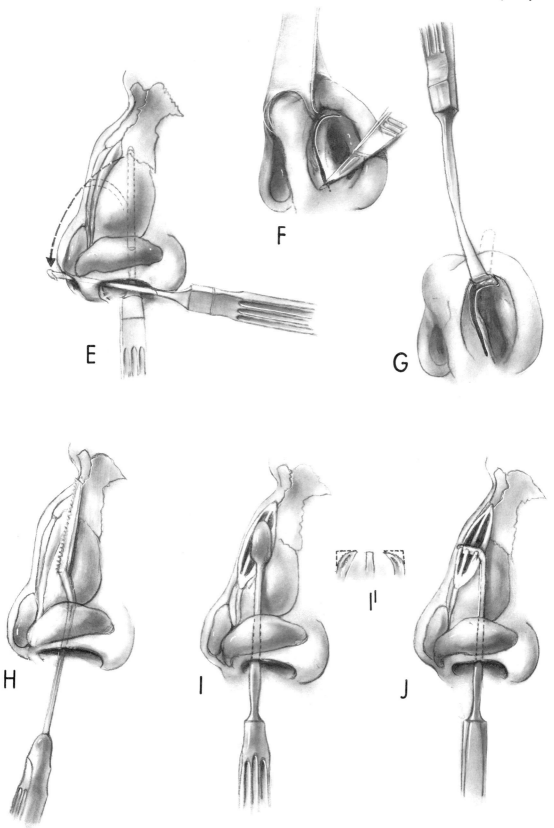

E

F

G

H

I

I'

J

RHINOPLASTY (*Continued*)

K   Any remaining attachments of the lateral cartilages to the septum are transected with scissors close to the septum.

L   The distal or lower margin of the septum is now delivered into one naris and a triangular section of cartilage with overlying mucoperichondrium is excised with scissors. The shape of this excised section depends on the relationship of the nasolabial angle (90 degrees). It is important to evaluate carefully the amount of shortening necessary to correct the existing deformity. This may be done by raising the tip along a fixed ruler and measuring the distance between the two points. Remember that excising an extra amount of the distal margin of the septum is no assurance of a properly raised tip; it is catastrophic if too much is excised.

L¹   The septal angle or tip of the septum is then rounded with a #15 blade knife. A small section of mucoperichondrium is also trimmed back from this angle to prevent any untoward bulkiness at the tip.

M
M¹   As the tip is raised and the nose shortened, there is usually a protrusion of the lower end of the lateral cartilage through the intercartilaginous incision. This is excised.

A schematic drawing showing the portion of lateral cartilage excised in the previous step. Again do not shorten this cartilage any more than is necessary.

It is usually necessary to excise two triangular wedges of bone, one on either side of the septum at its juncture with the nasal bones. This step may be done at this stage of the operation or concomitantly with the "outfracturing" of the lateral bony nasal wall (*U*, plate 74).

N   Using a narrow osteotome, a cut is made close to the septum.

O   With the same osteotome, another cut is made close to the edge of the nasal bone. In such fashion, a wedge of bone is hopefully outlined and freed. (This wedge of bone is removed with a hemostat. The same procedure is performed on the opposite side.)

P   The two wedges of bone removed.

Q   To expose the nasal (anterior) process of the maxilla for the lateral osteotomy, an incision is made in the pyriform recess which lies at the inferior margin of the nasal process. This incision is so directed that it leads to the periosteum on the external surface of this inferior bony margin.

Plate 73   The Nose and the Nasopharynx

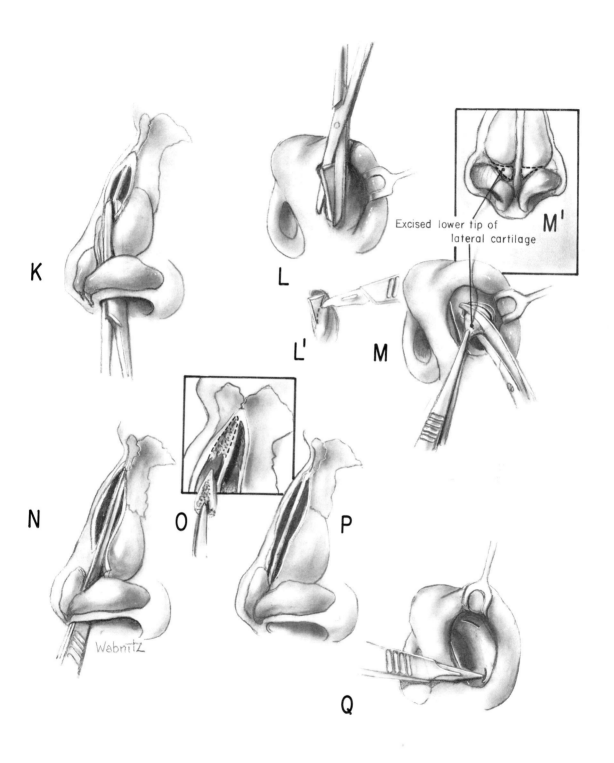

K

L

L'

M

M'

Excised lower tip of
lateral cartilage

N

O

P

Q

Wabnitz

RHINOPLASTY (*Continued*)

R First a Joseph knife and then a periosteal elevator is inserted through the incision in the pyriform recess and the periosteum is elevated along the base of the nasal (frontal) process of the maxilla up to its suture line with the frontal bone at the region of the inner canthus of the eye. This tunnel is as close to the base or origin of the nasal process as possible except that superiorly it is anterior enough so that the medial palpebral ligament is not detached. This ligament is attached to the nasal (frontal) process of the maxilla in front of the lacrimal groove.

S Using a narrow retractor or curved saw protector, the bayonet saw is inserted through the subperiosteal tunnel. This is done with the same care as depicted in step G when the saw was inserted for excision of the hump.

T Keeping as close to the base or origin of the nasal (frontal) process of the maxilla as possible, this bone is sawed through at right angles to the body of the maxilla. An attempt is made to remove the "sawdust" with small scoops. The entire procedure is now repeated on the opposite side. An alternate method is the use of an osteotome or small circular saw (see plate 75, steps B, C and D).

U The next step consists in the "outfracturing" of these two lateral bony frames, each consisting of the nasal bone and nasal process of the maxilla. This maneuver aids in the ultimate narrowing of the nasal bridge since it usually establishes a clean fracture line along the region of the suture line between this lateral frame and the frontal bone. The outfracturing is accomplished by the insertion of an osteotome between the septum and the nasal bone. Several slight taps on the osteotome are made and then, using the septum as a fulcrum, the osteotome is moved laterally, thus pushing the nasal bones outward. Beware of a green stick fracture. Some surgeons do not outfracture.

V The lateral nasal frame on each side, which is now quite mobile, is fractured inward by pressure with the operator's thumbs. If mobility is incomplete on one side or the other, a Walsham nasal forceps or heavy needle holder is used to grasp this lateral nasal frame and "outfracture" it again. The "infracturing" is repeated. The bridge of the nose is again evaluated for any rough or sharp edges which now may be rounded to a pleasing contour.

W Before the transfixion sutures are placed, evaluation of the hanging septum is made. This consists of an excessively deep columella made up of folds of skin and broad medial crura of the alar cartilages. An elliptical section of both skin and cartilage is excised as depicted by the dotted lines. The two transfixion sutures of 3-0 nylon are then inserted, being certain that there is good coaptation of the septal angle with the cartilages of the tip. These are through and through sutures joining septum with mucoperichondrium and columella with skin. They are usually staggered so that when they are tied they will tend to raise the columella and thence the tip. A problem may arise consisting of an eventually dropped tip after these sutures are removed. To minimize this complication, buried sutures of 5-0 nylon can be placed. Then sutures are not removed.

Plate 74   The Nose and the Nasopharynx

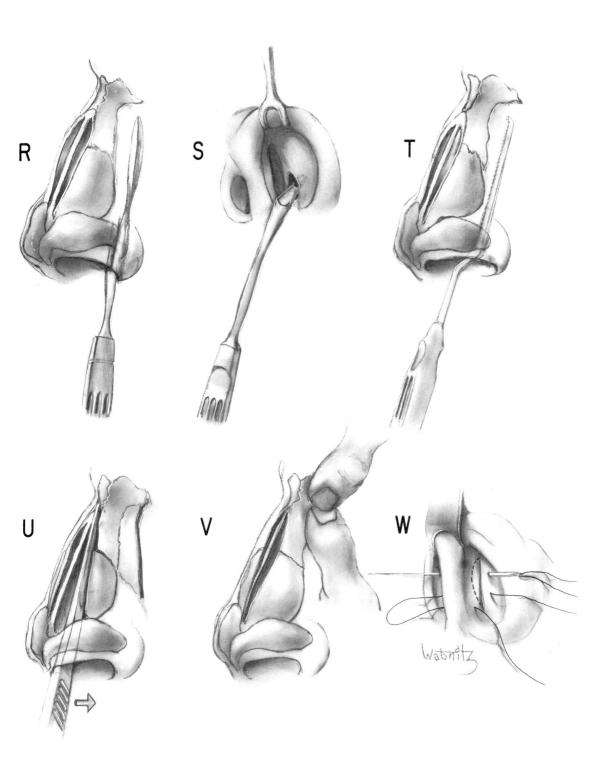

R

S

T

U

V

W

Wabnitz

RHINOPLASTY (*Continued*)

Rhinoplasty Dressing

X   Nasal packing of one half inch strip gauze impregnated with an antibiotic ointment or liquid Furacin is then gently and rather loosely inserted into the nose. A small plastic tube can be inserted along the floor of the nose on each side for breathing purposes. Some surgeons eliminate any intranasal packing.

   The skin is cleansed with hydrogen peroxide and water, dried and then coated with tincture of benzoin or Betadine. Narrow strips of adhesive are then applied with one or two strips placed around the tip and the superior portion of the columella and then pinched at the tip (see plate 76, step *D*).

Y   A thin layer of lint, cottonoid material or Telfa is placed over this adhesive dressing. Then a splint composed of a dental mold compound or soft malleable metal is used as an additional external protection. This external splint is held in place with adhesive strips as shown. Five to seven days later, the splint is removed.

RHINOPLASTY ALTERNATE TECHNIQUES

A   Removal of the dorsal hump, especially if small, can be performed entirely with an osteotome along the solid line. A Hilger guarded osteotome is ideal for this purpose. Deepening of the nasofrontal angle at the glabella can also be achieved by use of an osteotome along the dotted line.

B   The lateral osteotomy can be accomplished with a guarded osteotome inserted in the pyriform recess. Depicted is the relationship of the lacrimal groove (the site of the lacrimal sac) to the osteotomy. Although the proximity is striking, evidence of any significant and lasting damage has not been substantiated (Flowers and Anderson, 1968).

C   Another technique for lateral osteotomy is the use of a small power-driven Seltzer saw.

D   Close-up of Seltzer saw.

E   Cross section of correct (*1*) and incorrect (*2*) planes for the lateral osteotomy. The horizontal osteotomy facilitates support for the transected bone. The arrow shows the lack of support for the transected bone when the osteotomy is oblique (after Aufricht, 1943 and 1961 and Converse, 1964).

Complications

   1. Dropped tip.
   2. Broad nasal base.
   3. Prominent basal frontal angle.
   4. Saddleback deformity.

Plate 75   The Nose and the Nasopharynx

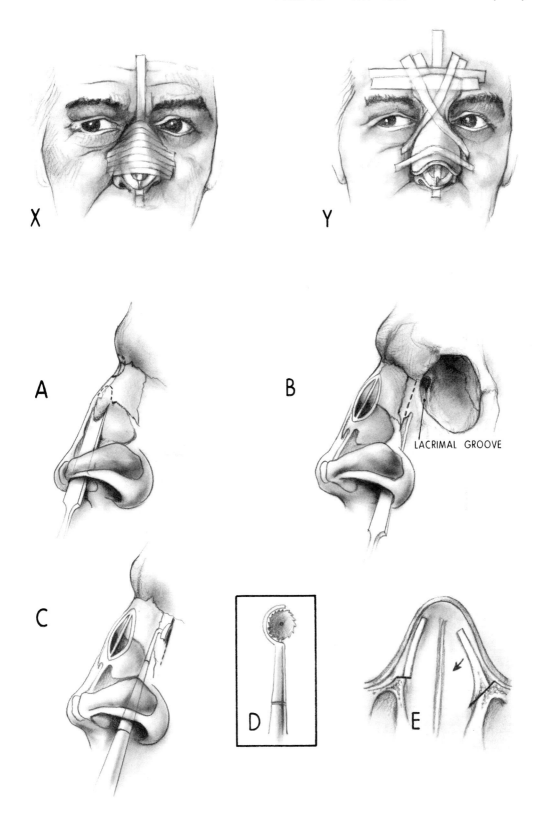

X

Y

A

B

LACRIMAL GROOVE

C

D

E

CORRECTION OF BROAD NASAL TIP
(Conservative Method)

Highpoints

1. Elevate perichondrium on both surfaces of medial portion of lateral crura of alar cartilage to be excised.
2. Excise cartilage along medial and upper edges of lateral crura.
3. Be conservative in amount of cartilage excised.
4. The anterior or rim incision (1) must be made at the free margin of the lateral crus and not at the margin of the nares.

A   The dotted lines enclose the medial and upper portion of the lateral crus to be excised.

B   Three incisions are made in the roof of the vestibule. The posterior incision (2) is the intercartilaginous incision between the lateral and alar cartilages as done in the standard rhinoplasty. The anterior incision (1) is along the lower margin of the alar cartilage known as the rim incision. The cartilage between these two incisions is separated subperichondrially on both surfaces. The medial incision (3) is made close to the septum and carried through the alar cartilage. External finger pressure over the alar cartilage aids in exposure and helps deliver the alar cartilage into the incision. During this maneuver, the cartilage is "turned upside down."

C   The medial and upper edges of the lateral crus of the alar cartilage are trimmed very conservatively. It is much safer to excise too little rather than too much cartilage; otherwise, a pinched tip will result.
   The same procedure is repeated on the opposite side.

D   Supportive narrow strip adhesive is utilized to coapt the cartilages by pinching the adhesive with a clamp.

Plate 76   The Nose and the Nasopharynx

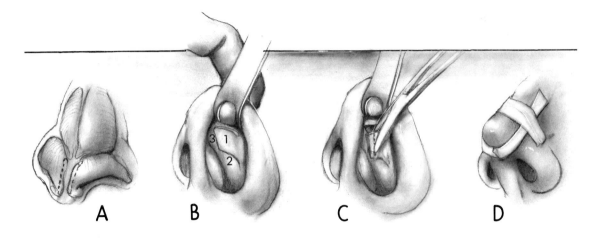

A   B   C   D

ADDITIONAL NASAL TIP PROCEDURES

Highpoints

1. Same as under conservative method (plate 76).
2. If the dome of the lateral crus or the underlying perichondrium and skin of the vestibule are cut through completely, extreme care must be taken to prevent overriding of the cut edges of the cartilage.

E   As in the previous conservative method, two initial incisions (Safian, 1935) are made. The anterior or rim incision (*1*) along the edge of the free margin of the lateral crus extending to the medial crus must not be along the extreme edge of the nares; otherwise, this soft tissue will contract and form a pinched or notched area. Another posterior incision (*2*) is the intercartilaginous incision (between the upper or posterior edge of the lateral crus of the alar cartilage and the quadralateral or upper lateral cartilage). This is the same incision made in the standard rhinoplasty.

F   Using straight or angulated scissors, the soft tissue is separated subperichondrially along the outside, presenting portion of the dome of the lateral crus and of the medial crus of the alar cartilage. The locations of the initial incisions are shown and numbered as in step *A*.

G   The dome is exposed. This is the site of the incision for resection of a portion of the cartilage. Again, it is emphasized that conservation of cartilage is recommended, since if too much cartilage is excised, a pinched tip will result which is impossible to correct.

Several modifications can be performed.

H   Depicted is a complete transection through the dome and underlying perichondrium and vestibular skin. The desired amount of cartilage and underlying soft tissue is then excised along the dotted line. This technique is indicated mainly in very broad and bulbous tips. Care must be taken so that there is no subsequent overriding of the cut ends of the cartilage or displacement of either the medial or lateral crura. This error may cause distortion of the columella.

I   A less radical type of cartilage incision is made as depicted. Here the underlying soft tissue is neither incised nor excised. It will be noted that the cartilage excised is along the posterior or upper border of the cartilage with a small rim of cartilage left intact along the anterior or lower border (rim) of the cartilage.

J   Depicted is the amount of cartilage excised according to Brown and McDowell (1958).

K   Depicted is the amount of cartilage excised according to Goldman (1952) and Fomon (1960).

Complications

1. Pinched tip.
2. Narrowed nares causing airway obstruction.
3. Distortion and twisting of columella.

Plate 76 Continued   *The Nose and the Nasopharynx*

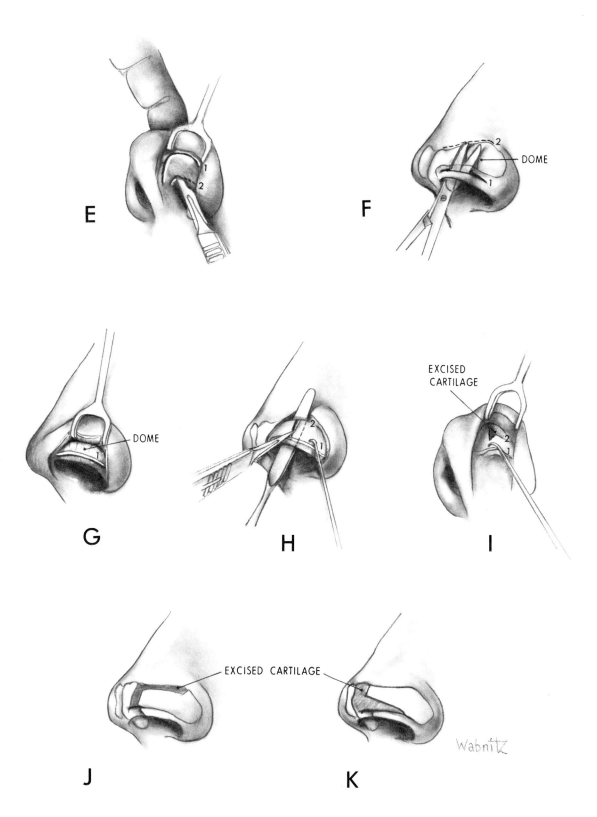

E

F   DOME

G   DOME

H

I   EXCISED CARTILAGE

J   EXCISED CARTILAGE   K

Wabnitz

COLUMELLAR GRAFT FOR COLLAPSED NASAL TIP

There are two main causes of a collapsed nasal tip. Type one is entirely due to lack of septal support and is associated with a retracted columella. The second type is due to a congenitally shortened columella associated with lack of septal support. In either case a columellar cartilage graft is necessary.

Columellar grafts are also used in total and subtotal nasal reconstruction.

Technique of obtaining a section of costochondral cartilage is shown on plate 22.

TYPE I

Highpoints

1. Graft can be autogenous cartilage, bone or Silastic.
2. Place graft anterior to medial crura of alar cartilages.
3. Cartilage graft should have layer of perichondrium attached.

A Through an incision made anterior to the medial crura of the alar cartilages, a tunnel is developed down to and anterior to the anterior nasal spine. The tunnel is extended upward into the bulk of the nasal tip but not so far that the end of the cartilage graft will be noticed subcutaneously.

B A thin strut of cartilage with attached perichondrium or Silastic is then inserted in this tunnel. An anchor mattress suture of 4-0 nylon is placed through the base of the graft and brought out through the skin of the columella. This suture is tied over a small rubber or plastic bootie. The lateral incision is approximated with fine sutures.

TYPE II

Highpoints

1. Lengthen skin of columella.
2. Cartilage graft should have layer of perichondrium attached.

C Collapsed nasal tip due to congenitally short columella. During previous surgery, the septum was shortened in an attempt to correct the deformity. There is an associated lack of cartilage support.

D Skin incisions to lengthen the skin of the columella and expose the area for a cartilage graft.

E The soft tissue of the columella is freed and reflected upward. The medial crura of the alar cartilages are included in this columellar flap. The distal end of the septum is exposed if present.

F After a tunnel is opened down to and anterior to the anterior nasal spine, a slitlike pocket is made in the bulk of the nasal tip. An anchor suture of 4-0 chromic catgut or 5-0 nylon secures the upper end of the cartilage graft. This suture is buried and remains.

G Additional sutures of 4-0 or 5-0 chromic catgut are placed to support the graft. These sutures grasp a portion of the perichondrium of the septal cartilage on either side. They straddle the graft but are not placed through the graft.

H Two or three of these straddling sutures are utilized. They are entirely buried and remain.

I The lateral margins of the upper lip defect are first approximated with deep sutures of 4-0 or 5-0 chromic catgut. The skin is closed with 5-0 nylon. The usual rhinoplasty splint and nasal packing with Furacin strip gauze are used. The upper lip is best immobilized with adhesive and the patient should be kept on liquids until healing occurs.

Following any graft, primary healing may be delayed. The patient should be kept on antibiotics and liquids with the upper lip immobilized. Secondary healing occurs usually within seven to 10 days.

Complications

1. Absorption of cartilage or bone graft.
2. Rejection of Silastic graft.
3. Dislocation of any type of graft.

Plate 77   The Nose and the Nasopharynx

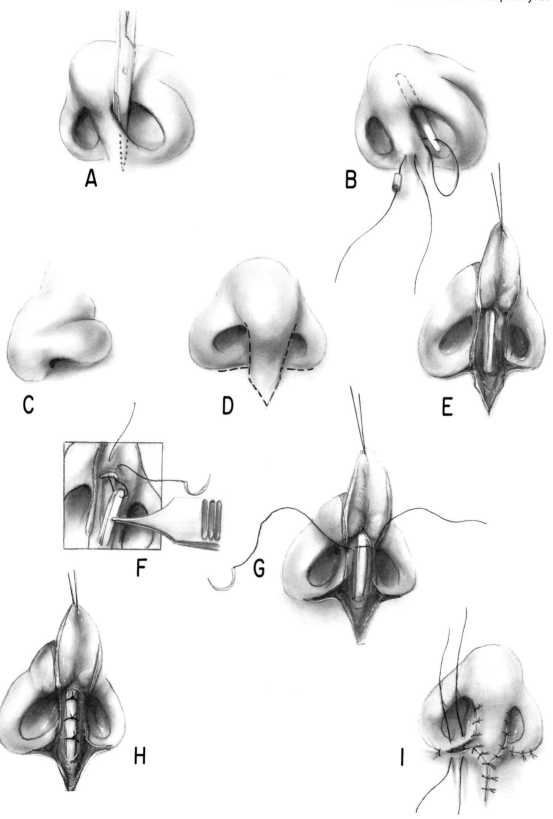

A

B

C

D

E

F

G

H

I

CORRECTION OF NASAL DEFORMITY IN CLEFT LIP

FIRST STAGE

Highpoints

1. May require two or more stages especially if a rhinoplasty is indicated.
2. Realign anterior nasal spine.
3. Realign and straighten septum.
4. Realign columella.
5. Correction of alar naris by rotation of alar cartilage on side of cleft.

A   The nasal deformity is characterized by marked flattening of the ala nasi on the side of the previously repaired cleft lip with the naris oval opening in more of a horizontal than a normal vertical position. The columella is angulated off the midline to the normal side and collapsed. The nasal septum is deviated to the normal side causing obstruction. There may be a coexisting cleft of the upper alveolar ridge, associated with a flattening and depression of the maxilla and the floor of the nasal vestibule in the region of this alveolar defect. The malposition of the deformed alar cartilage is shown in the dotted lines as compared with the normal alar cartilage. The arrows indicate the malrelationship of the nares.

B   An incision is made in the midportion of the upper gingivobuccal sulcus along the solid line leaving sufficient mucosa on the alveolar side for easy closure.

C   The anterior nasal spine and bony floor of the nose are then exposed. The defect of the alveolar ridge on the right side is seen to be part and parcel of the depression of the floor of the nose on the same side. The periosteum of the nasal spine is not elevated.

D   Using an osteotome the nasal spine and a portion of its base are mobilized. The base is included since additional length is required when the spine is realigned to the midline. This midline area is the edge of the depressed floor of the nose on the right side. The mobilization is continued posteriorly along the base of the septum slightly beyond the area of deviation.

E   The anterior nasal spine is realigned slightly to the right of center (slight overcorrection). This position is maintained with one or more 3-0 or 4-0 chromic catgut or 4-0 nylon sutures placed through the periosteum of the anterior nasal spine and through the floor of the nose on the right side. This suturing may follow the additional steps, to be mentioned later, to straighten and mobilize the septum.

F   To further straighten the septum, if necessary, two incisions are made in the septum —
F¹   one on either side. Each incision is through the cartilage but through only one side of the mucoperichondrium. The incisions are staggered and placed so that the septum is hinged on the opposing mucoperichondrium. A small vertical strip of cartilage is excised if the cartilage binds or buckles when straightened (see plate 66).

   Depending on the degree of deformity of the nasal septum at its anterior end, additional steps may be necessary. To realign the anterior end of the septum, an incision is made between the upper lateral and alar cartilages on each side and a transfixion incision is made as in a standard rhinoplasty (steps *E* and *F*, plate 72) across the dorsum of the septum and down the anterior end of the septum. The upper lateral cartilages are freed from the septum on either side (step *K*, plate 73). The septum is now entirely free and is easily shifted to a position slightly to the right of the midline — slightly overcorrected.

   If the deformity of the anterior end of the septum is minimal, the previous steps are bypassed and the procedure continues on plate 80, step A. If the previous steps are required, it may be best to stage this rotation and elevation of the alar cartilage as shown on plate 80.

Plate 78   The Nose and the Nasopharynx

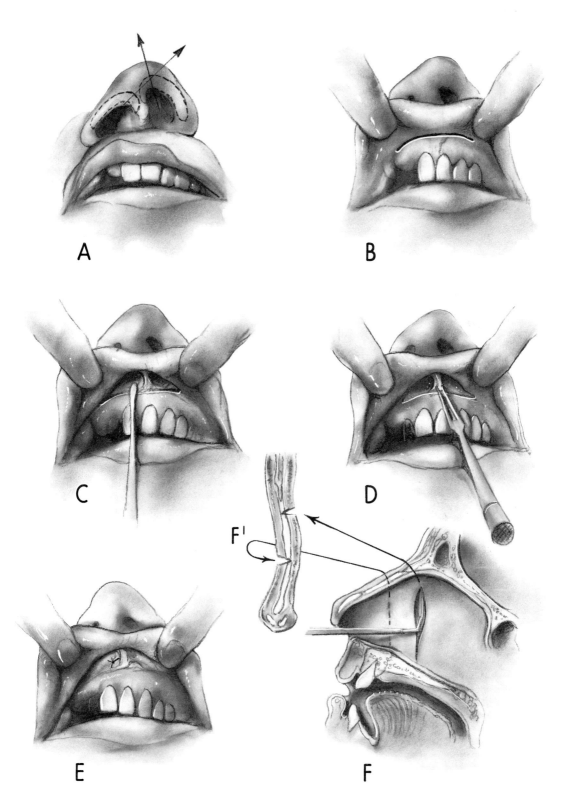

A

B

C

D

E

F

F'

CORRECTION OF NASAL DEFORMITY
IN CLEFT LIP (*Continued*)

SECOND STAGE

This stage is performed four to six weeks after the first stage if rhinoplasty is indicated or if realignment of anterior end of septum requires additional correction.

Highpoints

1. Standard rhinoplasty as indicated.
2. Rotation of naris on side of cleft (Berkeley, 1959).
3. Use excised "hump" from standard rhinoplasty as cartilage and bone graft to the floor of vestibule on side of cleft as indicated.
4. Revise scar of cleft lip if necessary with modified Z-plasty.

Since there may be an associated nasal hump, a standard rhinoplasty is first performed (see plates 71 to 74). The excised hump is saved.

A   An incision is made along the solid lines mobilizing the entire right alar nasi with the medial crus and dome of the cartilage and the skin of the juxtaposed cheek. A small triangle of tissue is excised in the nasolabial area to realign the skin edges (Blair). The base of the alar nasi is mobilized as another triangle (Young, 1949).

A¹   The incision is carried over the lateral side of the nasal tip (Joseph).

B   To build up the defect in the floor of the vestibule, the excised hump from the dorsum of the nose is inserted in the incision as an autogenous bone and cartilage graft. Several sutures of 3-0 chromic catgut are placed deep to the floor of the nose to secure this bone and cartilage graft. The alar nasi is rotated medially and superiorly over the graft and sutured to the columella. Any excess skin and mucous membrane are excised.

C   If necessary, the old scar of the cleft lip is excised. Small lateral and medial incisions are made to widen the upper lip.

D   The lip closure consists in the interdigitation of the margins as a modified Z-plasty.
   If additional realignment or lengthening of columella is required, this can be performed at a later date (see plate 81).

Plate 79   The Nose and the Nasopharynx

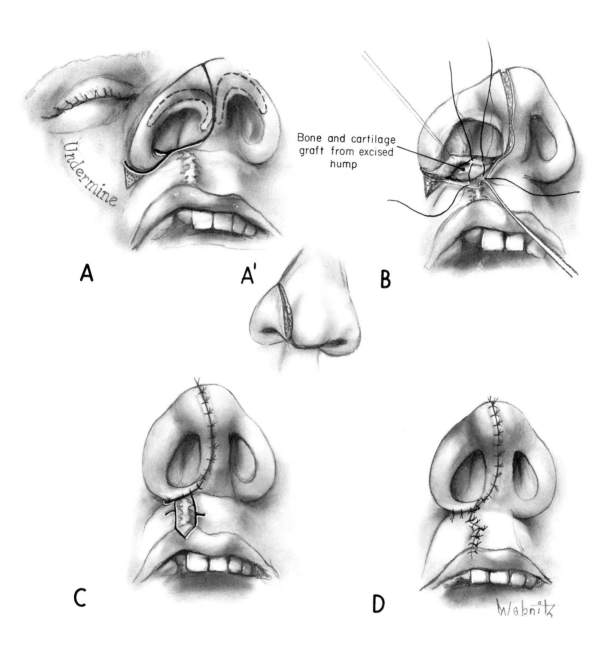

Bone and cartilage
graft from excised
hump

Undermine

A

A'

B

C

D

Wabnitz

NARES AND COLUMELLA PROCEDURES

Correction of Bulbous and Flattened Nasal Tip

A   An ellipse of skin and subcutaneous tissue is excised.

B   Closure with fine nylon.

Lengthening of Skin of Columella

C   Using the principle of conversion of a **V** incision into a **Y** closure, the skin of the columella is lengthened. The entire tip of the nose may require mobilization by a transfixation incision as in a rhinoplasty (see plate 72, step *E*). Further support may necessitate the use of cartilage strut (see plate 78).

D   The upper columella flap is raised and all skin edges are approximated with fine nylon.

Shortening of Columella

E   The skin of the entire columella is mobilized by a through and through incision. A small section of skin is excised and the skin margins are approximated.

Narrowing a Flared Naris

F   A flared naris often accompanies a complete cleft lip and is corrected by the excision of a triangular piece of skin along the floor of the nose. Only skin is excised since there is usually a deficiency of subcutaneous tissue.

G   Approximation to the base and side of the columella. At times the entire lip may require revision.

Correction of Pinched Naris

H   This deformity is corrected by a simple Z-plasty. The lower edge of the ala is freed while a flap is developed in the nasolabial fold.

I   The ala exchanges places with the nasolabial flap. One or two deep sutures help secure the ala. The skin margins are then approximated.

Straightening a Slanted Columella

J   This deformity usually is associated with the so-called harelip nose and when this is the case a complete rhinoplasty is necessary (plate 79). The skin of the columella, however, is corrected by utilization of a Z-plasty. The upper flap is in line with the slanted columella whereas the lower flap is placed so that its right margin is to the right of center. In this manner, when the flaps are exchanged, there is a tendency to slight overcorrection.

K   The flaps are exchanged and skin margins approximated.

For enlargement of nares with Z-plasty see plate 93, steps *G*, *H* and *I*.

Plate 80 The Nose and the Nasopharynx

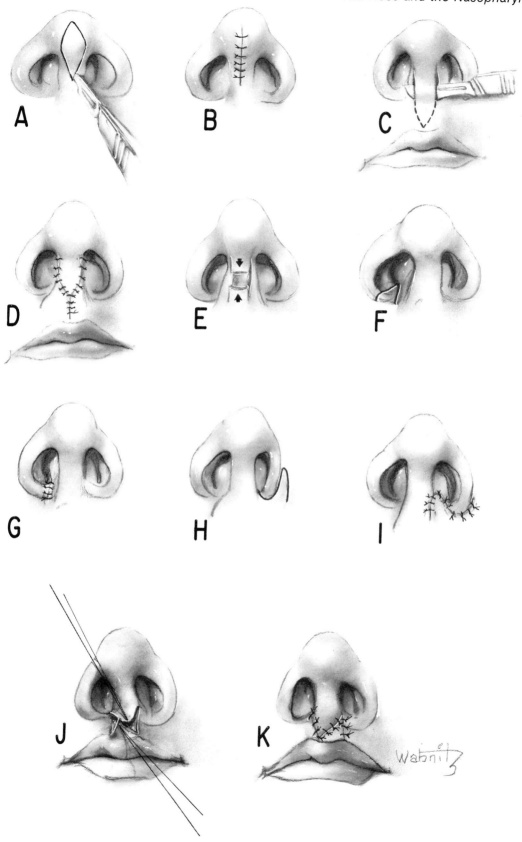

NASOFACIAL FLAPS

1. Skin on nose is so fixed and inelastic that simple closure is virtually impossible. Rotating or advanced flap or skin graft is necessary.
2. Rotating flaps include same adipose tissue.

A   For lesions in the nasofacial sulcus, advanced flaps usually suffice. A wide elliptical incision is carried down to the periosteum or perichondrium and the lesion excised.

B   The angular artery and vein are separately ligated.

C   The lateral skin flap is widely undermined. If closure is still difficult, the lower portion of the lateral flap is advanced upward as depicted by the arrow. The dog-ear at the superior margin is excised (dotted triangle). Several deep sutures are placed as shown in the insert (C^1).

D   The skin is approximated with 5-0 nylon.

E   A skin incision is made as outlined.

F   The lesion has been excised and the rotating flap is swung toward the defect. The lateral border of the donor site is mobilized. This facilitates closure of the donor site. Any dog-ear (**X**) at the superior margin of the donor site is excised.

G   Several deep sutures of 5-0 white silk or catgut are used. The skin is approximated with 5-0 nylon. A dog-ear at **Y** may require excision.

H   If the lesion is somewhat larger and lower on the nose, the reverse type of rotating flap is used.

I   The technique is identical to the preceding procedure. **X** in step *H* and **Y** refer to possible dog-ears which may require excision.

Plate 81   The Nose and the Nasopharynx

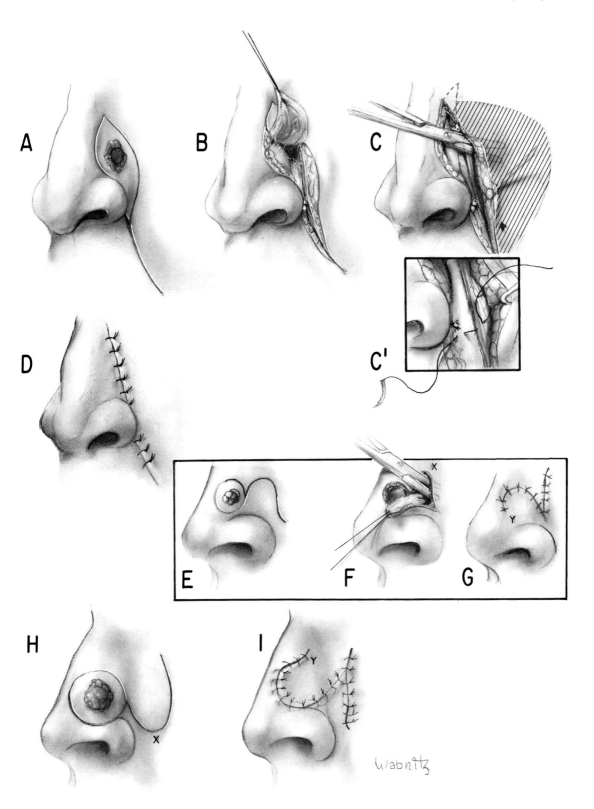

SEPTAL FLAP FOR EXTERNAL NASAL DEFECT
(After De Quervain; Kazanjian)

Through and through defects, surgical or traumatic, of the external nasal framework can be reconstructed in a number of ways: forehead flaps (plates 90 and 122), sickle or scalping flaps (plate 9), local turn-in flaps (plate 92) and arm flaps (plate 89). The choice depends on a number of factors such as size and location of defect and age of patient. In the older patient some type of forehead or scalp flap is preferred, while in the younger patient the use of a forehead flap is hardly justifiable because of the residual cosmetic deformity of the forehead. In the elderly an arm flap is contraindicated because of the danger of deltoid bursitis (supraspinatus tendonitis).

Depicted is a septal flap which avoids both of the previous criticisms. The septal flap, however, results in a permanent septal perforation which is associated with crusting, bleeding and possible chronic ulcerations along the margins of the perforation.

Highpoints

1. Full thickness septal flap.
2. Leave adequate support along bridge of nose and at columella.
3. Second stage utilizing full thickness skin graft or local flap.

A   Shown is a full thickness defect of the external nasal framework. The dotted lines represent the area to be trimmed or excised.

B   Superior-based septal cartilage flap, including both sides of the mucoperichondrium.

C   Cross-sectional view depicting the superior-based septal flap. The edges of the defect are trimmed along the dotted lines.

D   The flap is swung into the defect and sutured into position. The coapting *edges* of the flap are denuded of mucous membrane to facilitate adequate approximation to the edges of the defect.

At a later stage the remaining portion of mucous membrane externally (but not the perichondrium) is excised and a full thickness graft from the retroauricular region is applied over the perichondrium (plate 86, steps A, B, C, D).

External covering can also be achieved with a rotation flap described in steps E and F.

E   Superior-based nasal flap is elevated and rotated into defect. A cheek flap formed by an incision along the nasolabial fold is mobilized to close the donor site. Any resulting dog-ear (**X**) is excised.

If a lesion is to be excised, a cotton-tipped applicator inserted into the nasal cavity will aid in affording counter pressure during the excision.

F   The completed closure using 5-0 nylon interrupted sutures.

This procedure is well suited for non through and through defects resulting from excision of basal cell carcinoma of the skin. Other modifications of this flap are depicted on plate 81.

Plate 82   The Nose and the Nasopharynx

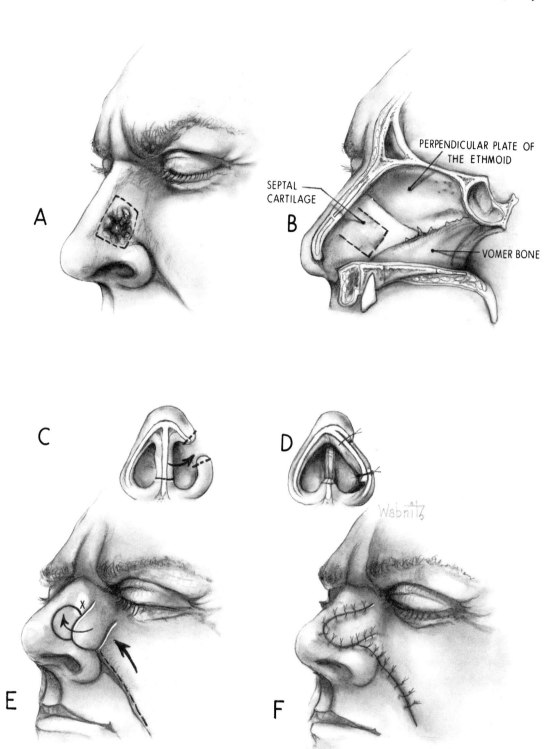

A

B

SEPTAL
CARTILAGE

PERPENDICULAR PLATE OF
THE ETHMOID

VOMER BONE

C

D

E

F

Wabnitz

EXCISION AND RECONSTRUCTION OF ALA NASI

Highpoints

1. Through and through excision of all malignant lesions.
2. Nasolabial turn-in flap forms inner nasal lining and skin covering.
3. If any question regarding adequate circulation, operation is performed in stages.

A Outline of skin incision for resection of lateral portion of ala nasi and nasolabial turn-in flap. The complete thickness of the ala nasi is resected along with a portion of the alar cartilage. The width of the turn-in flap should be slightly wider than the defect, especially at the site where it is folded on itself.

When the nasolabial flap is elevated and folded, if there is any question regarding adequate circulation, a delay is effected by returning the flap to its own bed for 10 to 14 days. The edges of the alar defect are closed by approximation of the inner nasal lining to the skin edges.

B The nasolabial flap is turned in and folded on itself with the approximation of its raw surface.

One or more sutures are placed within the nares to secure the end of the flap to its own base. Through and through sutures or a two-layer closure is used to approximate the edges.

C If the flap is large, a through and through mattress suture is placed in the middle of the flap over a rubber or plastic bootie. This type of suture, if the flap was made sufficiently wide, will tend to roll the fold in, simulating the natural roll of the ala nasi.

The nasolabial donor site is closed in two layers by advancement of the cheek. Furacin-soaked cotton is firmly packed in the naris for support and pressure. External pressure is achieved with similar material.

Another modification is the splitting of the distal end of the flap — one portion to form the ala nasi, the other portion to close a defect of the floor of the nose or the upper lip (Krizek and Robson, 1973).

Plate 83   The Nose and the Nasopharynx

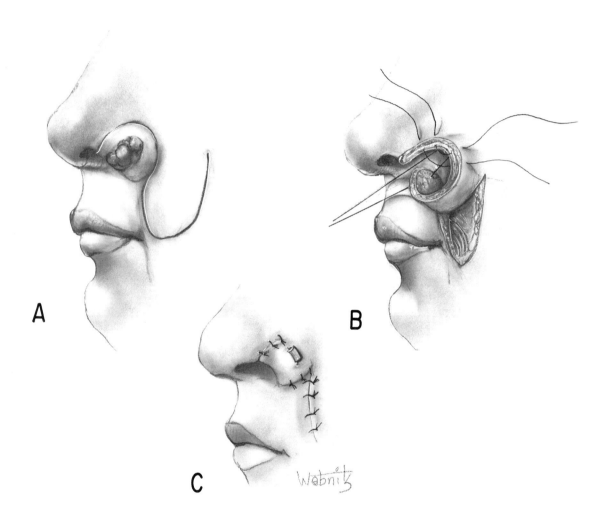

A

B

C

Wabnitz

RESECTION OF TUMOR OF TIP OF NOSE
(After Iverson and Martin, 1957)

Most lesions in the region of the nasal tip can be excised and the defect covered with a full thickness skin graft (see plate 86).

Highpoints

1. Adaptable for moderately large lesions in patients with drooping or elongated nasal tip.
2. Underlying cartilage can be excised.
3. Closure follows technique of nasal tip elevation and shortening of the nose as in rhinoplasty (see plates 71, 72 and 73).

A   The area excised is depicted by the oval incision. Underlying cartilage can be excised if necessary.

B   An incision is made intranasally between the lateral (upper) and alar cartilages bilaterally using a #11 blade knife. The incision is carried upward to start the separation of the lateral cartilage from its perichondrium.

C   The separation of the lateral cartilage from its perichondrium is continued using a Joseph knife up to the nasal bone. The lateral extent of the resected area is shown by the dotted line.

D   After the previous steps are completed, on the opposite side the so-called transfixion incision of a rhinoplasty is performed. It is modified in that only the distal portion of the transfixion incision is necessary. A #11 blade knife is inserted between the distal end of the septum and the columella, thus making a through and through incision which is extended downward to the base of the columella.

Plate 84   The Nose and the Nasopharynx

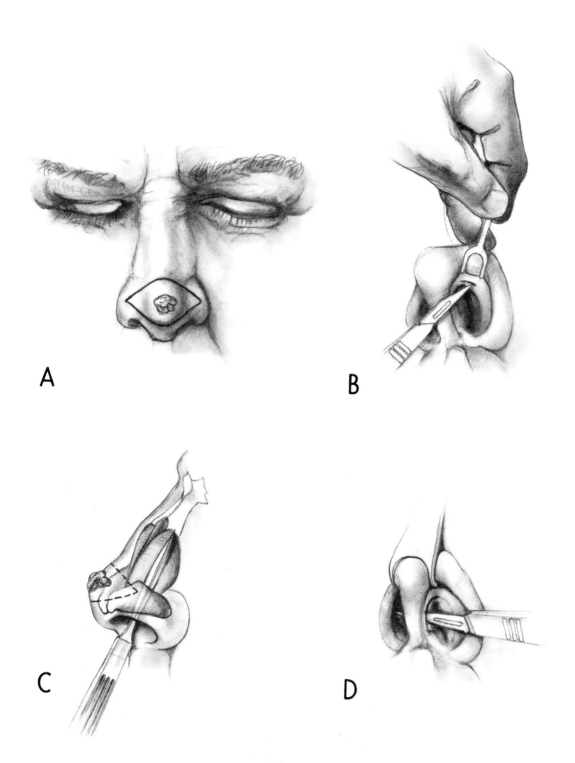

A

B

C

D

RESECTION OF TUMOR OF TIP OF NOSE (*Continued*)

E   The distal end of the septum is delivered into the left naris and a triangular section of septal cartilage with overlying mucoperichondrium is excised with scissors. This shortens the nose and raises the nasal tip, thus facilitating closure of the defect.

F   As the tip is raised and the nose is shortened, there is usually a protrusion of the lower end of the lateral cartilage through the intercartilaginous incision. This is excised. If the attachment of the lateral cartilages to the septum inhibits the raising to the tip, these attachments are transected (see step *K*, plate 73).

G   Two or three transfixion sutures of 3-0 or 4-0 nylon are utilized to approximate the columella to the distal end of the septum. These are placed in staggered fashion so as to raise the nasal tip.

H   The skin incision is then closed with fine nylon sutures.

I   If skin closure is under too much tension, a superior nasal flap is elevated with the excision of a triangle of skin bilaterally (Burow's triangle).

J   The completed closure with the superior-based nasal flap pulled downward.

Plate 85   The Nose and the Nasopharynx

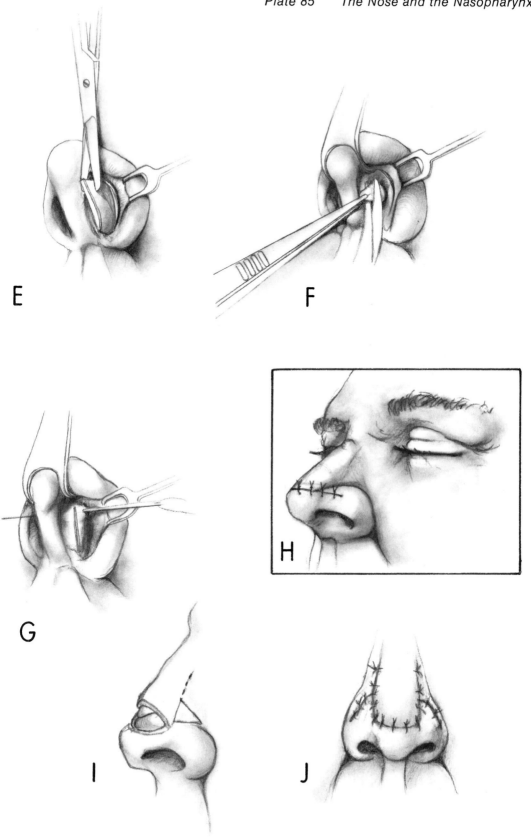

E

F

G

H

I

J

FULL THICKNESS GRAFT TO NOSE

Indications

1. Basal cell carcinoma of the nose.
2. Large benign skin lesions.
3. Skin loss from trauma.

Highpoints

1. Take graft first when lesion is basal cell carcinoma.
2. Excise to perichondrium when lesion is basal cell carcinoma.
3. Pressure dressing.
4. Avoid use of forceps on graft.
5. More radical excision usually necessary in squamous cell carcinoma.

A   After determination of the size of the defect using an outline of methylene blue (alcohol solution), a full thickness layer of skin is excised from the retroauricular region. All adipose tissue is removed from the graft. The donor site defect is closed primarily by undermining the posterior skin border.

B   The lesion is then excised. If it is thought to be malignant, biopsy may be by-passed and wide excision is done as a primary procedure. In such cases deep excision and frozen section are mandatory. A stay suture rather than forceps is used for traction. Absolute hemostasis is necessary.

C   The full thickness graft is secured with 5-0 nylon with moderate tension on the graft. At least four of these sutures are left long to be used to hold the dressing in place. No incisions are made in the graft.

D   After all serum and blood are gently extruded from beneath the graft, a cotton pressure dressing is applied. The long sutures are tied over the dressing. The cotton has been previously soaked in liquid Furacin surgical dressing, the excess liquid having been pressed out and the cotton molded to appropriate size and shape.

    The first dressing is done in seven to 10 days.

E
F   The same technique is used as in the previous procedure. The excision is carried down to the periosteum when the lesion is basal cell carcinoma.
G

    For composite graft from ear to nose, see plate 87.

Plate 86   The Nose and the Nasopharynx

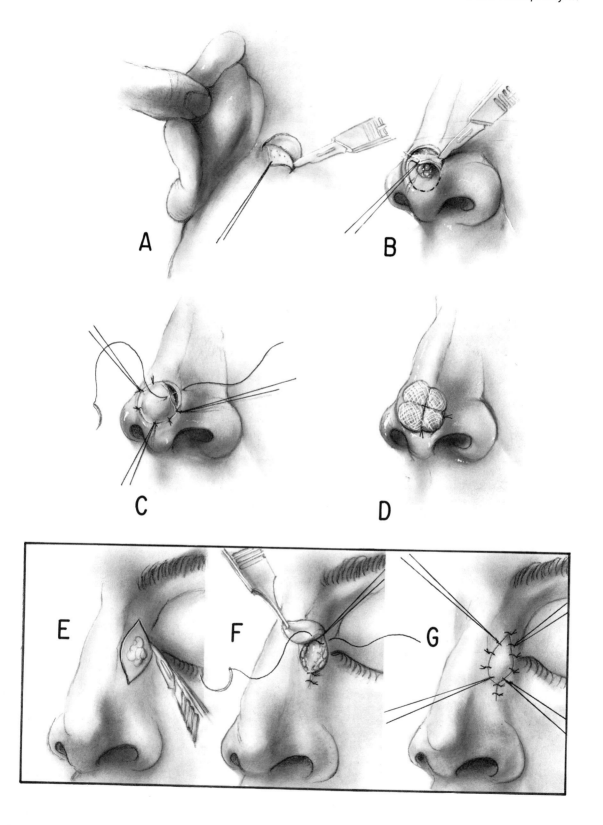

COMPOSITE GRAFT FROM EAR TO NOSE

Highpoints

1. Graft consists of two layers of skin with a layer of cartilage in between.
2. Good blood supply at recipient site.
3. Very delicate care for graft—no forceps.
4. All edges of graft should be less than 1 cm from blood supply of the recipient area.

Anesthesia

General or local—if local, no solution is injected into the graft or recipient area.

A A liberal incision is made along the alar defect to a point where there are a good blood supply and adequate thickness. This is most important. A narrow rim of scar tissue may even be excised if necessary.

B The donor site is chosen along the edge of the helix of the ear at a site that corresponds to the normal ala. A pattern of the defect is then cut out of a piece of discarded suture or knife blade wrapper or sterile chamois. Using 5 per cent alcoholic solution of methylene blue, the pattern is traced on the donor site.

C With a 6-0 silk suture through an edge of the graft, a #11 blade knife is used to cut the helix. No forcep is placed on the graft; the cut is clean and deliberate.

D The recipient site is clean and edges sharp.

E Using 6-0 silk sutures, the anterior edges of skin are first approximated with very delicate care.

F The graft is then gently everted using a cotton-tipped applicator. The posterior skin edges are approximated.

G The completed graft is supported internally with cotton soaked with Furacin liquid. Externally, cottonoid also impregnated with Furacin is placed, over which loose cotton is laid. A splint of dental molding compound is then applied over this dressing to protect the graft.

H If the defect in the helix is long, a posterior auricular skin flap is elevated, turned and used to close the defect.

I Several weeks later the flap is severed along the dotted line. This flap should be as wide as the hairline permits so that a rolled edge of skin may simulate the removed helix.

J
K When the alar defect is narrower, a wedge of the helix is removed. If the defect at the donor site is short in length, it also may be converted into a wedge to facilitate primary closure.

L The wedge defect is easily closed. The cosmetic result is excellent.
   The first dressing may be delayed to the fifth or seventh day and then a similar dressing applied. Alternate sutures are removed at the tenth to fourteenth day. The remaining sutures are removed in two to three days.

If the defect is large, a two-stage composite graft is used. A first graft is placed which is no wider than 1 cm at any one point. Three to four months later a second composite graft is placed alongside the first graft.

Composite grafts may also be used for small defects of the columella.

Complications

1. Partial or complete loss of graft.
2. Deformed donor site with larger grafts when primary closure is attempted without a posterior auricular skin flap.

Plate 87   The Nose and the Nasopharynx

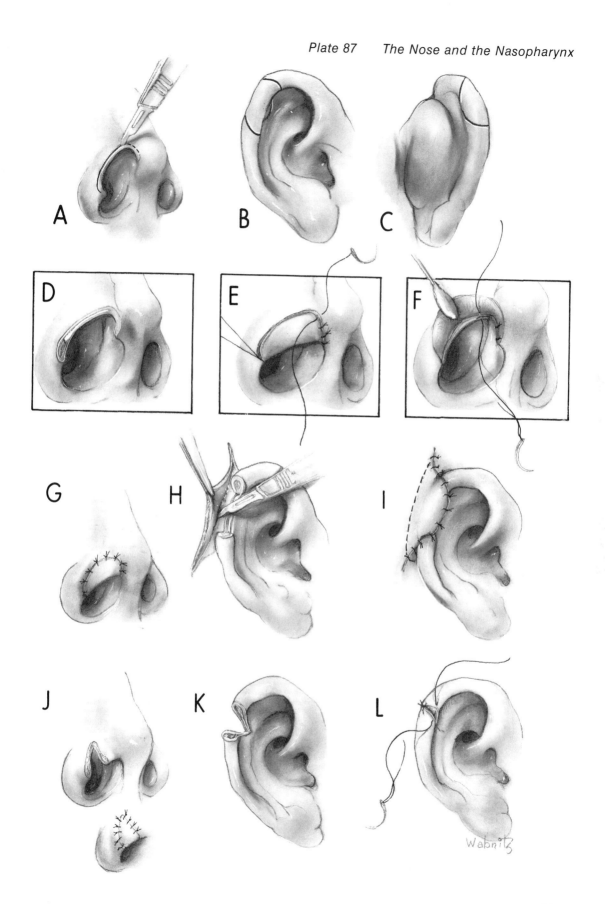

RECONSTRUCTION OF NOSE WITH ARM FLAP

Highpoints

1. In young persons, an arm flap is preferred over a forehead flap since it avoids a forehead scar.
2. Arm flaps should be avoided in the elderly and those with bursitis.
3. Allow for 30 per cent shrinkage of graft.
4. Allow additional length for folding over to form columella and ala nasi—this may eliminate necessity of cartilage graft at tip.
5. Remove all subcutaneous fat from graft. See also plate 121.

A   The nasal defect consists in the loss of the entire right ala nasi, the nasal tip and portion of the columella and left ala nasi.

B
C   With the nasal defect primarily on the right side, the left arm is used as the donor site. A piece of chamois or other suitable material is used as a form to outline the size of the defect. An allowance is first made for 30 per cent shrinkage and another allowance is made for the length of the pedicle during transfer. The widest portion of the graft is at its base, since that will be used to form the ala nasi by turning in the edges. As a rule of thumb, this should be 7.5 cm wide, while the free or distal end should be about 5 cm wide. The length is from 12 to 15 cm. These measurements may have to be modified depending on the defect, but remember it is better to err with too large a graft than too small a one.

    The arm is then placed in position as in *D* and the outline form transferred to the donor site. The angle of the flap is approximately 30 degrees from the horizontal with the base toward the axilla. An area free of hair is desirable in which the texture of the skin simulates that of the remaining nose.

    Full thickness skin cleared of all subcutaneous adipose tissue is then elevated as a bipedicle flap; two weeks' delay ensues. Some surgeons will prefer a single pedicle flap as the first delaying procedure, with complete elevation of the distal or free end at this stage. If the bipedicle technique is used, after two weeks the distal or free end is severed. Another two weeks of delay—now we have a single pedicle flap in either case—and the entire flap is elevated and returned to its bed and left there until most of the edema has regressed. This takes two to four weeks.

D   The flap is now ready for transfer. The flap is elevated and split thickness or dermal graft (free of hair) covers both the donor site and the raw surface of the flap except for edges along the distal end which will be sutured to the nasal defect. It is well to use catgut sutures on this distal end since the grafted surface will form the lining of the nose and be inaccessible for suture removal. The edges of the nasal defect are trimmed to expose normal healthy tissue. A generously bared area is important to receive and nurture the flap. By the same token, any portion of the split thickness skin which lines the flap must be incised and any section must be excised that comes in contact with a bared area of the recipient site.

E   The arm and forearm are immobilized in a plaster posterior molded splint. Circular plaster then is used to secure the forearm and arm to the head and shoulders and anchored to the thorax. All pressure points and areas of contact should be well padded previously.

F   Transection of the pedicle is begun at the end of two weeks. This is done in stages during the next week by transecting one third at first, another third in three days and the final third in three or four more days. Sufficient length is allowed for turn in flaps to form the edges of the nares and columella.

G   The nares and columella are shaped after the edema has completely subsided (plate 92, steps *D*, *E* and *F*). Final tailoring of these structures depends on defects. The columella will probably require a strut of autogenous cartilage for support. The extent

(Text continued on opposite page.)

Plate 88   The Nose and the Nasopharynx

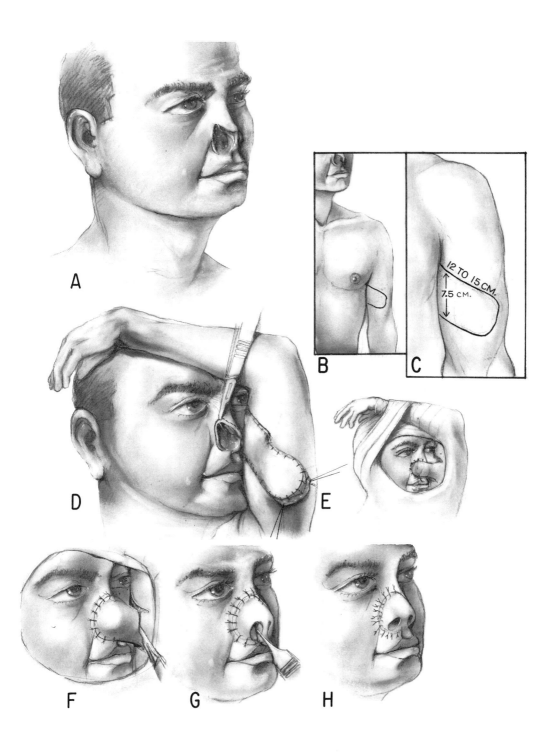

H   of the defect along the bridge and whether or not there is sufficient septal cartilage
will govern the need for another cartilage graft to support the bridge. The nares will
most likely require a Z-plasty at the apices to shape both a functional airway and
natural external contour (plate 92, steps *G, H* and *I*).

NASAL RECONSTRUCTION WITH LATERAL FOREHEAD FLAP

Highpoints

1. Plan forehead flap in such a manner that the returned pedicle and other rotated scalp flaps will cover the forehead donor site. Careful preoperative evaluation of hairline in men and hairdressing styles in women will aid in this planning.
2. Delay flap three times and before transfer wait until there is minimal edema.
3. That part of the flap to form the nose should include skin only, while the pedicle includes muscle and galea.
4. Line the future new nose flap with split thickness or dermal skin graft or local turn-in flaps from remaining nose or face (see plate 91).
5. A drawback is a scar on the forehead—unfavorable in a young patient. See also plate 121.

A   The flap is outlined using the measurements depicted as a rule of thumb. The extent of the defect will change these measurements. Allow about 15 per cent for shrinkage. At this stage only the upper and lower skin margins are incised, leaving both ends intact. Along the pedicle portion, the incision is made down through the galea while at the distal end, which will form the future nose, only skin is incised. This permits a better blood supply for the pedicle and at the distal end there is only full thickness skin, thus avoiding a bulky future nose. At the end of two weeks, the skin of the distal end is shaped and incised with flares to form the nares and a projection to form the columella. It is not necessary to undermine the flap completely, since there is no significant blood supply from the periosteum.

B   Two weeks later the entire flap is elevated, swung into position and evaluated regarding length. If additional length is needed, the upper or lower incision is extended at the base of the pedicle. Possibly only the galea need be incised, thus preserving the precious blood vessels. If desired and if the color of the flap is satisfactory, the lining for the future nose may now be grafted using split thickness skin only where necessary. At the same time, the opposing donor site is grafted with thick split thickness skin. The entire flap is then returned and sutured along its bed. The two skin grafts are now face to face. The only drawback may be the collection of some fluid at these graft sites.

C   After the edema has subsided—this may take up to two months—the flap is transferred. The columella is formed by folding over the projecting end of the flap and applying one or two mattress sutures with rubber or plastic booties. Be sure the skin is cleaned of all adipose tissue during this and the next step. The bare forehead donor site is covered with split thickness skin. A relatively slender, strong strip of bone can act as a bridge support secured at the glabella and as a cantilever attached to the tip (Millard, 1967).

D   The alae nasi are formed by turning in the edges and using mattress sutures with booties.

E   If a skin graft lining was not used in step *B*, a lining split thickness skin graft is now applied and held in place with several fine catgut sutures. In any case, the flap must have bare areas at its point of contact with the recipient areas. In turn, these recipient areas should be carefully freshened and broadened if necessary to furnish adequate arterial supply and venous return for the flap. This step is very important.

F   After three to four weeks, the flap is divided in **V** fashion (see plate 92, steps *A, B* and *C*). If desired, this division may be staged over a period of one week. The remaining portion of the flap is then returned to the forehead, removing the unwanted skin graft. The top wing of the **V** on the returned flap may be rotated downward to meet the lower wing.

Complications

1. Bulky and edematous at nares, causing airway obstruction.
2. Kinking of flap, causing vascular obstruction.

Plate 89   The Nose and the Nasopharynx

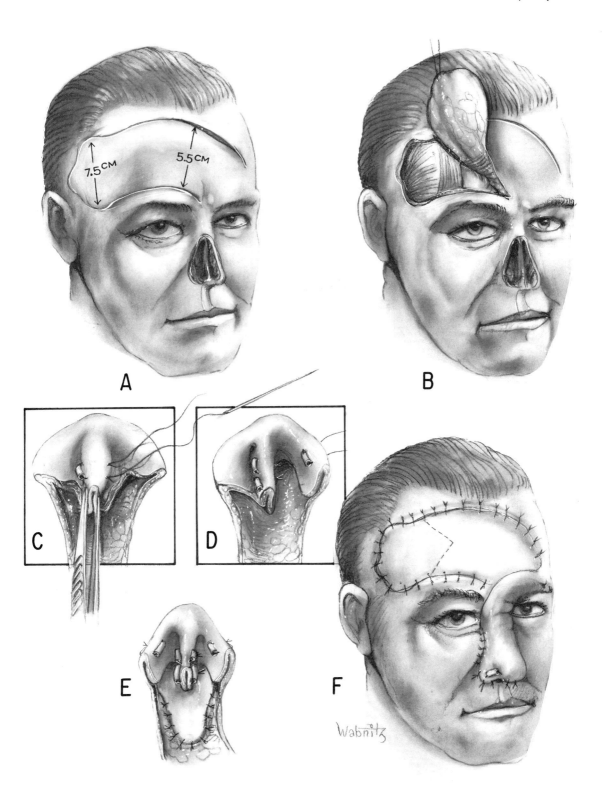

A

B

C

D

E

F

Wabnitz

NASAL RECONSTRUCTION WITH COMBINED
SCALP AND FOREHEAD FLAPS

THE SICKLE FLAP—*A* AND *B*

The technique of elevation, delay, shaping and skin grafting is similar to that for the forehead flap described in detail on plate 89.

Stages

1. Elevate flap between the two ends.
2. Two weeks later the distal or forehead end is transected.
3. Three weeks later the entire flap is elevated and returned to its bed. At this stage a split thickness graft may be inserted as the lining of the future nose.
4. Six to nine weeks later—after the edema has subsided—the flap is rotated into position over the nasal defect.
5. Three to four weeks later the pedicle is transected in **V** fashion. This may be staged over a one week period.
6. Two to four weeks later refinement of the grafted nose is begun (see plate 92).
7. Blood supply is from superficial temporal and posterior auricular arteries.

THE "SCALPING" FLAP (CONVERSE, 1959)—*C, D, E* AND *F*

The main difference in technique with this type of flap is that it can be swung either at the initial stage or with only one delay. If used for reconstruction following subtotal or total nasal resection for carcinoma, the flap is outlined and edges incised at the time of the resection. Although immediate reconstruction with transfer of the flap is more common, a delay of one or more weeks may be preferred. This delay serves several purposes. Time is allowed for permanent histologic sections to be evaluated regarding adequacy of the resection for the carcinoma. This basic principle in the surgery of a malignant tumor, especially when the nasal mucosa is involved, is sound even though frozen section may have been used. Delay also allows skin grafting for the lining of the flap. Turn-in flaps at the site of the defect are not recommended in the surgery for a malignant tumor, since extension of disease at a later date may be masked.

During this delay, the raw areas at the site of the nasal defect are covered with split thickness skin.

C
C¹ The flap is outlined and incised as depicted. The details of size and shape are as shown in plate 89, step *A*. The distal end does not include the frontalis muscle which is left in place, as is done in the other forehead and scalp flaps (plate 89, step *B*). This minimizes the occurrence of a bulbous nose. The remainder of the flap includes all layers down to the periosteum. Hence, the frontalis muscle is split at the medial border of the free distal end so that it can be included in the base of the flap.

D The entire flap is elevated and folded on itself, thus covering the major portion of the raw area of the flap. If any raw area remains, especially in the region where the flap crosses the brow and that portion of the nose which is intact, split thickness skin is used for cover. This is most important since any raw area is susceptible to infection and troublesome drainage. The donor site is likewise skin grafted.

E The flap in position. The distal end forming the nose is shaped as in steps *C*, *D* and *E* of plate 89.

F The pedicle is transected in **V** fashion in three to four weeks, in stages if necessary. The final shaping follows the technique shown in plate 92.

When the flap is returned to the scalp, an attempt is made to adjust it so that a minimal forehead defect results.

Complications

1. Problems in shaping the alar nasi.
2. Nasal obstruction.

Plate 90   The Nose and the Nasopharynx

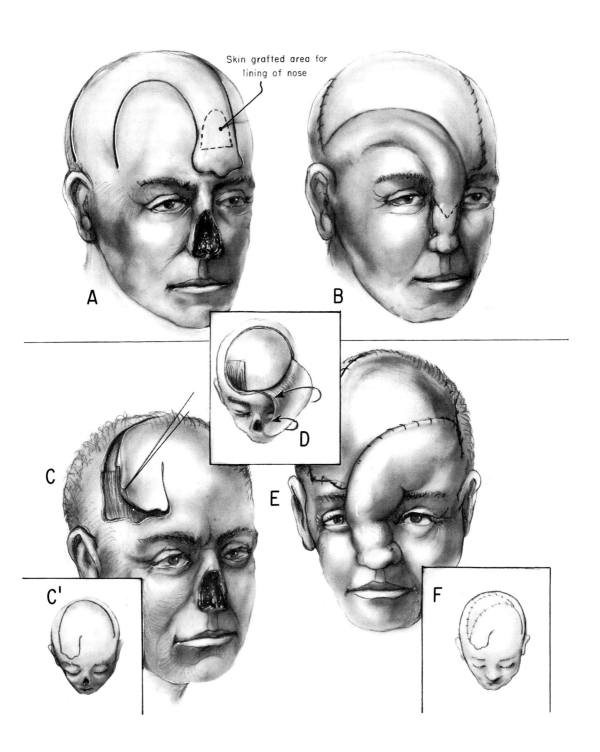

Skin grafted area for lining of nose

A

B

C

C'

D

E

F

NASAL TURN-IN FLAPS

Indications

In total or subtotal loss of the nose, local turn-in flaps serve as skin lining for the nasal cavity. The outer covering is obtained from an arm, forehead or scalp flap. Cartilage grafts are usually necessary for large defects.

A   Four turn-in flaps are elevated and made as thin as possible. One flap above is brought down from the bridge. One flap below is turned up from the lip for the columella. Two lateral flaps are outlined and reflected from the nasolabial regions.

B   These flaps are then sutured to one another with 4-0 chromic catgut. If structural support is believed necessary, cartilage grafts are placed on the flaps. One strip is used for the bridge with or without a hinged portion for columella support. Cartilage grafts can also be placed for support of the ala nasi. A portion of the nasolabial defect and lip defect may be closed by advanced flaps. An arm, forehead or scalp flap is now used for external cover (see plates 88, 89, and 90).

Complications

1. Absorption of cartilage grafts.
2. Contracture with nasal obstruction.

Plate 91   The Nose and the Nasopharynx

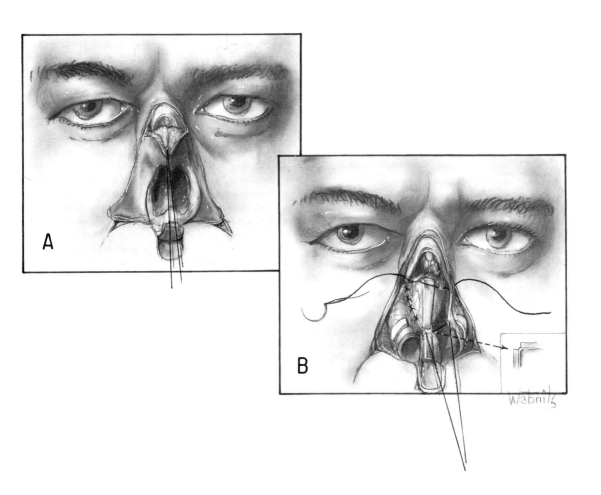

TRANSECTION OF FOREHEAD AND SCALP PEDICLE IN NASAL RECONSTRUCTION

A   The pedicle of a forehead or scalp flap used for the reconstruction in subtotal or total loss of the nose is transected in three to four weeks in one or two stages. The method of Penn is ideal since it acclimates the graft to the remaining portion of the nose. A **V** type of incision is used as depicted.

B   The **V** incision is bevelled on the undercut so that a smooth approximation is facilitated along the dorsum (bridge) of the nose.

C   The completed approximation results in a **T** closure.

REVISION OF NASOLABIAL FOLD AND ALA NASI IN NASAL RECONSTRUCTION

D   Following subtotal or total nasal reconstruction, the lateral borders of the new nose usually require revision. The superior portion of the nasolabial fold may be retracted and too deep. The ala nasi may be too bulky. An incision is made as depicted.

E   Any excess subcutaneous tissue is excised at the lateral border of the ala nasi.

F   The superior portion of the nasolabial fold is reapproximated with everting mattress sutures while the lateral borders of the ala nasi are reapproximated with simple sutures. If deepening of this lateral border is necessary, these sutures grasp the underlying tissue or even the periosteum. This will tend to invert and deepen the lateral sulcus.

ENLARGEMENT OF NARES WITH Z-PLASTY

Proper shaping of the nares at the time of flap reconstruction is not always satisfactory. Revision is done at another stage using a modified Z-plasty (Joseph). Such a deformity may also be congenital and is corrected in the same fashion.

G   A triangular flap of skin is first elevated with its base on the columella. Excess subcutaneous tissue is excised.

H   The lower flap is freed by an incision along the septum and then raised and sutured to the rim of the ala nasi.

I   The first flap is now swung in against the septum and sutured in place. The same steps are repeated on the opposite side. The nares are then firmly packed with Furacin-soaked cotton.

For other nares and columella procedures see plate 80.

Plate 92   The Nose and the Nasopharynx

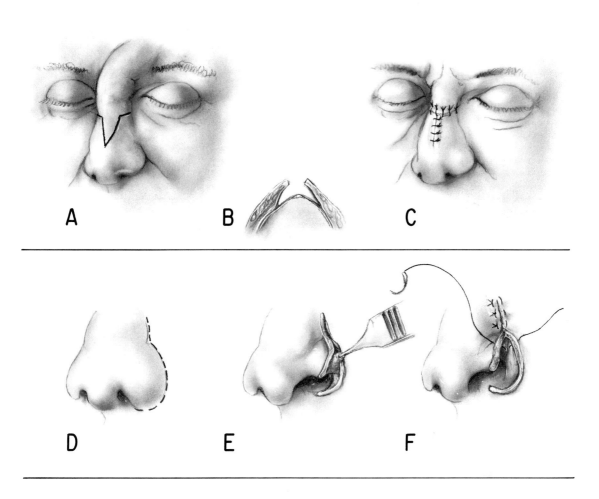

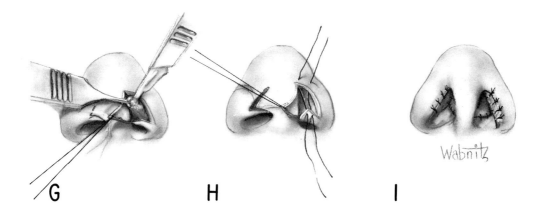

RESECTION OF NASAL SEPTUM FOR CARCINOMA
(LATERAL RHINOTOMY APPROACH)

Highpoints

1. Wide resection of septum with adjacent floor of nose.
2. Electrosurgical cutting knife to aid in control of hemorrhage when transecting mucous membrane.
3. Adequate visualization. Usually requires lateral rhinotomy to evaluate gross extent of tumor, especially in reference to floor of nose. For small lesions, centrally located, septum with both layers of mucoperichondrium can be resected through intact nares.
4. If possible, leave anterior and dorsal strut of septal cartilage for nasal support. This must not be done if adequate resection of safe margins around tumor would be jeopardized. Support then is achieved with autogenous cartilage or bone grafts (see plates 22 and 77) or Silastic strut.

A   A lateral rhinotomy incision is made extending along the nasofacial sulcus. When the lower edge of the nasal (frontal) process of the maxilla is reached, the incision is extended into the nasal cavity. The lateral nasal and angular vessels, branches of the external maxillary artery and tributaries of the anterior facial vein, should be identified above and below and be ligated. The lateral attachment of the ala nasi is completely mobilized by swinging the incision into the floor of the nose.

B   The nasal flap is rotated upward and medially. With the septal lesion located anteriorly or distally on the septum, such a flap suffices for visualization. For more posteriorly located tumors, however, a lateral bone flap is developed. This is performed by transection of the base of the nasal process of the maxilla and transection of its superior attachment along the same plane as the horizontal suture line of the lateral nasal bone. This is demonstrated in plate 95, step *F*.

C   Additional exposure, if necessary, is gained by transection of the columella at its base. An incision is then made posterior to the columella, the exact location depending on the anterior extent of the tumor. In the tumor pictured, no septal cartilage remains anterior. The only cartilages in the columella then are the two medial crura of the alar cartilages. With an electrocautery knife, the incision is extended around the septal angle at the tip of the nose and upward along the dorsal aspect of the septum. This incision is through and through, and, if possible, a strut of septal cartilage is preserved along the bridge of the nose for support. Preservation of any nasal supporting cartilage must *not* be done at the expense of adequate resection of the tumor. In situations in which no anterior or dorsal cartilage strut is preserved, cartilage or bone grafts or Silastic is used either at the time of the primary operation or at a second stage (see plate 77).

D   The septal incision has been carried across the posterior aspect down to the floor of the nose. This will entail removal of a portion of the perpendicular plate of the ethmoid and the vomer bones. Care must be exercised in high posterior resections that the cribriform plate of the ethmoid, which is continuous with the perpendicular plate, is not inadvertently fractured, with resultant opening into the anterior cranial fossa. Obviously extension of disease in this region may require elective removal of a portion of the cribriform plate. The dural leak if small may be handled by the use of a piece of Gelfoam held in place with Furacin-soaked gauze. Massive doses of antibiotics are used to prevent meningitis. Local Bacitracin may also be used.

Using an osteotome, the inferior portion of the septum is now freed by transecting the crest of the maxillae anteriorly and, if posterior resection is indicated, the crest of the palatine bone. If the tumor has extended further along the floor of the nose, an entire section of the midportion of the maxillae will require resection (see plate 31).

E   The completed resection. An anterior cartilage graft (see plate 22) with an attached piece of perichondrium is inserted in the columella. The inferior end is placed near

(Text continued on opposite page.)

Plate 93   The Nose and the Nasopharynx

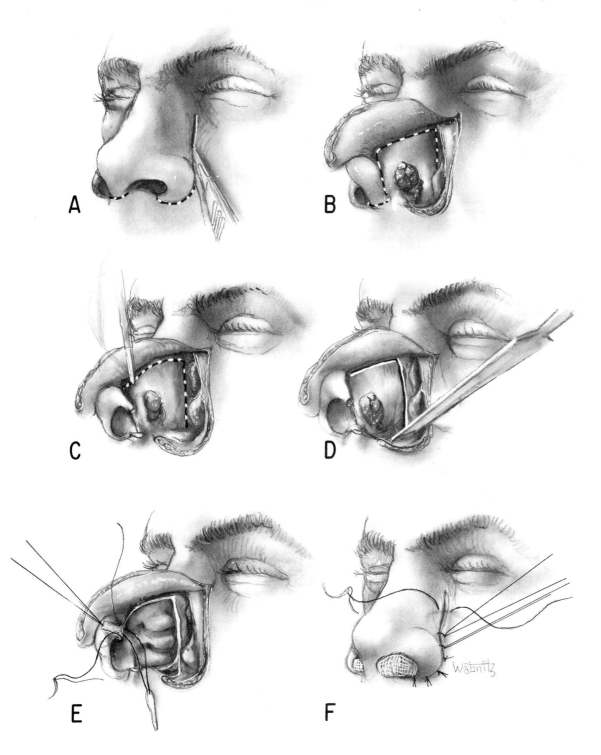

the anterior nasal spine. It is important that the mucocutaneous edges be closed behind the cartilage graft so that it becomes completely covered.

F   All skin edges are approximated after the nasal cavity is packed with Furacin-soaked one half inch strip gauze.

TOTAL RESECTION OF NOSE FOR CARCINOMA

Highpoints

1. Unusually wide resection of external framework.
2. Careful evaluation of internal extent of disease.
3. Wide resection of nasal septum and columella.

A
B   The skin incision is outlined. The entire columella is excised and the incision encompasses the base of the nasal septum to the floor of the nasal cavity.

C   The excision is begun from the lateral edge of one naris so that there is adequate visualization to determine the extent of the septal invasion by the neoplasm.

D   After both lateral walls of the nose have been sectioned, excision of the columella and nasal septum is begun. Liberal margins are resected. Stay sutures are used on the specimen to avoid use of clamps or forceps which might fragment the tumor and cause implants.

E   Whereas the cartilage is easily transected with a knife, the bony septum, nasal bones and nasal processes of the maxillae if encompassed in the resection may require bone cutting forceps.

F   The nasal cavity is packed with Furacin-soaked or antibiotic-impregnated gauze strips.

G   Split thickness skin is used to cover all bare areas; sutures are used only along the skin margins. A pressure dressing of Furacin-soaked cotton is applied. Cosmetic appearance is provided for by a prosthesis or forehead flaps (see plates 89 and 90).

Plate 94   *The Nose and the Nasopharynx*

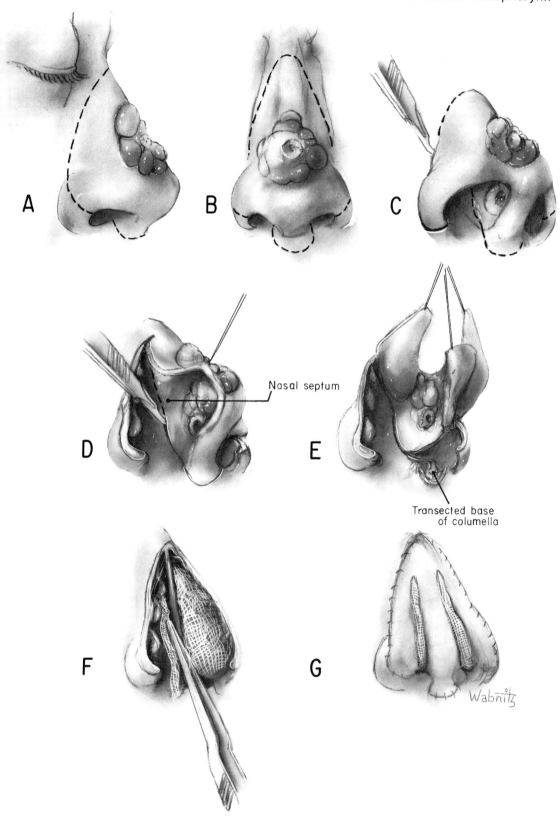

A

B

C

D

Nasal septum

E

Transected base
of columella

F

G

Wabnitz

RESECTION OF NASAL GLIOMA—EXTERNAL ETHMOID APPROACH

Highpoints

1. A nasal glioma is a space-occupying expansile lesion, histologically usually benign, arising from congenital central neural elements. It is an encephalocele and not a neoplasm.
2. There may be a connection with the intracranial cavity and hence removal may cause a dural defect with leakage of cerebrospinal fluid and danger of meningitis unless recognized.
3. In view of possibility of dural defect, any nasal polypoid mass in newborn must be considered a glioma until proved otherwise.
4. Intracranial extent of glioma is evaluated by air studies according to signs and symptoms.
5. If intracranial portion is large and especially if a large dural defect is anticipated, initial surgical attack is transcranial. However, dural defects are usually handled easily through an adequate transnasal approach. Important point is to recognize them and treat them accordingly.
6. Two stage procedures may be necessary when initial diagnosis is obscure.

A Rhinoscopic view of the polypoid mass which is the intranasal portion of the glioma. The overlying covering is normal appearing nasal mucosa which arises from the ethmoid region.

B The external appearance of the glioma present in this four-month-old child since birth. It resembles a dermoid cyst. Nasal gliomas may be either external or internal or both.

   The dotted and solid lines represent the skin incision. The excess skin is left attached to the glioma. The incision is that of an external ethmoid approach.

C Medial and lateral skin flaps are developed. A 0.5 cm diameter (external) pedicle of gliomatous tissue is seen extending through a smooth, well rounded defect in the nasal bone and nasal (frontal) process of the maxilla.

D The inferior margin of the nasal bone and nasal process of the maxilla are exposed and an incision is made along this margin to elevate the periosteum.

E The external portion of the glioma has been removed for simplicity of exposure and working space. Since it is not a neoplasm, this technique is permissible. In a staged procedure, this may conclude the first stage for diagnostic purposes and further evaluation.

   With a nasal freer, the periosteum is elevated over and under the nasal process of the maxilla.

F A lateral osteotomy is performed with a small curved chisel up to the bony defect. From this point, the chisel is directed horizontally across the superior suture line of the lateral nasal bone to the midline. This forms a periosteal bone flap which is attached in the midline along the dorsum of the nasal septum.

Plate 95   *The Nose and the Nasopharynx*

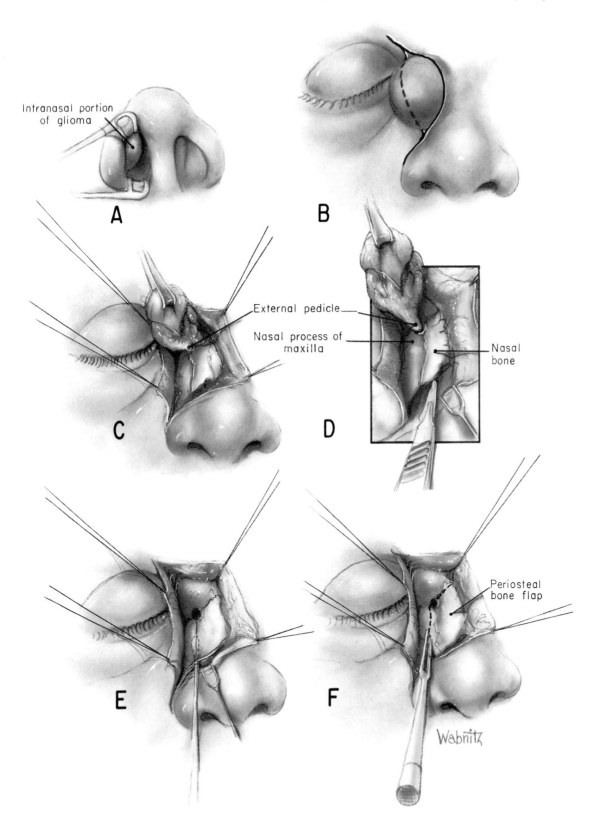

Intranasal portion
of glioma

A

B

External pedicle

Nasal process of
maxilla

Nasal
bone

C

D

E

Periosteal
bone flap

F

Wabnitz

RESECTION OF NASAL GLIOMA — EXTERNAL
ETHMOID APPROACH (*Continued*)

G   The periosteal bone flap is swung medially along its hinged attachment to the septum. The intranasal portion of the glioma is seen extending from the ethmoid labyrinth covered with nasal mucosa and attached to the septum. With sharp dissection along the mucosal reflection on the septum and careful blunt dissection in the ethmoid region, mobilization is begun.

H   As the glioma is dissected, another (internal) pedicle becomes exposed, extending through the roof of the ethmoid labyrinth into the anterior cranial fossa. The middle and inferior turbinates are not involved.

I   The entire intranasal glioma and as much of its pedicle as possible are removed. There is a small dural defect through which cerebrospinal fluid leaks. A patch of Gelfoam is placed over the dural defect.

J   Furacin-soaked or antibiotic-impregnated one fourth inch strip gauze is inserted through the nares and placed firmly against the Gelfoam to keep the latter in place.

K   The periosteal bone flap is turned back into position and fixed with periosteal sutures of 4-0 chromic catgut.

L   The skin is approximated with interrupted 5-0 nylon. Massive doses of penicillin and a broad spectrum antibiotic are used until all evidence of cerebrospinal fluid leak has ceased. Bacitracin is used locally on the packing.

Plate 96   The Nose and the Nasopharynx

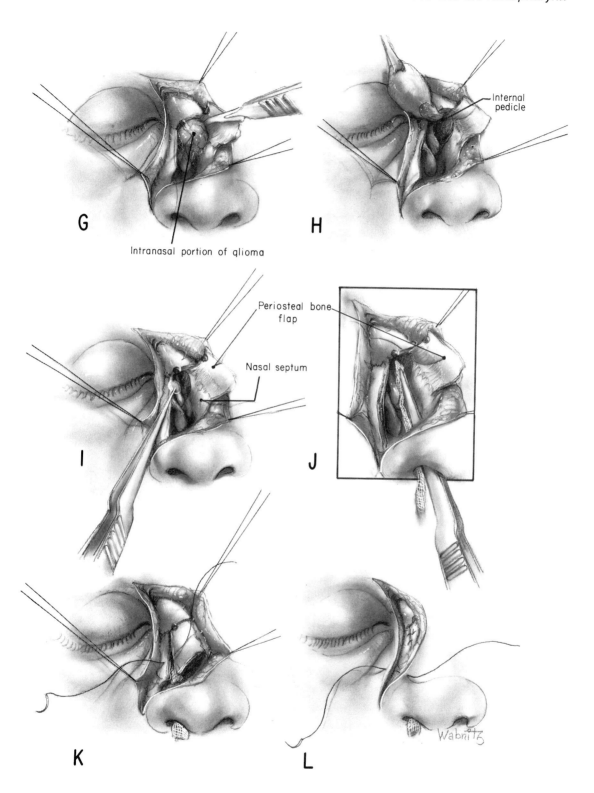

G

Intranasal portion of glioma

H

Internal pedicle

I

Periosteal bone flap

Nasal septum

J

K

L

Wabnitz

EXCISION OF RHINOPHYMA

Rhinophyma is thought to be the final stage of acne rosacea. It is a benign nodular swelling consisting of dilated blood vessels. Between the nodules are fissures of varying depths containing greatly increased numbers and sizes of sebaceous glands.

Highpoints

1. Do not expose cartilage.
2. Preserve rim of nares.
3. Grafting usually speeds recovery, although the skin will regenerate if remnants of the epidermis remain.

A   The hyperplastic sebaceous glands, fibrous tissue and involved skin are planed down to the desired size without injury to the perichondrium.

B   If the area to be grafted is large, split thickness skin is taken from the clavicular area and sewn tightly in place once the bleeding has been controlled.

Plate 97   The Nose and the Nasopharynx

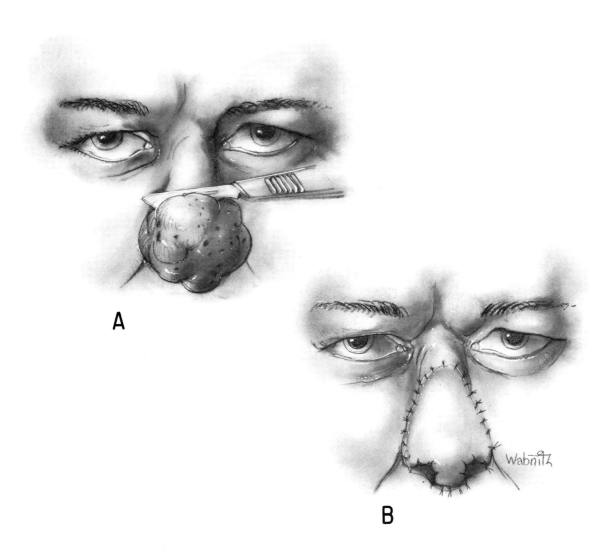

A

B

BIBLIOGRAPHY

Allen, G. W.: Ligation of the internal maxillary artery for epistaxis. Laryngoscope 80:915–923, 1970.

Anderson, J. R.: New approach to rhinoplasty. Arch. Otolaryng. 93:284–291, 1971.

Apostal, J. V., and Frazell, E. L.: Juvenile nasopharyngeal angiofibroma: A clinical study. Cancer 18:869–878, 1965.

Ardran, G. M., and Kemp, F. H.: The nasal and cervical airway in sleep in neonatal period. Amer. J. Roentgen. 108:537–542, 1970.

Aretsky, P. J., Freund, H. R., Kantu, K., and Polisar, I. A.: Chondrosarcoma of the nasal septum. Ann. Otol. 79:382, 1970.

Badib, A. O., Kurohara, S. S., Webster, J. H., and Shedd, D. P.: Treatment of cancer of the nasal cavity. Amer. J. Roentgen. 106:824–829, 1969.

Bartels, R. J., O'Malley, J. E., Baker, J. L., and Douglas, W. M.: Naso-ocular clefts. Plast. Reconstr. Surg. 47:351–353, 1971.

Batsakis, J. G.: Mucous gland tumors of the nose and paranasal sinuses. Ann. Otol. 79:557, 1970.

Bayon, P. J.: The Stevens nasal balloon: Further experience with its use in the management of epistaxis. Eye Ear Nose Throat Monthly 44:74–77, 1965.

Becker, O. J.: Problems of septum in rhinoplastic surgery. Arch. Otolaryng. 53:622–639, 1951.

Beinfield, H. H.: Bilateral choanal atresia in the newborn. Arch. Otolaryng. 73:659–661, 1961.

Beinfield, H. H.: Closure of choanal atresia opening explained. Arch. Otolaryng. 83:480–481, 1966.

Beinfield, H. H.: Surgery for bilateral bony atresia of the posterior nares in the newborn. Arch. Otolaryng. 70:1–7, 1959.

Beinfield, H. H.: Surgical management of bony choanal atresia of the posterior nares. Instruction Section, Trans. Amer. Acad. Ophthal. Otolaryng., 1965.

Beinfield, H. H.: Surgical management of complete and incomplete bony atresia of the posterior nares (choanae). Amer. J. Surg. 89:957–963, 1955.

Berger, D. S., Fletcher, G. H., Lindberg, R. D., and Jesse, R. H., Jr.: Elective irradiation of the neck lymphatics for squamous cell carcinomas of the nasopharynx and oropharynx. Amer. J. Roentgen. 111:66–71, 1971.

Berkeley, W. T.: The cleft-lip nose. Plast. Reconstr. Surg. 23:567–575, 1959.

Bloom, S. M.: Rhinoplasty in adolescence. Arch. Otolaryng. 92:66–70, 1970.

Bocca, E.: Transpharyngeal approach to nasopharyngeal fibroma. Ann. Otol. 80:171, 1971.

Bordley, J. E., and Longmire, W. P.: Rhinotomy for exploration of the nasal passages and the accessory nasal sinuses. Ann. Otol. 58:1055, 1949.

Brown, J. B., and McDowell, F.: Skin Grafting. 3d ed. Philadelphia, J. B. Lippincott Company, 1958. Chapter 13.

Brunk, A.: A new case of unilateral osseous choanal occlusion: An operation through the palate. Z. Ohrenheilk. 59:221, 1909.

Bryce, D. P., and Crysdale, W. S.: Nonhealing granuloma: A diagnostic problem. Laryngoscope 79:794–805, 1969.

Butler, R. M., Nahum, A. M., and Hanafee, W.: New surgical approach to nasopharyngeal angiofibromas. Trans. Amer. Acad. Ophthal. Otolaryng. January–February, 1967.

Chandler, J. R.: Iatrogenic cerebrospinal rhinorrhea. Trans. Amer. Acad. Ophthal. Otolaryng. 74:576–584, 1970.

Cinelli, J. A.: Lengthening of nose by a septal flap. Plast. Reconstr. Surg. 43:99–101, 1969.

Cocke, E. W., Jr.: Transpalatine surgical approach to the nasopharynx and the posterior nasal cavity. Amer. J. Surg. 108:517–525, 1964.

Conley, J., Healey, W. V., Blaugrund, S. M., and Perzin, K. H.: Nasopharyngeal angiofibroma in the juvenile. Surg. Gynec. Obstet. 126:825–837, 1968.

Converse, J. M.: Corrective plastic surgery of the nose. In Jackson, C., and Jackson, C. L. (eds.): Diseases of the Nose, Throat and Ear. 2d ed. Philadelphia, W. B. Saunders Company, 1959.

Converse, J. M.: Surgical elongation of the traumatically foreshortened nose. The perinasal osteotomy. Plast. Reconstr. Surg. 47:529–546, 1971.

Converse, J. M.: The surgical treatment of facial injuries. Proc. Roy. Soc. Med. 38:811, 1942.

Crawford, H. H., Horton, C. E., and Adamson, J. E.: Composite earlobe grafts for one-stage reconstruction of facial defects. Plast. Reconstr. Surg. 42:51–57, 1968.

Davison, F. W.: Intranasal surgery. Laryngoscope 79:502–511, 1969.

Denecke, H. J., and Meyer, R.: Plastic Surgery of Head and Neck, Corrective and Reconstructive Rhinoplasty. Berlin, Springer-Verlag, 1967.

Dingman, R. O., and Claus, W. C.: Use of composite ear grafts in correction of the short nose. Plast. Reconstr. Surg. 43:117–124, 1969.

Doyle, P. J.: Approach to tumors of the nose, nasopharynx and paranasal sinuses. Laryngoscope 78:1756–1762, 1968.

Doyle, P. J., and Paxton, H. D.: Combined surgical approach to esthesioneuroepithelioma. Trans. Amer. Acad. Ophthal. Otolaryng. 75:526–531, 1971.

Duncan, R. B., and Briggs, M.: Treatment of uncomplicated anosmia by vitamin A. Arch. Otolaryng. 75:116, 1962.

Durisch, L. L., Jr., and Frable, M. A.: A surgical solution for posterior epistaxis. Surg. Gynec. Obstet. 133:669–670, 1971.

Eller, J. L., Roberts, J. F., and Ziter, F. M. H., Jr.: Normal nasopharyngeal soft tissue in adults: A statistical study. Amer. J. Roentgen. 112:537–541, 1971.

Fairbanks, D. N. F., and Chen, S. C. A.: Closure of large nasal septum perforations. Arch. Otolaryng. 91:403–406, 1970.

Farrior, R. T.: Corrective surgery of the nasal framework. J. Florida Med. Ass. 45:276–289, 1958.

Farrior, R. T., and Connolly, M. E.: Septorhinoplasty in children. Otolaryng. Clin. N. Amer. 3:345–364, 1970.

Fearon, B., and Dickson, J.: Bilateral choanal atresia in the newborn: Plan of action. Laryngoscope 78:1487–1499, 1968.

Flake, C. G., and Ferguson, C. F.: Congenital atresia in infants and children. Ann. Otol. 73:458–473, 1964.

Flowers, R. S., and Anderson, R.: Injury to the lacrimal apparatus during rhinoplasty. Plast. Reconstr. Surg. 42:577–581, 1968.

Fomon, S.: Cosmetic Surgery. Philadelphia, J. B. Lippincott Company, 1960.

Freeman, B. S.: Reconstructive rhinoplasty for rhinophyma. Plast. Reconstr. Surg. 46:265–268, 1970.

Gerughty, R. M., Hennigar, G. R., and Brown, F. M.: Adenosquamous carcinoma of the nasal, oral and laryngeal cavities — A clinicopathologic survey of ten cases. Cancer 22:1140–1155, 1968.

Goldman, I. B.: Maxillofacial triad and its correction with special reference to nasal septum. J. Int. Coll. Surg. 17:157–180, 1952.

Gorney, A. J.: Illustrations for septum surgery in the twisted nose. Instruction Section, Trans. Amer. Acad. Ophthal. Otolaryng., 1962.

Hagan, P. J.: Posttraumatic anosmia. Arch. Otolaryng. 85:85, 1967.

Henderson, G. P., Jr., and Patterson, C. N.: Further experience in treatment of juvenile nasopharyngeal angiofibroma. Laryngoscope 79:561–580, 1969.

Hinderer, K.: Fundamentals of Anatomy and Surgery of the Nose. Birmingham, Aesculapius Publishing Company, 1971.

Hiranandani, L. H.: Nasopharyngeal angiofibroma. Rev. Laryng. (Bordeaux) 86:733–746, 1965.

Hiranandani, N. L., Jr.: Treatment of chronic vasomotor rhinitis with clinicopathological study of vidian nerve section in 150 cases. J. Laryng. 80:902–932, 1966.

Hutter, R. V. P., Lewis, J. S., Foote, F. W., Jr., and Tollefsen, H. R.: Esthesioneuroblastoma. A clinical and pathological study. Amer. J. Surg. 106:748–753, 1963.

Jereb, B., Anggard, A., and Baryd, I.: Juvenile nasopharyngeal angiofibroma. Acta Radiol. 9:302–310, 1970.

Johnson, N. E.: Revision surgery of nasal septum. New York J. Med. 71:2300–2302, 1971.

Johnson, N. E.: Septal surgery and rhinoplasty. Trans. Amer. Acad. Ophthal. Otolaryng., September–October, 1964.

Kaplan, G., Rubenfeld, S., and Gordon, R. B.: Unusual manifestations of carcinoma of the nasopharynx. A case report. Cancer 24:781–785, 1969.

Katz, A., and Lewis, J. S.: Nasal gliomas. Arch. Otolaryng. 94:351–355, 1971.

Kazanjian, V. H., and Converse, J. M.: Surgical Treatment of Facial Injuries. 2d ed. Baltimore, The Williams & Wilkins Company, 1959.

Kirchner, J. A., Yanagisawa, E., and Crelin, E. S., Jr.: Surgical anatomy of the ethmoidal arteries. Arch. Otolaryng. 74:382–386, 1961.

Kremen, A. J.: Surgical management of angiofibroma of the nasopharynx. Ann. Surg. 138:672, 1953.

Krizek, T. J., and Robson, M. C.: The split flap technique in head and neck reconstruction. Presentation at Society of Head and Neck Surgeons and American Society for Head and Neck Surgery, May 1973.

Lehman, J. A., Jr., Garrett, W. S., Jr., and Musgrave, R. H.: Earlobe composite grafts for the correction of nasal defects. Plast. Reconstr. Surg. 47:12–16, 1971.

Lewis, J. S.: Sarcoma of the nasal cavity and paranasal sinuses. Ann. Otol. 78:778, 1969.

Lewis, J. S., Hutter, R. V. P., Tollefsen, H. R., and Foote, F. W., Jr.: Nasal tumors of olfactory origin. Arch. Otolaryng. 81:169–174, 1965.

Lin, H.-S., Lin, C.-S., Yeh, S., and Tu, S.-M.: Fine structure of nasopharyngeal carcinoma with special reference to the anaplastic type. Cancer 23:390–405, 1969.

Loeb, H. W.: Operative Surgery of the Nose, Throat and Ear. Vol. II. St. Louis, C. V. Mosby Company, 1917.

Lofgren, R. H.: Surgery of the Pterygomaxillary Fossa. Arch. Otolaryng. 94:516–524, 1971.

Longacre, J. J., Mayfield, F. H., Lotspeich, E. S., Kahl, J. B., Wood, R. W., Munick, L. H., and Chunekamrai, D.: Combined transoral, transcervical and transosseous team approach to tumors of the nasopharynx and pharyngeal region. Amer. J. Surg. 110:644–648, 1965.

Lowe, R. S., Robinson, D. W., Ketchum, L. D., and Masters, F. W.: Nasal gliomata. Plast. Reconstr. Surg. 47:1–5, 1971.

MacComb, W. S.: Juvenile nasopharyngeal fibroma. Amer. J. Surg. 106:754–763, 1963.

Mair, W. S., and Johannessen, T. A.: Nasopharyngeal tuberculosis. Arch. Otolaryng. 92:392–393, 1970.

Martin, H.: Surgery of Head and Neck Tumors. New York, Hoeber-Harper, 1957.

Martin, H., Ehrlich, H. E., and Abels, J. C.: Juvenile nasopharyngeal angiofibroma. Ann. Surg. 127:513–536, 1948.

Millard, D. R., Jr.: Hemirhinoplasty. Plast. Reconstr. Surg. 40:440–445, 1967.

Millard, D. R., Jr.: Total reconstructive rhinoplasty and a missing link. Plast. Reconstr. Surg. 37:167–183, 1966.

Miller, D., Goldman, J. M., and Goodman, M. L.: Etiologic study of nasopharyngeal cancer. Arch. Otolaryng. 94:104–108, 1971.

Miller, W. E., Holman, C. B., Dockerty, M. B., and Devine, K. D.: Roentgenologic manifestations of malignant tumors of the nasopharynx. Amer. J. Roentgen. 106:813–823, 1969.

Montgomery, W. W., Lofgren, R. H., and Chasin, W. D.: Analysis of pterygopalatine space surgery–1970. Presented at 73d Annual Meeting of Amer. Laryng. Rhinol. Otol. Soc., Hollywood Beach, Florida, April 1970.

Ommaya, A. K., Di Chiro, G., Baldwin, M., and Pennybacker, J. B.: Nontraumatic cerebrospinal fluid rhinorrhoea. J. Neurol. Neurosurg. Psychiat. 31:214–225, 1968.

Owens, H.: Observations in treating seven cases of choanal atresia by the transpalatine approach. Trans. Amer. Laryng. Rhinol. Otol. Soc. 295:312, 1951.

Parisier, S. C.: Correction of deviated nose. Arch. Otolaryng. 92:60–65, 1970.

Pearson, B. W., MacKenzie, R. G., and Goodman, W. S.: The anatomical basis of transantral ligation of the maxillary artery in severe epistaxis. Laryngoscope 79:969–984, 1969.

Pearson, C. M., Kline, H. M., and Newcomer, V. D.: Relapsing polychondritis. New Eng. J. Med. 263:51–58, 1960.

Penn, J.: Kiel-bone implants to the chin and nose. Plast. Reconstr. Surg. 42:303–306, 1968.

Perez, C. A., Ackerman, L. V., Mill, W. B., Ogura, J. H., and Powers, W. E.: Cancer of the nasopharynx. Factors influencing prognosis. Cancer 24:1–17, 1969.

Pilapil, V. R., Day, L. H., and Watson, D. G.: Cor pulmonale resulting from chronic nasopharyngeal obstruction.

Potter, G. D.: The pterygopalatine fossa and canal. Amer. J. Roentgen. 107:520–525, 1969.

Pressman, J. J.: Nasopharyngeal angiofibroma. Arch. Otolaryng. 76:167–173, 1962.

Quain, R.: The Anatomy of the Arteries of

the Human Body and Its Applications to Pathology and Operative Surgery. London, 1844.

Rees, T. D.: Nasal plastic surgery in the Negro. Plast. Reconstr. Surg. 43:13–18, 1969.

Rosen, L., Hanafee, W., and Nahum, A.: Nasopharyngeal angiofibroma, an angiographic evaluation. Radiology 86:103–107, 1966.

Rulon, J. T., Brown, H. A., and Logan, G. B.: Nasal polyps and cystic fibrosis of the pancreas. Arch. Otolaryng. 78:192–199, 1963.

Safian, J.: Corrective Rhinoplastic Surgery. New York, Paul B. Hoeber, 1935.

Sanchez-Casis, G., Devine, K. D., and Weiland, L. H.: Nasal adenocarcinomas that closely simulate colonic carcinomas. Cancer 28:714–720, 1971.

Sardana, D. S.: Nasopharyngeal fibroma. Arch. Otolaryng. 81:584–588, 1965.

Saunders, W. H.: Septal dermoplasty for control of nose bleeds caused by hereditary hemorrhagic telangiectoma. Trans. Amer. Acad. Ophthal. Otolaryng. 64:500–506, 1960.

Saunders, W. H.: Septal dermoplasty—Its several uses. Laryngoscope 80:1342–1446, 1970.

Schaeffer, J. P.: Embryology, development and anatomy of the nose, paranasal sinuses, nasolacrimal passageways and olfactory organ in man. Philadelphia, Blakiston, 1920.

Schiff, M.: Juvenile nasopharyngeal angiofibroma. Laryngoscope 69:981–1016, 1959.

Singleton, G. T., and Hardcastle, B.: Congenital choanal atresia. Arch. Otolaryng. 87:620–625, 1968.

Snyder, G. B.: Rhinoplasty in the Negro. Plast. Reconstr. Surg. 47:572–575, 1971.

Stark, R. B., and Frileck, S. P.: Conchal cartilage grafts in augmentation rhinoplasty and orbital floor fracture. Plast. Reconstr. Surg. 43:591–596, 1969.

Thomsen, K. A.: Surgical treatment of juvenile nasopharyngeal angiofibroma. Arch. Otolaryng. 94:191–194, 1971.

Uchida, J.-I.: A new approach to the correction of cleft lip nasal deformities. Plast. Reconstr. Surg. 47:454–458, 1971.

Unno, T., Nelson, J. R., and Ogura, J. H.: The effect of nasal obstruction on pulmonary, airway and tissue resistance. Laryngoscope 78:1119–1139, 1968.

Walike, J. W., and MacKay, B.: Nasopharyngeal angiofibroma: Light and electron microscopic changes after stilbestrol therapy. Laryngoscope 80:1109–1121, 1970.

Weddell, G., MacBeth, R. G., Sharp, H. S., and Calvert, C. A.: The surgical treatment of severe epistaxis in relation to the ethmoidal arteries. Brit. J. Surg. 33:387–392, 1946.

Williams, H. J.: Posterior choanal atresia. Amer. J. Roentgen. 112:1–11, 1971.

Wright, W. K.: General principles of lateral osteotomy and hump removal. Trans. Amer. Acad. Ophthal. Otolaryng. 65:854–816, 1961.

Wynn, S. K.: Primary nostril reconstruction in complete cleft lips. The round nostril technique. Plast. Reconstr. Surg. 49:56–60, 1972.

Young, F.: The surgical repair of nasal deformities. Plast. Reconstr. Surg. 4:59, 1949.

5. THE FACE

ANATOMY OF FACIAL AND SCALP MUSCLES

A   Depicted are the primary muscles of facial expression and major blood vessels. The reader is referred to the publications by Thomas S. Walsh, Jr. in the bibliography regarding the ligation of the feeder vessels in the treatment of giant strawberry nevi.

B   Depicted is a frontal section of the head showing the layers of the scalp, skull and meninges (after Piersol, 1911).

Plate 98   The Face

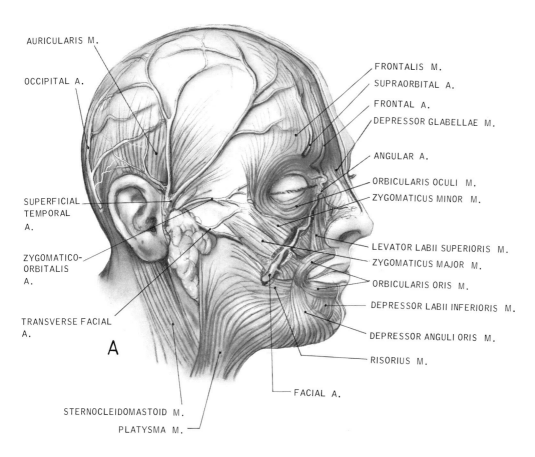

AURICULARIS M.

OCCIPITAL A.

SUPERFICIAL
TEMPORAL
A.

ZYGOMATICO-
ORBITALIS
A.

TRANSVERSE FACIAL
A.

FRONTALIS M.

SUPRAORBITAL A.

FRONTAL A.

DEPRESSOR GLABELLAE M.

ANGULAR A.

ORBICULARIS OCULI M.

ZYGOMATICUS MINOR M.

LEVATOR LABII SUPERIORIS M.

ZYGOMATICUS MAJOR M.

ORBICULARIS ORIS M.

DEPRESSOR LABII INFERIORIS M.

DEPRESSOR ANGULI ORIS M.

RISORIUS M.

FACIAL A.

STERNOCLEIDOMASTOID M.

PLATYSMA M.

A

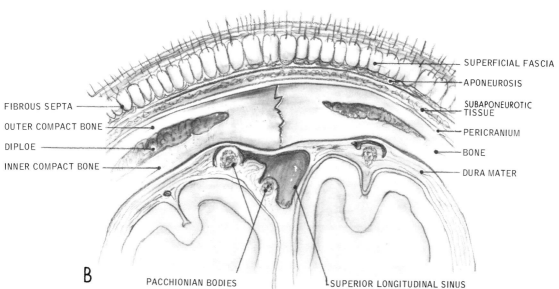

FIBROUS SEPTA

OUTER COMPACT BONE

DIPLOE

INNER COMPACT BONE

SUPERFICIAL FASCIA

APONEUROSIS

SUBAPONEUROTIC
TISSUE

PERICRANIUM

BONE

DURA MATER

B

PACCHIONIAN BODIES

SUPERIOR LONGITUDINAL SINUS

239

EXCISION OF SEBACEOUS CYST

A   The incision is outlined to include a wedge of overlying skin with the sebaceous duct involved. Even though the duct may not be apparent, the wedge of skin is always included.

B   The wedge of skin affords an excellent traction point for the cyst, while the capsule is dissected. The cyst is thus easily removed intact and the more viable skin edges ensure primary healing with a minimum of dimpling.

BASIC TECHNIQUE FOR EXCISION OF FACIAL LESIONS

C   The ellipse of skin excised always follows a natural skin crease.

D   The skin and subcutaneous tissue are cut in a plane at right angles to the skin. Forceps may be used on the specimen but should be avoided on the skin edges.

E   At least one margin is undermined adequately to prevent tension on the skin closure. This, plus the deep sutures, tends to maintain a fine scar. In this case, in the nasolabial fold only the lateral edge is mobilized to prevent distortion of the corner of the lips and mouth.

F   The deep or subcutaneous sutures of fine material, either 5-0 white silk or 5-0 chromic catgut, are placed so that the knots are buried. These sutures may grasp either the deep edge of dermis or superficial fascia, as the case may be.

G   5-0 or 6-0 nylon is used for the epidermis. Mattress sutures are utilized only when inversion occurs.

Plate 99   *The Face*

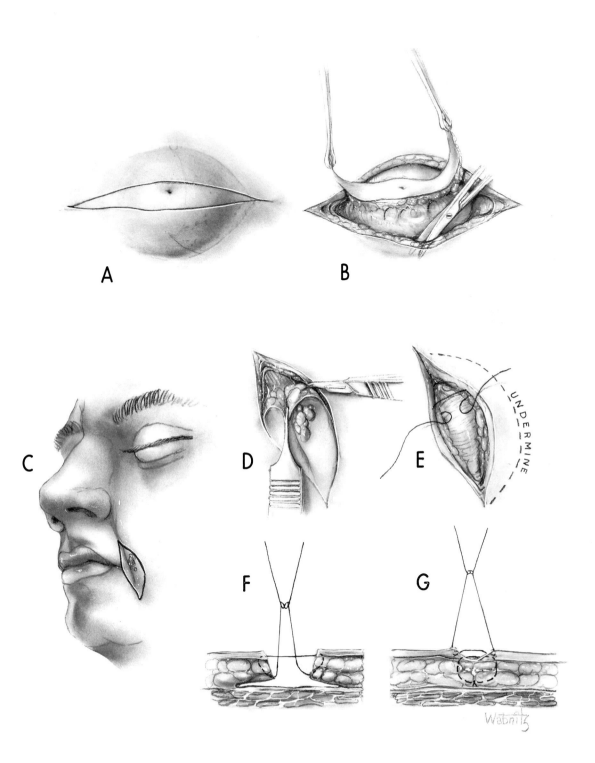

A

B

C

D

E

UNDERMINE

F

G

Wabnitz

EXCISION OF TUMORS OF SKIN OF FOREHEAD

Highpoints

1. Excision of all layers of scalp for malignant lesions.
2. Margins depend on type of tumor: basal cell requires 0.8 to 1 cm; squamous cell 1.5 to 2.0 cm beyond gross disease. Use frozen section on margin if in doubt.
3. Full thickness skin mobilization without muscle for advanced flaps to cover defect.

A Smaller lesions off the midline are excised as outlined, including skin, superficial fascia, galea and muscle. The galea is the tendinous aponeurosis which connects the occipitalis and frontalis muscles. The galea and muscles together form the epicranial layer. The line of cleavage is the subepicranial connective tissue space.

B A single, lateral, full thickness skin flap is mobilized. The underlying frontalis muscle and nerve are left intact except in the area excised when the tumor is malignant.

C The lateral flap is advanced and sutured in place using several subcuticular sutures of 4-0 chromic or 5-0 white silk and 5-0 nylon sutures for the skin.

D When the lesion is larger or in the midline, a shield-shaped excision is used with bilateral advanced flaps. Again the tissue is excised through the subepicranial space.

E Bilateral full thickness flaps are elevated, preserving the frontalis muscle and nerve.

F Closure is in similar fashion.

Plate 100   The Face

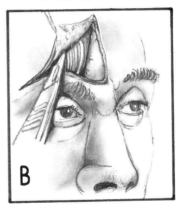

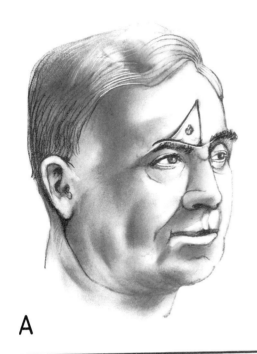

A

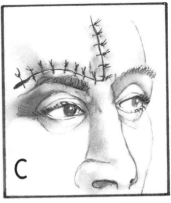

B

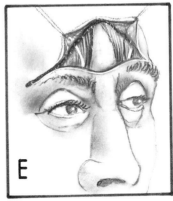

C

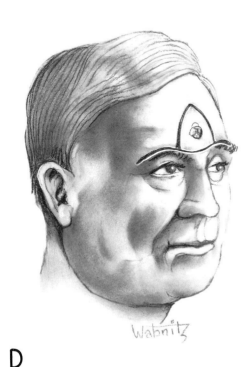

D

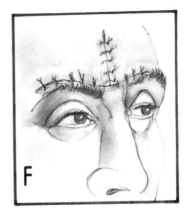

E

F

Wabnitz

243

EXCISION OF BASAL CELL CARCINOMA
OF SKIN OF TEMPLE

Highpoints

1. Wide excision to deep fascia.
2. Liberal mobilization of skin flaps.

A
A¹   The skin incision is made as outlined. The upper edge is slightly concave and the lower edge convex.

B   If compatible with adequate excision, a branch of the temporal division of the facial nerve is preserved at the inner angle of the operative site. At other areas, the excised tissue is carried down to the temporal fascia. Branches of the superficial temporal artery are ligated. Undermining is mainly carried out on the lower skin flap. This plane (E) is through the subcutaneous tissue, superficial to the fascia overlying the parotid gland.

C   A minimum of undermining is done on the upper flap. Here the plane (E) is superficial to the temporal fascia.

D   Two layer closure is used with 5-0 white silk buried and 5-0 nylon for the skin.

E   Depicted is the cross-sectional anatomy.

EXCISION OF SQUAMOUS CELL CARCINOMA
OF SKIN OF TEMPLE

F   When the tumor is bulkier or is a squamous cell carcinoma, the area excised must be wider and deeper. Closure is then achieved by raising a more extensive face flap with a postauricular incision. As the flap is rotated upward, the postauricular dog-ear is excised.

Plate 101   The Face

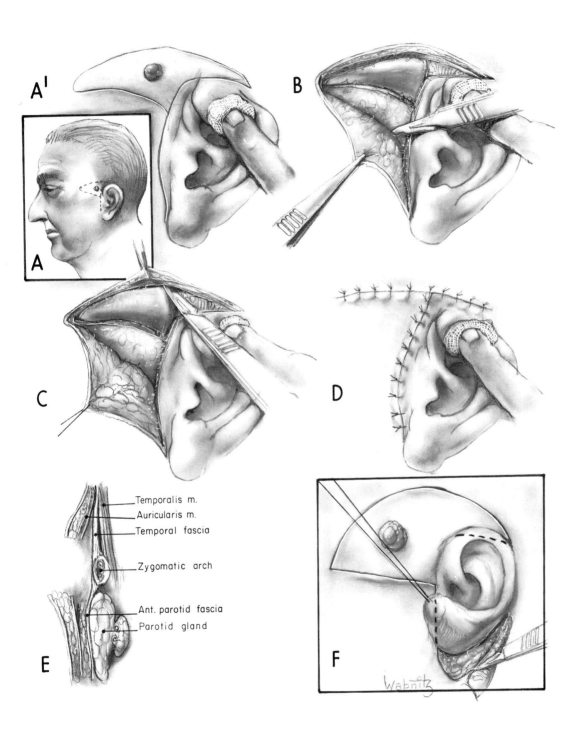

A'

A

B

C

D

E

Temporalis m.
Auricularis m.
Temporal fascia

Zygomatic arch

Ant. parotid fascia
Parotid gland

F

Wabnitz

TEMPORAL SCALP ROTATION FLAP
(After Mustardé, 1969)

The design of the flap must take into account the shifting of the hairline and traction on the eyebrow. Injury to the facial nerve must be avoided by any flaps which are used to cover the operative defect. The zygomatic branch to the orbicularis occuli muscle is the important one and usually this will not be injured if the lines of incision are above a horizontal line drawn from the lateral canthus of the eye. Above this level is the temporal branch to the forehead.

Highpoints

1. Adequate deep and wide resection of lesion if malignant — no regard for facial nerve.
2. However, do not injure zygomatic branch with flap incision.
3. Avoid traction superiorly on eyebrow — flap must be well mobilized and long.

Correct Method

A Depicted is lesion with area of resection and large scalp flap. When this flap is rotated, there will be minimal upward pull on the eyebrow. The amount of hairline advanced on to the forehead at the temple will be quite acceptable. Note the back cut which adds to the length of the flap.

Incorrect Method

B A poorly devised flap which is short and almost vertical.

C The result is an objectionable upward distortion of the eyebrow and noticeable drop in hairline on a conspicuous area of the forehead.

CHEEK FLAP ROTATION (After Mustardé, 1969)

D
E A lesion inferior to the lower lid on the cheek has been excised, including a small triangle of skin-stippled area below the resected area to facilitate a closure without the formation of a dog-ear. Also prevented is downward tension of the lower lid preventing ectropion.

A cutback incision (dotted line) may be necessary to afford greater length to the flap and to avoid tension. The cheek flap only involves skin and subcutaneous tissue, thus avoiding the branches of the facial nerve.

Plate 102   The Face

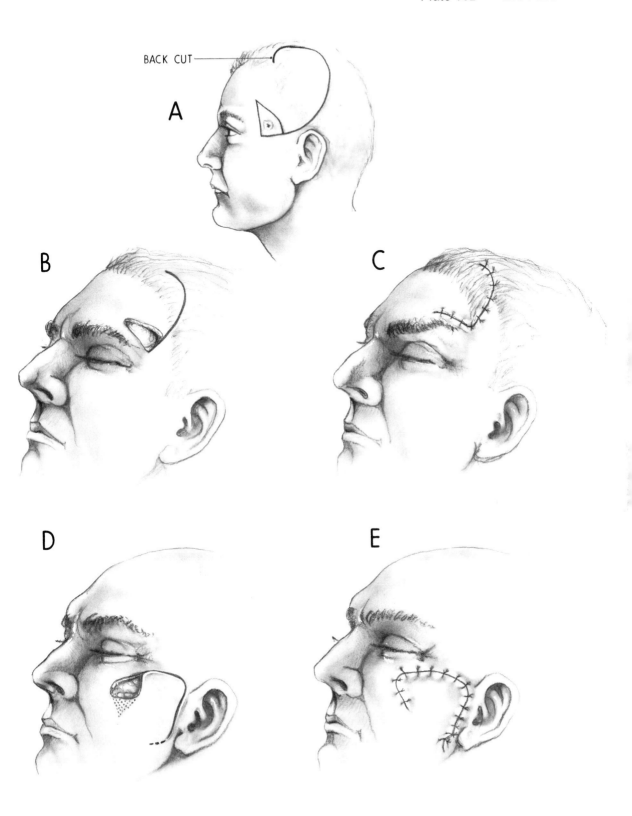

BACK CUT

A

B

C

D

E

EXCISION OF TUMORS OF CHEEK

Highpoints

1. Adequate mobilization and extent of cheek flap to prevent ectropion.
2. When elevating flap, preserve branches of facial nerve to orbicularis oculi muscle.

A   Tumor below lower lid close to nasolabial fold. Area of excision outlined. Cheek flap elevation shown in stippled area. The horizontal portion of the flap incision is just above the level of the lateral canthus. A back cut is shown if necessary (dotted line).

B   The completed procedure. If directly in the nasolabial fold, this lesion can be managed with a local flap or split thickness epidermal graft (plates 81, *A* to *D* and 86, *E*, *F* and *G*) or a midline forehead flap (plate 121, step *D*).

C
D   Tumor is smaller and located more laterally. Area of excision is outlined, with stippled area indicating lateral cheek flap. If there is undue tension, the cheek flap is extended as in steps *A* and *B*.

Plate 103   The Face

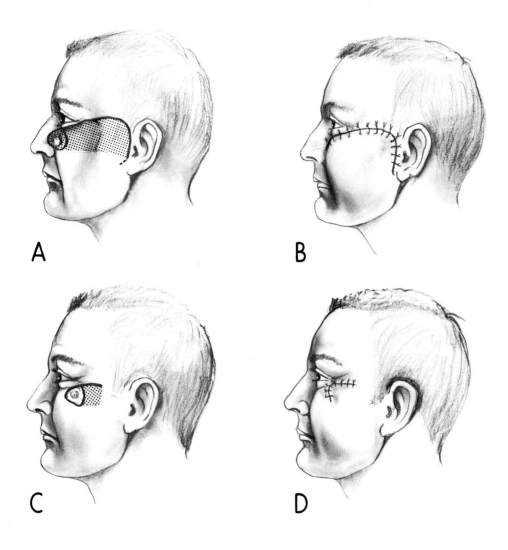

A

B

C

D

FASCIAL SLINGS FOR FACIAL PARALYSIS

Facial nerve paralysis should be initially managed at the source, whether it be Bell's palsy or traumatic or surgical section of the nerve.

Bell's palsy. Its etiology and pathologic anatomy are disputed. However, edema with compression of the facial nerve in its bony canal appears quite evident. Whether or not an intratemporal bone decompression of the facial canal should be performed and, if so, when is beyond the scope of this atlas. However, conservative management, consisting of steroids, antibiotics and proteolytic enzymes, is commenced immediately. Frequent evaluation of the progress of the impaired physiology is followed with electric stimulation. Apparently, weak sinusoidal stimulation has been found to be of some help. The same can be said for a light massage of the facial muscles. Both of these latter forms of therapy should be delayed until any present local edema or tenderness, which is rare, disappears. This same regimen is followed after parotid surgery when temporary paresis occurs. After a nerve graft, the electrical stimulator only is used. When wound healing is complete, light massage and electrical stimulation are used. A Hilger stimulator may be used. Galvanic stimulation of the muscles themselves has also been utilized by the patient himself. Such a stimulator may be economically constructed from dry cells.

If the nerve is lacerated, immediate repair is performed, preferably using magnification (an operation microscope is excellent) and 6-0 to 8-0 nonabsorbable suture material.

A nerve graft is described on plate 254.

Occasionally, drooping of the side of the face occurs following a radical maxillectomy when the major portion of the malar (zygoma) bone is removed. The fascial sling operation described is of distinct help. Stage I is not necessary, the fascial sling being attached to the muscle and the dermis (using a fine white nonabsorbable suture) at the lowest point of the droop through a small skin incision. The other end of the fascia is fixed in the temporal region as in Stage II. It is performed in one stage. The drooping or sagging of the cheek under the eye is also aided.

Another aspect of facial paralysis is the theory that spontaneous recovery occurs in a significant number of patients. Martin and Helsper (1960) believe there is cross innervation via the trigeminal nerve, and Conley has published data relative to a circuitous route of crossed innervation.

When the facial paralysis is ascertained to be permanent—a waiting period of up to nine months is justified—a fascial sling procedure can be performed to provide static support for the drooping face, especially for the corner of the mouth. The problem relative to closing the eye, especially during sleep, to protect the cornea is believed better helped by performing a tarsorrhaphy (plate 161) rather than by extension of the sling procedure to include the orbicularis oculi muscle.

Highpoints

1. Two basic features of the problem:
   a. Static suspension.
   b. Dynamic action.
   In the operation described, static suspension is involved.
2. Two stages:
   a. Fascia implanted at orbital region.
   b. Sling from first stage to temporal region.
3. Fascia support at oral cavity only on paralyzed side, slightly crossing midline.
4. Autogenous fascia.
5. No procedure is 100 per cent perfect and may not be lasting. Inform the patient of this.

Stage 1 (From Ragnell, 1968; after May, 1970)

A Depicted is one method of obtaining autogenous fascia from fascia lata. A fascia stripper is used to obtain a piece of fascia 0.6 cm wide and 18 cm long. Superiorly, the fascia lata is in two layers; inferiorly, the two layers fuse to form the iliotibial band.

(Text continued on opposite page.)

Plate 104   The Face

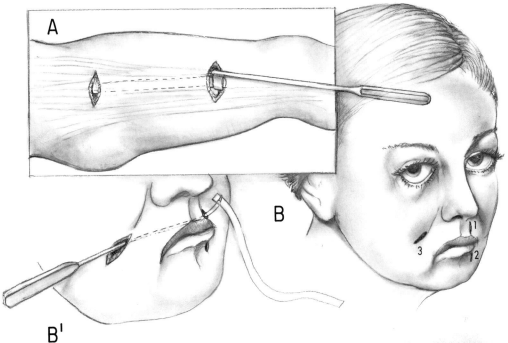

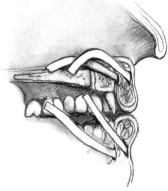

Stage I (*Continued*)

B Three small incisions are made: (1) just lateral to the philtrum column on the normal side; (2) opposite #1 on the lower lip; and (3) lateral to the commissure on the paralyzed side in or close to the nasolabial fold.

B[1] Using a fascia carrier, one end of the fascial strip is passed from the lateral incision (3, step *B*) in a plane between the oral mucous membrane — do not perforate it — and the paralyzed orbicularis oris muscle of the upper lip out through the muscle of the normal side at incision 1 in step *B*. The fascia strip, locking the normal muscle, is

B[2] then passed back laterally between the paralyzed muscle and the subcutaneous tissue to the point of beginning (incision 3). The position of this doubled-back fascia is depicted in sagittal section in step *B²*, including the same maneuver on the lower lip.

The four ends of the fascial strip are then tightened, care being taken not to make them too tight for fear of stenosis. If the patient wears dentures, these must be in place at this moment. These ends are then tied together or sutured with 4-0 Tevdek. The wounds are closed and sealed with collodian.

FASCIAL SLINGS FOR FACIAL PARALYSIS (*Continued*)

Stage II (Several months later)

C By direct exposure a wider (1 to 1.5 cm) and longer (15 cm) piece of fascia lata is removed and used as the sling. The previous lateral incision 3 in step *B* is opened and the ends of the previously placed fascia are localized. Another incision is made in the temporal region with a pre-auricular extension if a rhytidectomy (face lift) is also planned. The temporal fascia is exposed. A subcutaneous tunnel is then made connecting the two incisions. A long slender clamp or fascia carrier can be used for this purpose.

D The lower end of the fascia is then passed around the loop formed by the fascia placed in stage I and sutured with 4-0 nonabsorbable material. Redundant skin may be excised and then the dermis on the lateral skin wound (rolled edge) is approximated to the fascia with fine white nonabsorbable sutures. This wound is left open until the operation is completed so as to view the resulting effect with tension on the sling.

E The fascial sling is then drawn upward through the temporal incision so as to slightly overcorrect the deformity. The fascial end is then passed through two incisions in the temporal fascia as depicted and sutured securely in place with 4-0 Tevdek. The skin incisions are closed with 5-0 nylon.

A collodian dressing is used as extensively as possible. Supportive Kling dressing is used for as long as possible — one month. The patient should avoid chewing and excessive talking for at least one to two weeks.

F The completed operation schematically depicting the location of the fascial strips. Also shown are modifications of fascial strips placed around the eye. These latter strips can be secured around the medial canthal ligament. An alternate approach to achieving narrowing of the palpebrae fissure is the performance of a lateral canthoplasty (plate 161).

Complications

1. Disruption of sutures holding sling.
2. Wound infection. Since facial paralysis may be associated with mastoid disease, be sure the ears are "dry."
3. Some sag may be expected over the years.

Ragnell (1968) performs a vastly different second stage in that he affixes one end of a fascial sling to the transected upper end of the coronoid process and the other end to the zygomatic arch. The reader is referred to his original article (see bibliographical entry) and to May's Plastic and Reconstructive Surgery (3rd ed.).

If warranted, as time goes by, excision of additional skin along the nasolabial fold is performed.

Conley advises exploration of the facial nerve if there has been a possible history of injury and transection. If feasible, a transposition graft utilizing the hypoglossal nerve is then performed. He prefers this prior to any sling type of operation, almost regardless of the time elapsed since injury.

Another method of dynamic reconstruction preferred by Bernstein is the use of three muscle flaps from the masseter muscle and two or three from the temporalis muscle to the oral region and the orbital region, respectively.

Plate 105   *The Face*

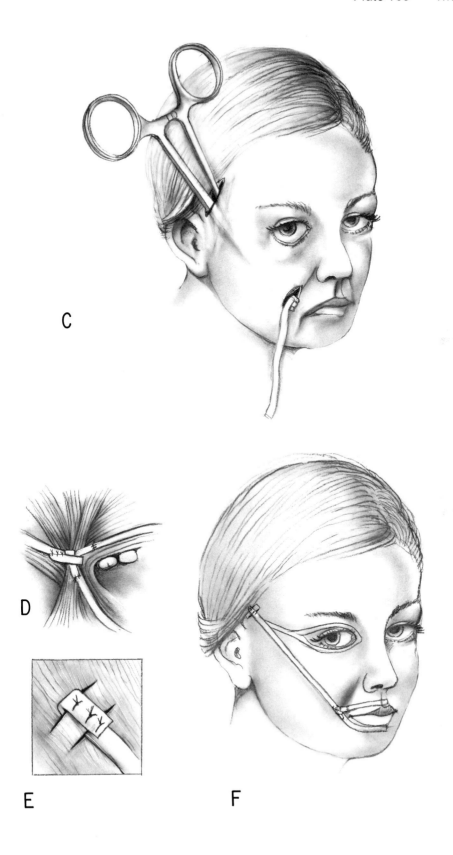

C

D

E

F

TRIGEMINAL NEURALGIA (Tic Douloureux)

The usual initial treatment for trigeminal neuralgia is local block of the involved nerve with a suitable local anesthetic. This is followed by the injection of 1 or 2 cc of 90 per cent alcohol. If this therapy fails, section and avulsion of the involved nerve are performed under local anesthesia. The more commonly involved branches of the trigeminal nerve are depicted. In all patients with trigeminal pain, disease in the paranasal sinuses and naso-pharynx must be excluded. Glaucoma also is ruled out.

A Location and distribution of supraorbital (*1*), frontalis (*2*), supratrochlear (*3*), infra-trochlear (*4*) and infraorbital (*5*) nerves.

B The surgical approach to these nerves is demonstrated through three incisions. One or all nerves are exposed and sectioned depending on the clinical picture. The eye-brow is never shaved. The approach to the infraorbital nerve is depicted in detail on plate 28, steps *A, B* and *C*.

C Details of the technique of section and avulsion of the supraorbital and frontalis nerves are depicted. The same technique applies to all the other nerves.
The orbicularis oculi muscle fibers are split.

D Using nerve hooks, the nerves are mobilized.

E Clamps are placed proximally and distally and the nerve is transected.

F By twisting the clamps, both proximal and distal ends are avulsed.

For pain distribution along the lateral side of the tongue or lower lip, an intraoral block and injection of the lingual nerve or inferior dental nerve are performed. Various techniques to block the maxillary division of the trigeminal nerve in the pterygopalatine (sphenomaxillary) fossa as it leaves the skull through the foramen rotunda have been de-scribed. Medical management, using Tegretal, has also been utilized. Serious side effects of this drug may occur. Regardless of the manner of treatment, relief may be only tempo-rary. The reader is referred to Hollinshead (see Suggested Library) for an anatomic de-scription of the problem.

Resection of portions of the lingual and inferior dental nerves has been performed intra-orally. The lingual nerve is exposed at the posterior floor of the mouth, while the inferior alveolar nerve is exposed on the lateral aspect of the oropharynx, overlying the mandibular foramen on the inner surface of the mandible.

Plate 106   The Face

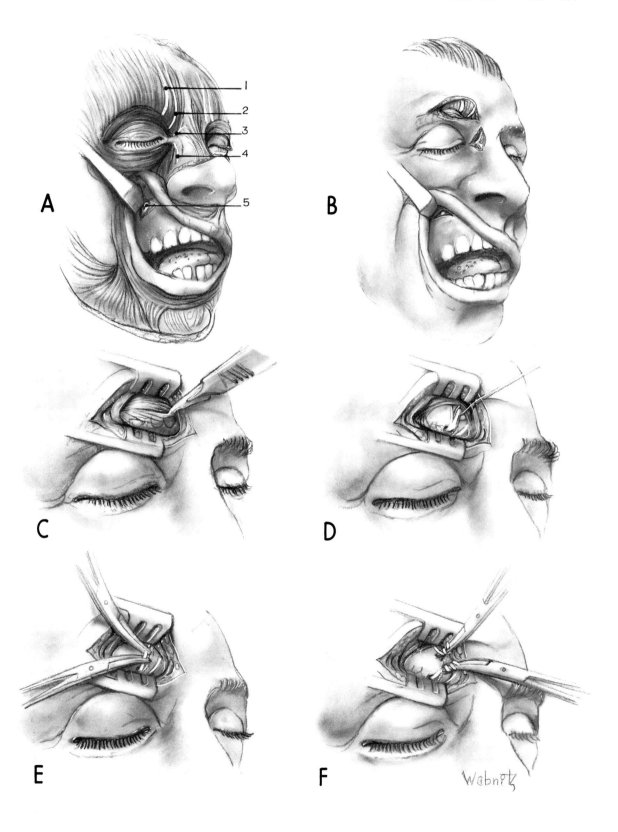

INCISION AND DRAINAGE OF ABSCESSES OF FACE

Highpoints

    1. All intraoral and intranasal abscesses are simply drained with no anesthesia or topical or local anesthesia. General anesthesia is contraindicated unless an endotracheal tube is used.

    2. Abscesses at or near cartilage should be drained early.

    3. Massive systemic antibiotics.

A   *Septal Abscess.* A vertical incision is made to the most dependent point. Postoperatively, vasoconstrictor nose drops with or without sulfathiazole are used. Drain is optional.

B
C   *Abscess of Upper Lip.* A horizontal incision is made in the presenting mass on the inner aspect of the lip.

D   A rubber tissue drain is sewn in place with nylon.

E   *Abscess of Lower Lip.* An incision is made along the vermilion border. If there are multiple abscesses, a separate incision is made on the opposite side and connected under the lip.

F   A through and through drain is used with the two incisions.

Complications

    1. Cavernous sinus thrombosis.

    2. Chondritis if cartilage is involved, with possible slough of cartilage.

Plate 107   The Face

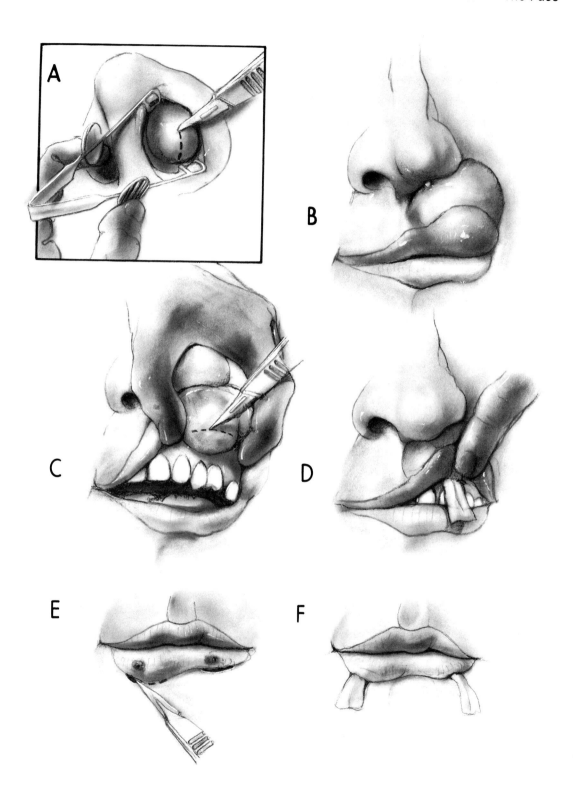

BIBLIOGRAPHY

Adour, K. K.: Facial paralysis: Treatment response in 403 consecutive cases. Trans. Amer. Acad. Ophthal. Otolaryng. 75:1284–1301, 1971.

Alford, B. R., Weber, S. C., and Sessions, R. B.: Neurodiagnostic studies in facial paralysis. Ann. Otol. 79:227–233, 1970.

Anderson, J. R.: The face lift operation and the otolaryngologist. Laryngoscope 81:866–872, 1971.

Assor, D.: Basal cell carcinoma with metastasis to bone. Cancer 20:2125–2132, 1967.

Bingham, H. G., and Lichti, E. L.: The doppler as an aid in predicting the behavior of congenital cutaneous hemangioma. Plast. Reconstr. Surg. 47:580–583, 1971.

Blatt, I. M., and Freeman, J. A.: Bell's palsy III: Further observations on the pathogenesis of Bell's palsy and the results of chorda tympani neurectomy. Trans. Amer. Acad. Ophthal. Otolaryng. 73:420–438, 1969.

Caron, A. S., Hajdu, S. I., and Strong, E. W.: Osteogenic sarcoma of the facial and cranial bones. A review of forty-three cases. Amer. J. Surg. 122:719–725, 1971.

Catlin, D., McNeer, G., and Das Gupta, T.: Melanoma of the skin of the head and neck. The American Cancer Society 16:19–25, 1966.

Chakravorty, B. G.: Association of trigeminal neuralgia with multiple sclerosis. Arch. Neurol. 14:95–99, 1966.

Coleman, C. C., Jr., and Hoopes, J. E.: Complex carcinomas of the skin of the head and neck and their surgical treatment. Amer. J. Surg. 108:558–564, 1964.

Coletta, D. F., Haentze, F. E., and Thomas, C. C.: Metastasizing basal cell carcinoma of the skin with myelophthisic anemia. Cancer 22:879–884, 1968.

Conley, J. J.: Treatment of facial paralysis. Surg. Clin. N. Amer. 51:403–416, 1971.

Conley, J., Healey, W. V., and Stout, A. P.: Fibromatosis of the head and neck. Amer. J. Surg. 112:609–614, 1966.

Edgerton, M. T., and Wolfort, F. G.: The dermal-flap canthal lift for lower eyelid support. A technique of value in the surgical treatment of facial palsy. Plast. Reconstr. Surg. 43:42–52, 1969.

Edgerton, M. T., Udvarhelyi, G. B., and Knox, D. L.: The surgical correction of ocular hypertelorism. Ann. Surg. 172:473–496, 1970.

Farrior, R. T.: Implant materials in restoration of facial contour. Laryngoscope 76:934–954, 1966.

Farrior, R. T.: Reconstructive surgery for the middle one-third of the face. Eye Ear Nose Throat Monthly, October, November, and December 1965 and January 1966.

Gaisford, J. C., and Hanna, D. C.: Facial pedicle flap reconstruction: Immediate repair after surgical excision. Amer. J. Surg. 108:514–516, 1964.

Georgiade, N. G., Matton, G. E., and Kessel, F.: Facial burns. Plast. Reconstr. Surg. 29:648–657, 1962.

Gorlin, R. J., and Cohen, M. M., Jr.: Frontometaphyseal dysplasia. A new syndrome. Amer. J. Dis. Child. 118:487, 1969.

Griffith, B. H., Monroe, C. W., and McKinney, P.: A follow-up study on the treatment of keloids with triamcinolone acetonide. Plast. Reconstr. Surg. 46:145–150, 1970.

Guerrero-Santos, J., Ramíez, M., and Espaillat, L.: Treatment of facial paralysis by static suspension with dermal flaps. Plast. Reconstr. Surg. 48:325–328, 1971.

Guilford, F. R.: Surgical consideration in disorders of the horizontal and vertical portions of the facial nerve. Ann. Otol. 79:241, 1970.

Hirshowitz, B., and Mahler, D.: Unusual case of multiple basal cell carcinoma with metastasis to the parotid lymph gland. Cancer 22:654–657, 1968.

Jobe, R. P., and Briggs, R. M.: Marking the surgical specimen in skin neoplasm excision. Surg. Gynec. Obstet. 126:1325–1326, 1968.

Jongkees, L. B. W.: The timing of surgery in intratemporal facial paralysis. Laryngoscope 79:1557–1561, 1969.

Kettel, K.: Danish Otolaryngological Society Symposium: Management of peripheral facial palsies. Arch. Otolaryng. 81:441–546, 1965.

King, G. D., and Salzman, F. A.: Keloid scars. Analysis of 89 patients. Surg. Clin. N. Amer. 50:595–598, 1970.

Lampe, I., and LaTourette, H. B.: Management of hemangiomas in infants. Pediat. Clin. N. Amer. 6:511–528, 1959.

Martin, H., and Helsper, J. T.: Spontaneous return of function following surgical section or excision of the seventh cranial nerve in the surgery of parotid tumors. Ann. Surg. 151:538, 1960.

Masson, J. K., and Soule, E. H.: Desmoid tumors of the head and neck. Amer. J. Surg. 112:615–622, 1966.

Masters, F. W., Robinson, D. W., and Simons, J. N.: Temporalis transfer for lagophthalmos due to seventh nerve palsy. Amer. J. Surg. 110:607–611, 1965.

May, M.: Facial paralysis, peripheral type: A proposed method of reporting. Laryngoscope 80:331–390, 1970.

McCabe, B. F.: Management of hyperfunction of the facial nerve. Ann. Otol. 79:252, 1970.

McCoy, E. G., and Boyle, W. F.: Reinnervation of the facial muscles following extratemporal facial nerve resection. Laryngoscope 81:1–7, 1971.

McGovern, F. H.: Chorda tympani neurectomy for Bell's palsy. Arch. Otolaryng. 92:189–190, 1970.

Mohs, F. E.: Chemosurgery for facial neoplasms. Arch. Otolaryng. 95:62–67, 1972.

Mohs, F. E.: Chemosurgery for the microscopically controlled excision of skin cancer. J. Surg. Oncol. 3:257–267, 1971.

Mustardé, J. C.: Repair and Reconstruction in the Orbital Region. Edinburgh, E. & S. Livingstone, Ltd., 1969.

Phelan, J. T., and Milgrom, H.: The use of Mohs' chemosurgery technique in the treatment of skin cancers. Surg. Gynec. Obstet. 125:549–560, 1967.

Piersol, G. A.: Human Anatomy. 3rd ed. Philadelphia, J. B. Lippincott Company, 1911.

Pilney, F. T., Broadbent, T. R., and Woolf, R. M.: Giant pigmented nevi of the face: Surgical management. Plast. Reconstr. Surg. 40:469–474, 1967.

Poppen, J. L.: An Atlas of Neurosurgical Techniques. Philadelphia, W. B. Saunders Company, 1960.

Pressman, J. J., Berman, W., and Simon, M. B.: Primary repair of defects following a surgical removal of tumors of the face. Arch. Surg. 79:921–938, 1959.

Pulec, J. L.: Facial nerve grafting. Laryngoscope 79:1562–1583, 1969.

Ragnell, A.: Experience with dynamic and static reconstruction in cases of facial paralysis. Scand. J. Plast. Reconstr. Surg. 41:343, 1968.

Rees, T. D., Rhodes, R. D., and Converse, J. M.: Palliation of facial paresis. Amer. J. Surg. 120:82–88, 1970.

Robinson, J. R., and Pou, J. W.: Bell's palsy: A predisposition of pregnant women. Arch. Otolaryng. 95:125–130, 1972.

Sachatello, C. R., and McSwain, B.: Regression of cutaneous capillary hemangioma. Amer. J. Surg. 116:113–114, 1968.

Spira, M., Gerow, F. J., Hardy, S. B., and Beall, A. C., Jr.: Windshield injuries of the face. J. Trauma 8:513–526, 1968.

Strahan, R. W., and Calcaterra, T. C.: Otolaryngologic aspects of mycosis fungoides. Laryngoscope 81:1912–1916, 1971.

Symposium on Facial Pain Issue. Headache 9, 1969.

Thomas, M. L., and Andress, M. R.: Angiography in angiomas of the face. Amer. J. Roentgenol. 112:332–338, 1971.

Tulenko, J. F., and Conway, H.: An analysis of sweat gland tumors. Surg. Gynec. Obstet. 121:343–348, 1965.

Walsh, T. S., Jr.: Giant strawberry nevi of the orbital arteries: Treatment of ligation. Surgery 65:659–667, 1969.

Walsh, T. S., Jr.: The dermal arteries of the neck and shoulder. Plast. Reconstr. Surg. 32:455–458, 1963.

Ziegler, J. L., Wright, D. H., and Kyalwazi, S. K.: Differential diagnosis of Burkitt's lymphoma of the face and jaws. Cancer 27:503–514, 1971.

6. GENERAL PURPOSE FLAPS

DELTOPECTORAL FLAP (After Bakamjian, 1965)

One of the most versatile flaps for reconstruction following major tissue loss in head and neck surgery is the deltopectoral flap (Bakamjian, 1965). It is a full thickness (including the fascia of the pectoral muscles) anterior chest wall flap medially based, with its blood supply from the first through the fourth perforator vessels and branches of the internal mammary artery.

Characteristics and Advantages

1. Usually not delayed.
2. Unilateral or bilateral.
3. Bilateral can be simultaneous.
4. Usual length reaches the tip of shoulder but can be extended behind the shoulder or inferior to the deltoid prominence or superior to the spine of the scapula.
5. Deltoid portion usually not hair-bearing. In the rare situation in which hair is present over the shoulder, the distal end of the flap can be dropped below the axillary fold which is not hair-bearing (Conley).
6. Flap is usually outside radiotherapy fields.
7. Excellent blood supply with dependent venous drainage.
8. Donor site is hidden, thus cosmetically acceptable.
9. Flap can be rotated deep or superficial to cervical flaps, depending on purpose.
10. Flap can be split longitudinally and distally and de-epithelialized proximally (Krizek and Robson, 1973).

Disadvantages

This requires a second stage to close an orocutaneous fistula unless an epithelial shave is performed. An epithelial shave is the removal of the epithelium of the flap where it comes in contact with the overlying cervical flap. The failure rate is 9 to 18 per cent (Bakamjian and Conley report less). If the flap is used to cover the carotid vessels, blowout of carotid is a hazard if the flap fails.

Highpoints

1. Ratio of base of flap to length of flap is of little concern.
2. Caution when elevating flap at base not to injure the perforator vessels. The flap includes the fascia of the pectoral muscles, excluding the thin musculature investing fascia.
3. Meticulous care in the handling of the flap.
4. Postoperative care to avoid kinking or compression of flap by dressing, drains, tubes or tape of the tracheostomy tube.
5. If the flap is to be passed beneath cervical flaps, the lower cervical incision must be horizontal and is usually the same incision as the superior incision of the flap.
6. Delay flap, if:
   a. Tissue turgor is poor.
   b. Presence of systemic disease, e.g., severe arteriosclerosis, diabetes or severe malnutrition.
   c. Excessive length—however, Bakamjian does *not* necessarily use this as a reason for delay.
7. Usually incise distal esophagus in vertical plane for 1 to 2 cm to enlarge the esophageal opening when the flap is used to reconstruct the esophagus.
8. Do not drape flap over the hardware which is used to stabilize the ends of resected mandible.

Types of Delay

1. Complete skin incision without elevation (preserves thoracoacromial vessels).
2. Complete skin incision with elevation and return (transects thoracoacromial vessels).
3. Partial skin incision:
   a. Leave small area along the axillary area for dependent venous drainage.
   b. Leave small area along superior margin near thoracoacromial vessels.

Plate 108   General Purpose Flaps

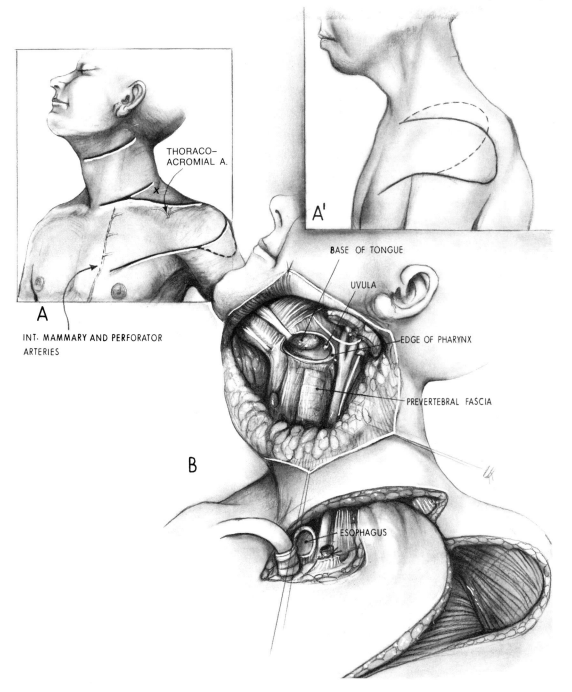

THORACO-
ACROMIAL A.

A'

BASE OF TONGUE

UVULA

EDGE OF PHARYNX

PREVERTEBRAL FASCIA

A

INT. MAMMARY AND PERFORATOR
ARTERIES

B

ESOPHAGUS

RECONSTRUCTION OF PHARYNGOESOPHAGUS

A   Skin incision outlined for a total laryngopharyngectomy and left radical neck dissection with immediate reconstruction using a deltopectoral flap. The dotted line at
the distal end of the flap depicts an extension of the flap below and behind the deltoid

A   prominence. A¹ depicts a more horizontal and posterior extension which is preferred.
The distal end of the flap can be extended superior to the spine of the scapula (dotted
line). This has the advantage of combining the cervical incision with the superior
flap incision throughout its entire length. This eliminates the small posterior triangular skin flap **X** in step A. The lower horizontal cervical incision (McFee) is the
same as the superior incision for the flap at its medial end.

B   The ablative surgery has been performed. The deltopectoral flap is elevated without
delay and gently passed beneath the bipedicle cervical flap.

RECONSTRUCTION OF PHARYNGOESOPHAGUS (*Continued*)

C   The distal end of the flap is approximated to the transected edge of the pharynx with interrupted or continuous nylon, chromic catgut or Dexon sutures. Although nylon causes the least tissue reaction, it can be troublesome since it does not absorb. If the distal end of the flap is curved superiorly, the posterior cervical triangular skin flap **X** is eliminated. This modification appears to be more desirable at this point in time. The knots should be buried if nylon is utilized. A feeding tube is passed along the inside of the flap.

    For shorter defects of the pharyngoesophagus, reconstruction can be achieved by a one stage operation utilizing a tongue flap and a dermal graft (see plate 329).

Plate 109   General Purpose Flaps

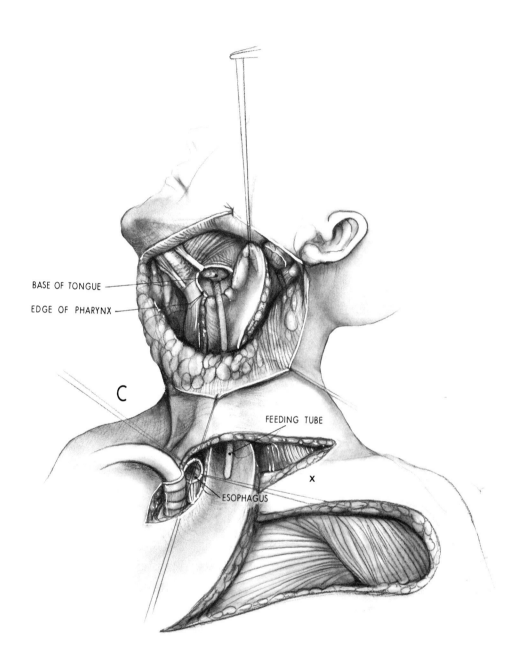

BASE OF TONGUE

EDGE OF PHARYNX

C

FEEDING TUBE

x

ESOPHAGUS

RECONSTRUCTION OF PHARYNGOESOPHAGUS (*Continued*)

D   The anastomosis of the distal end of the flap to the pharynx is completed and the flap is tubed. Depicted is the vertical line of closure of the flap, thus forming the tube with the skin surface as the lining of the new gullet. The feeding tube has been passed into the esophagus. The esophageal lumen is incised (along the dotted line) for 1 or 2 cm to enlarge the opening.

Plate 110   General Purpose Flaps

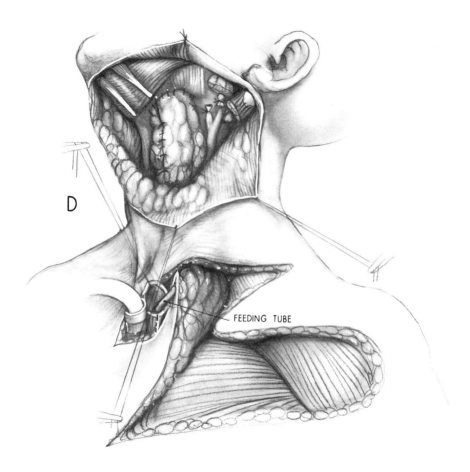

D

FEEDING TUBE

DELTOPECTORAL FLAP (*Continued*)

RECONSTRUCTION OF PHARYNGOESOPHAGUS (*Continued*)

E
F Anastomosis of the side of the tube flap to the end of the esophagus is performed using interrupted sutures. If nylon is used, the knots are buried.

G Completion of the anastomosis except for a most inferior portion which forms the fistula (arrow). Conley has performed an epithelial shave — removal of the epidermis — at this site and then closed the fistula at this initial stage. This could be hazardous. Usually closure of the fistula is performed some four to six weeks later.

Plate 111   General Purpose Flaps

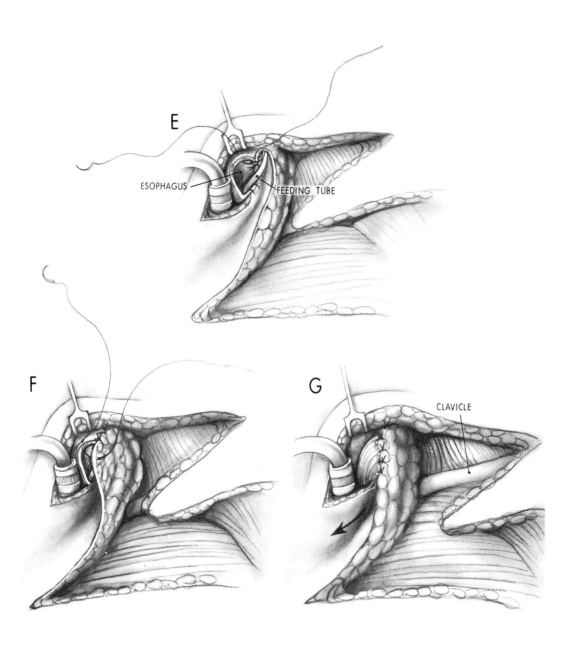

E

ESOPHAGUS   FEEDING TUBE

F

G

CLAVICLE

DELTOPECTORAL FLAP (*Continued*)

RECONSTRUCTION OF PHARYNGOESOPHAGUS (*Continued*)

H   The first stage reconstruction and the ablative surgery are complete. The fistula (arrow) is lateral to the tracheostome. The tube flap esophageal anastomosis with the feeding tube and the vertical closure of the flap to form the new gullet is "ghosted in" for clarification. A split thickness skin graft covers the donor site.

I   Four to six weeks later the second stage is performed to revise the lower anastomosis and thus close the fistula, as well as transect the flap and return the proximal unused portion of the flap to the chest wall. The previous anastomosis is exposed and the flap transected along the dotted line. The skin graft is partially elevated off the flap and chest wall.

J   Transection of the flap is completed along the dotted line and returned to the chest wall.

K   The original side-to-end anastomosis is now converted to an end-to-end anastomosis. The skin is then closed without wound drainage. A feeding tube is inserted and kept in place for about one week.

Plate 112   General Purpose Flaps

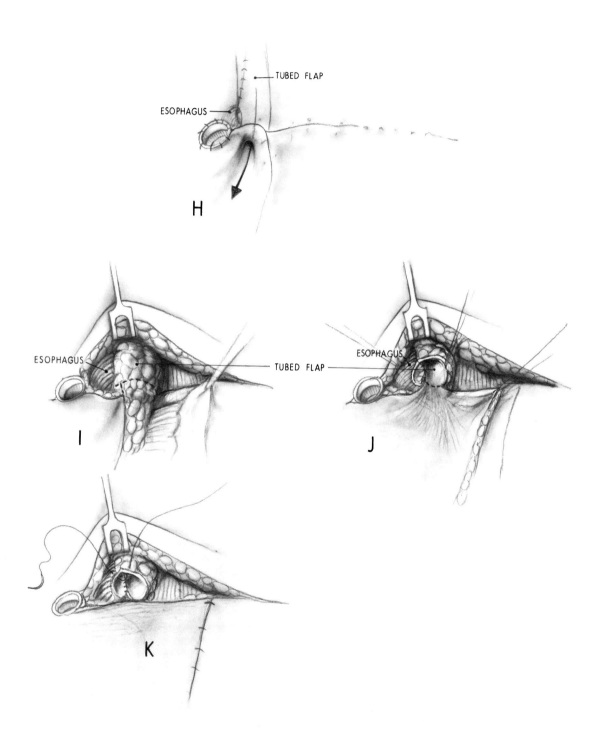

APPLICATIONS OF DELTOPECTORAL FLAP

The deltopectoral flap can be used to reconstruct the cervical esophagus (plates 108–112), intraoral defects, floor of mouth, tongue, skin of the neck, chin and face, wall of hypopharynx and oropharynx and covering for carotid artery and vascular grafts. It can also be combined with other flaps, e.g., apron flap (Haar, 1970). Bilateral deltopectoral flaps can also be utilized with one flap forming the inner lining and the other flap used as the outer skin covering. Several examples are depicted.

A   A deltopectoral flap is used to cover a large skin defect in the region of the chin following resection of a portion of the mandible and anterior floor of the mouth. The inner lining can be covered with the forehead flap brought intraorally under the detached zygomatic arch (plates 196 and 197). The lips are sutured together to temporarily prevent the lower lip from drooping (Bakamjian, 1969). The portion of the flap lying beneath the cervical flap can be de-epithelialized — an epithelial shave (Krizek and Robson, 1973) — thus eliminating a second procedure to return that portion of the deltopectoral flap to the donor site. This is a form of an island flap.

B   A long deltopectoral flap extending around the tip of the shoulder was delayed and then used to reconstruct a portion of the soft palate, lateral oropharyngeal wall and a portion of the base of the tongue. The flap is to be rotated on its long axis. This flap lies beneath the cervical flap of a radical neck dissection. After assurance of the viability of the deltopectoral flap, the overlying cervical bipedicle flap is resected and discarded. The fistula associated with this flap is then closed by using local turn-in flaps.

C   Another long deltopectoral flap is utilized to cover a large defect in the region of the parotid gland and face. The base of this flap is exterior to the cervical skin and is either tubed or bare under the area dressed with split thickness skin. After viability, the unused portion of the pedicle of the flap is returned to the chest wall if the pedicle has been tubed.

Plate 113   General Purpose Flaps

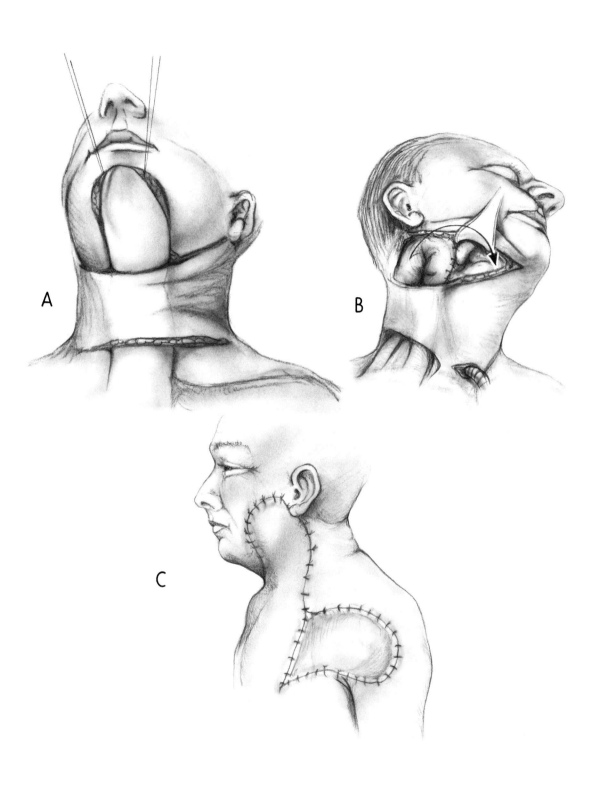

A

B

C

APPLICATIONS OF DELTOPECTORAL FLAP (*Continued*)

APRON FLAP

A   Depicted is an apron flap (Edgerton; Farr) elevated with a concomitant resection of the floor of the mouth, partial glossectomy and radical neck dissection. The mandible has been preserved according to the criteria reported by Marchetta. Farr (1969) extends the inferior dip of the apron flap below the clavicles. Tip necrosis can occur with such a long flap. **X** represents a superior extended deltopectoral flap which is usually preferred.

B   The apron flap has been brought into the floor of the mouth and sutured to the remaining tongue and gingiva, thus reconstructing the intraoral defect following a resection of the floor of the mouth and partial glossectomy, preserving the mandible. The apron flap donor site is now covered with a deltopectoral flap (Haar). This may be readily combined with a radical neck dissection.

   Although a deltopectoral flap can be used directly to reconstruct the anterior portion of the floor of the mouth, this combination with the apron flap has proved to be very adaptable. The forehead flap is somewhat more adaptable for reconstruction of the anterior floor of the mouth, while the deltopectoral flap is more adaptable for reconstruction of the posterior regions.

Complications

1. Nine per cent of deltopectoral flaps in our hands have lost viability.
2. A carotid artery blowout if flap loses viability when used to cover the vessel.
3. Serious aspiration may occur when flap is used in combined reconstruction. A laryngectomy could have been performed; however, the problem was simply solved by performing a permanent tracheostomy and total stripping and suture approximation of both vocal cords.
4. Dysphagia and pooling of food.
5. Most flaps do not have any muscular function; hence, there may be difficulty in swallowing and propelling food.

Plate 114   General Purpose Flaps

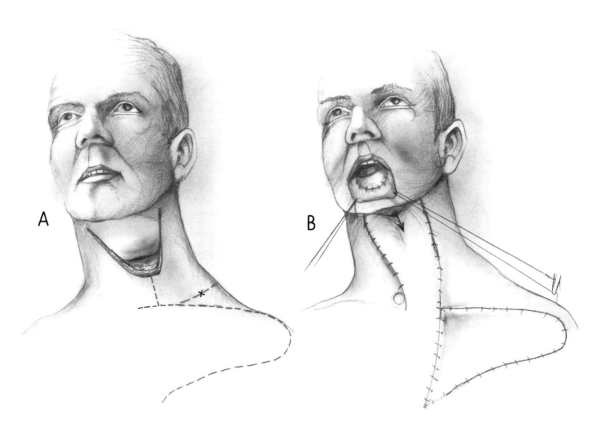

LATERALLY BASED CHEST FLAP (After Conley, 1960)

Highpoints

1. Usually not delayed.
2. Donor site cosmetically acceptable in male; not as adaptable in female because of the breast.
3. Donor site able to be covered with local advancement flaps or skin graft.

A   Pictured is a patient with two separate recurrences following a right jaw and radical neck resection for carcinoma of the floor of the mouth. One recurrence is in the submandibular region; the other involves soft tissue over the sternoclavicular area. Treatment consisted of planned preoperative super-voltage radiation therapy followed by surgical resection and immediate reconstruction using a bipedicle cervical flap combined with a laterally based chest flap. The areas of resection are outlined in solid lines which correspond to horizontal cervical skin incisions. Between the two areas of resection is a bipedicle horizontal cervical flap. The laterally based chest flap is outlined with the broken line. A vertical incision below the nipple is made to facilitate closure of the donor site. Both flaps are full thickness. The chest flap includes all soft tissue down to the level of the pectoral muscles.

The blood supply of this laterally based chest flap is:

1. Cutaneous branch, corocoid branch, transverse scapular artery.
2. Cutaneous branch, corocoid branch, thoracoacromial branch, axillary artery.
3. and 4. Cutaneous branch, deltoid branch, thoracoacromial branch, axillary artery (after Walsh, 1963).

The lateral thoracic artery may likewise contribute to the flap.

In faint outline are the inverted **Y-** or **H**-type neck dissection incisions from the original surgery. These are well healed and offer no problem for new flaps as planned.

B   The areas of local recurrence have been resected. The medial third of the clavicle can be removed if necessary. The upper bipedicle cervical flap is elevated and advanced upward. This advancement enlarges the lower defect which, however, will be easily closed by the laterally based chest flap.

C   The laterally based flap is elevated, including all soft tissue, to the level of the pectoral muscles. Its blood supply, laterally based, is preserved. The perforating vessels of the branches of the internal mammary artery medially are necessarily sacrificed. The flap is then rotated upward to close the lower cervical defect. The donor site is closed by advancing the inferior skin margins upward. A vertical incision is of some help in this maneuver. Hemovac tubes are inserted as depicted. If the donor site is too large, it is covered with a split thickness graft.

D   The completed procedure.

Plate 115   General Purpose Flaps

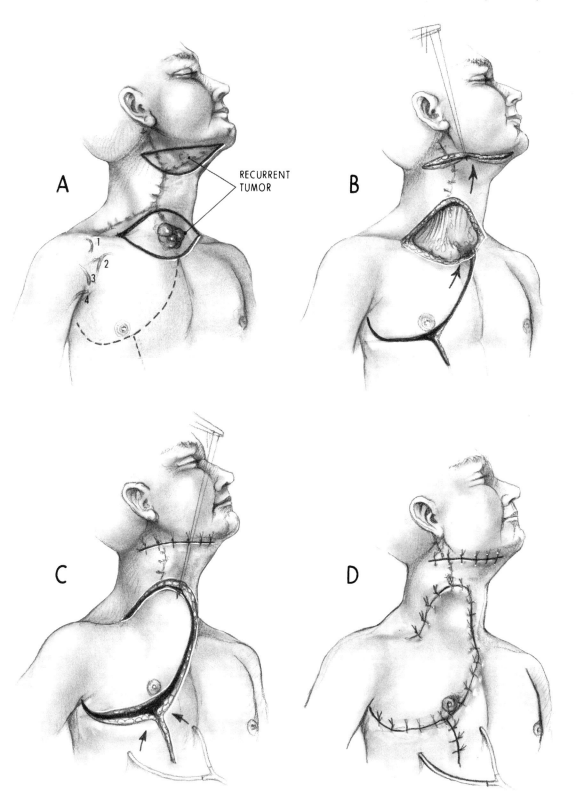

RECURRENT
TUMOR

A

B

C

D

NAPE OF NECK FLAP (After Corso, Gerold and Frazell, 1963)

Highpoints

1. Delay is recommended.
2. Flap may be lined with split thickness graft or not lined, depending on defect to be covered.
3. If a concomitant radical neck dissection performed, best to preserve posterior auricular and occipital arteries.
4. May be preferable to deltopectoral flap in females, since the latter type flap deforms the breast.
5. Useful in closing orocutaneous fistulae and defects of the side of the face and neck as well as palate and lateral oropharynx wall.

A   The arterial supply is superior via the posterior auricular and occipital arteries on the homolateral side. If there has been an interruption of these vessels during a radical neck dissection, the superior base of the flap can be widened to include the same group of vessels on the contralateral side. This, however, will limit the mobility of the flap to some extent. One of two types of delay is performed, depending on the type of defect to be covered.

Two-Stage Delay

B   If an extensively lined flap is necessary, e.g., with an orocutaneous fistula, and time is of little concern, a two-stage delay is performed by first making the two lateral parallel incisions and then lining the flap and the donor site with split thickness skin.

C   In 10 to 14 days, the inferior margin is transected. The excess split thickness on the flap lining is removed, leaving an island of skin corresponding to the size of the orocutaneous fistula as depicted. A portion of split thickness graft is left proximal to the dotted line of the flap if not tubed. If the flap is tubed, all split thickness skin is removed from the proximal portion of the flap. The edges of the fistula are cleared of granulation tissue and possibly some skin to afford a good base for the transposed flap. Occasionally, sufficient skin can be mobilized around the edge of the fistula to form a trap door-type turn-in flap to line the transposed flap. Usually this has not been successful and is not recommended because of a poor blood supply to the trap door flap. The flap is transected when blood supply and healing around the fistula is secured. This is some two to three months later. The remaining portion of the flap is returned to the donor site. A rubber-shod intestinal clamp or Huffman-Iowa clamp can be placed across the pedicle for 15 minutes to evaluate the adequacy of blood supply.

One-Stage Delay

D   A single step delay is achieved by simply incising around the entire flap as depicted. The flap is elevated to include the fascia of the underlying muscles and returned to the donor site. The area to be covered is a large skin defect overlying the side of the cheek.

E   In 10 to 14 days, the flap is swung into position and sutured in place. The original defect may have occurred along with a neck dissection. In such cases, the delay is done prior to the neck dissection so that the definitive surgery and the reconstruction are performed concomitantly.

F   After suitable healing has occurred, the flap is transected and the remaining portion returned to the donor site. The time interval may be from six to 12 weeks, depending on the estimated blood supply. Cross clamping the pedicle with a lightweight rubber-covered clamp can be performed to evaluate this blood supply as described under C. The histamine wheal test can also be used to evaluate the competency of the blood

(Text continued on opposite page.)

Plate 116   General Purpose Flaps

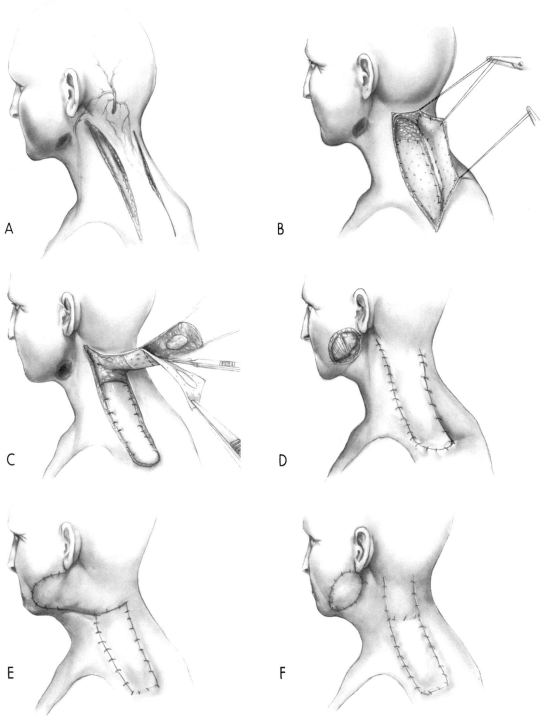

supply. This is performed by first occluding the blood supply at the base of the pedicle with clamps as described previously (C). Several areas just distal to the clamp and a comparable area on the opposite side of the body are scarified with a needle. A drop of 1:1000 histamine acid phosphate is then applied to each scarified area. If there is an adequate blood supply, a wheal will occur in both areas at about the same time, usually within eight minutes (after Conway, Stark and Joslin, 1951).

POSTERIOR SCAPULA FLAP

Highpoints

1. Indicated primarily in large basal cell or smaller squamous cell carcinoma of the skin located in a posterior lateral cervical region.
2. May be combined with radical neck dissection by utilizing a large cervical flap based anteriorly.
3. Wide and deep resection of lesion.
4. Non-delayed flap.
5. Wide base to scapula flap.

A   Triangular area with lesion to be excised. The blood supply of the scapula flap is from the superficial cervical and transverse cervical arteries arising from the subclavian artery. The dotted line depicts a superior extension which may be necessary to mobilize a superior occipital flap to aid in the closure. The blood supply of this flap is from the ascending branch of the occipital artery. The other solid lines are the incisions for the scapula flap and the cervical flap.

B   The lesion excised. It is well to obtain frozen sections to check the adequacy of the depth of resection if there is any question regarding deep extension. If so, remove underlying muscle. The larger scapular flap and smaller cervical flap are undermined and advanced.

C   The completed closure should be with minimum tension. One drawback to this type of closure is the three lines of closure at the apex. If the occipital portion is elevated and advanced, there will be four suture lines at the apex; this is a further drawback; a deltopectoral flap may be preferred (plate 108).

Plate 117   General Purpose Flaps

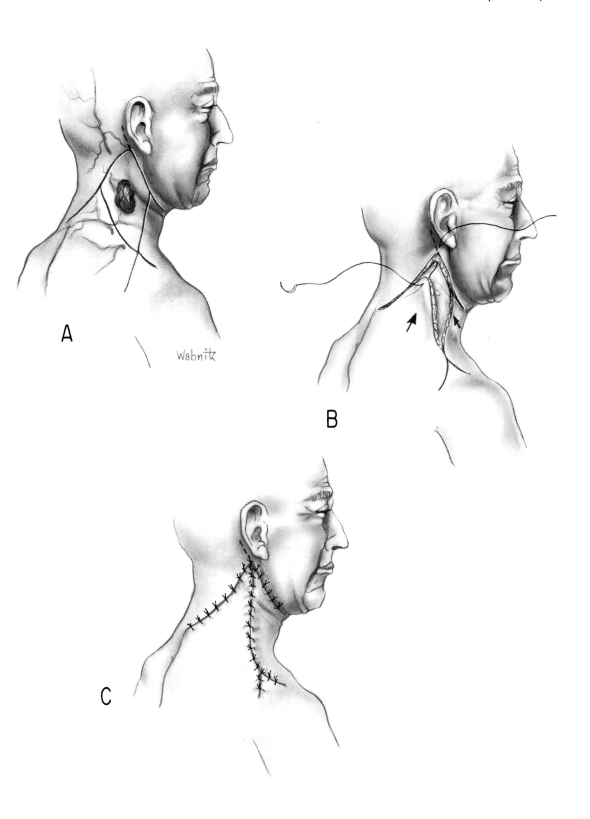

A

Wabnitz

B

C

FOREHEAD FLAP (Temporal Flap) (After McGregor)

General Data

The forehead flap and its modifications can be used for a large number of reconstruction procedures: cheek (inside and outside), floor of the mouth, nose, upper eyelid, chin covering for reconstructed mandible, portions of tongue and alveolar region. More often than not, it can be nondelayed if both the superficial and temporal and posterior auricular arteries are included in its base and not extended beyond the midline. It is best to delay the flap if it extends beyond the midline of the forehead, especially if a radical neck dissection is performed (Cramer and Culf, 1969). The flap may be in jeopardy if a radical neck dissection has been performed in which the feeding vessels of the external carotid artery have been sacrificed, although some surgeons report no difference at all (McGregor, 1963). Another problem is the cosmetic deformity. In younger patients, it is believed to be much less desirable especially in reconstruction procedures for tissue loss following trauma. Other flaps from the neck or pectoral region are much preferred. When using the forehead flap, less deformity is usually noted if the entire forehead is utilized. Split thickness skin graft taken from the anterior chest wall if practical is best for covering the donor site of the forehead. Numerous variations of forehead flaps are depicted in the following plates. Other varieties are on plates 89, 90, 119, 121, 195, 196, and 197. Remember not to cause more deformity than what is being reconstructed. For example, to use a forehead flap to reconstruct a palate is hardly justified when a prosthesis will serve the purpose.

Highpoints

1. Usually not delayed if posterior auricular artery and superficial temporal artery are included in the base and flap does not extend beyond the midline of forehead; otherwise, delay the flap especially with radical neck dissection.
2. Full thickness down to periosteum of skull (pericranium) including the frontalis muscle.
3. Use only nonhair-bearing portion of forehead for intraoral reconstruction. The base does include hair at the temporal region but this is later returned.
4. Some surgeons bring the flap through the cheek, via a separate incision well below the zygomatic arch. Care must be taken not to injure the facial nerve or the ducts of the parotid salivary gland. Others prefer to tunnel the flap through an incision either just above or just below the arch. The superficial temporal artery must not be injured.
5. The tunnel may be superficial or deep to the zygomatic arch. If deep, fracture the arch outward to avoid pinching of the base of the flap between the arch and the temporalis muscle.
6. When teeth are present, the flap can be pinched as it crosses the occlusion line.
7. Another serious point of jeopardy is the crossing of the flap over a Kirschner wire if there is undue tension or angulation.
8. The base can be returned in three to four weeks.

A The forehead flap is outlined. Note the contour follows the eyebrows and the forehead hairline. This is more pleasing cosmetically. The lower incision of the flap must not
A¹ extend beyond the level of the lateral canthus to avoid injury to the facial nerve.
   The dotted horizontal line depicts the incision through which the flap enters the oral cavity. A lower point of entrance can also be utilized. If so, do not injure the facial nerve or the parotid duct system.

B A tunnel is formed through an incision just below the zygomatic arch. This can be performed with Metzenbaum scissors or a large Kelly clamp. Effort must be made to avoid injury to the facial nerve and parotid salivary gland. The donor site and bare exposed area of flap are covered with split thickness skin. Skin from the anterior chest wall if not hairy is a good cosmetic cover. The dotted line indicates the intraoral position of the flap.

Plate 118   General Purpose Flaps

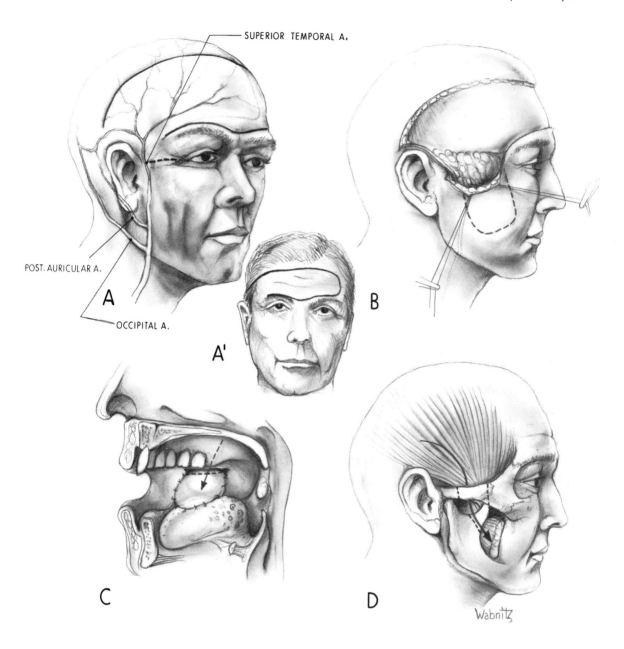

SUPERIOR TEMPORAL A.

POST. AURICULAR A.

A

OCCIPITAL A.

A'

B

C

D

Wabnitz

C   Distal end of the flap brought into intraoral defect and sutured in place with 3-0 or 4-0 nylon. It can be used to cover cheek, alveolar region, floor of mouth, tongue and somewhat posterior to tonsil region if wide enough. The arrow delineates the tunnel and a temporary fistula. The pedicle is sectioned along to the dotted line in three to four weeks and the base of the flap withdrawn from the tunnel and returned to the forehead or discarded.

D   An alternate tunnel is deep to the zygomatic arch which is fractured along the dotted line. (The coronoid process of the mandible may be likewise fractured if there is pressure on the flap.) This method of introduction is preferred by the author. The section of zygomatic arch is left attached to the overlying fascia and realigned after the base of the flap is returned.

RECONSTRUCTION OF CHEEK WITH FOREHEAD FLAP

This type of forehead flap with a lined skin graft surface is used for deep soft tissue and bony defects of the maxillary region. The flap must bridge the defect. A cavity simulating the antrum is thus reconstructed with dependent drainage. The problem in reconstruction is the ultimate viability of the flap, since the only source of blood supply is at the edges of the defect and the pedicle itself. The edges of the defect may be further compromised if the patient has received any radiation therapy. Hence the pedicle is preserved and not transected.

Highpoints

1. Preserve superficial temporal and posterior auricular vessels.
2. Forehead flap can be used with or without delay. Delay in this case is preferred.
3. Allow permanent drainage from antrum into oral cavity.
4. Base of defect is previously skin grafted.
5. Delay all forehead flaps if external carotid artery has been ligated.

A The skin incision as outlined includes the superficial temporal vessels. The dotted line indicates the inclusion of the posterior auricular artery which facilitates non-delay. In a male, hair-bearing scalp may be included, but in a female it should be excluded.

The defect consists of a loss of the entire anterior and lateral bony wall of the maxilla along with the overlying skin and muscles.

B The flap is full thickness, encompassing all soft tissue with muscle down to but not including the pericranium (periosteum of the skull). The flap is rotated nearly 180 degrees and swung over the defect. The distal end of the flap should easily overlap the farthest edge of the defect by 1 cm. The incisions mobilizing the flap are thus extended as necessary, being careful not to injure the main trunks of the superficial temporal vessels and posterior auricular vessels. At times only the galea aponeurosis need be released.

The posterior and medial walls of the defect have previously been covered with split thickness skin graft.

C After satisfactory mobilization, the flap is returned and sutured with continuous 5-0 nylon. The flap is delayed in this case because of the poor vascularity of the defect which was previously irradiated.

D In two to three weeks the flap is again elevated, rotated 180 degrees and swung over the defect. If any shrinkage has occurred, release incisions are again made with the same precautions. Now the inner side of the flap and the donor site are grafted with split thickness skin using slightly thicker skin for the forehead donor site. Be sure the donor sites for the split thickness skin are hairless, since hair in the new antrum is a nuisance because occasionally some hair will grow.

E The edges of both defect and flap are trimmed and freshened and very carefully approximated with fine interrupted sutures. If the soft tissue is scant at any edge on the defect, a wire suture through bone is used, being secured on the flap with a button

F or silicone disk so the flap is not injured. Since the entire undersurface of the flap has been previously covered with grafted skin, the base of the pedicle need not be tubed.

F¹ After two to three months go by, the dependent edge may be revised if it becomes rolled and edematous. This is done by undercutting and overlapping the edges or by using the fat flip flap of Millard (plate 122).

G The drainage tunnel from the new antrum is depicted in the gingivobuccal sulcus. The patient cares for this with daily irrigations.

Plate 119   General Purpose Flaps

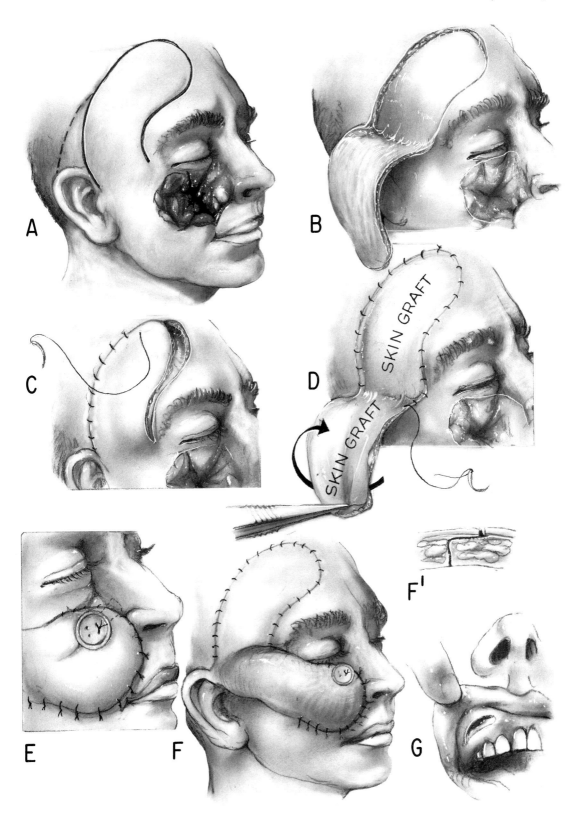

A

B

C

D

SKIN GRAFT

SKIN GRAFT

SKIN GRAFT

E

F

F'

G

RECONSTRUCTION OF CHEEK WITH FOREHEAD FLAP
(*Continued*)

H After four to six months, the pedicle of the flap is denuded of skin and buried. In this fashion the superficial temporal vessels are preserved and viability of the flap is assured. This is safer than transecting the pedicle since the only other source of blood supply is at the margin of the flap. These margins have a very poor blood supply because of previous irradiation. The outside layer of skin is elevated by sharp dissection from the pedicle. It is preserved at both ends and retracted with stay sutures.

I The inner layer of skin of the pedicle is dissected and discarded.

J The skin on the side of the face under which the vascular pedicle will be buried is now elevated with upper and lower skin flaps.

K The full thickness lower skin flap is elevated. The same technique is used on the upper flap.

L The pedicle is covered with the upper and lower flaps, using interrupted sutures of 5-0 nylon.

M The remaining defects are covered with portions of skin from the pedicle which are trimmed accordingly.

N Subcutaneous adipose tissue is removed from the distal portion as required to achieve a smooth surface.

This is a type of island flap with the vascular pedicle buried.

Plate 120   *General Purpose Flaps*

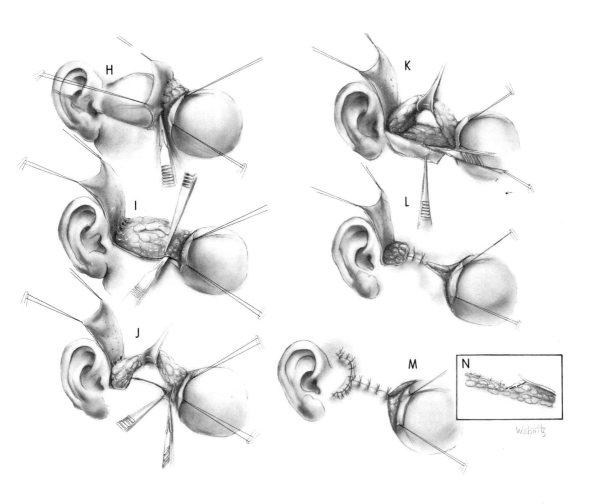

MIDLINE FOREHEAD FLAP (After Kazanjian, 1946)

Highpoints

1. Useful for full thickness defects of the nose including the ala and portions of the columella and cheek, especially below the eye.
2. May be lined with split thickness skin if necessary.
3. No delay.
4. Blood supply via both supratrochlear arteries with contribution from the dorsal nasal branches.
5. Extreme care must be exercised with incisions: the upper portions of the incisions are carried down to the periosteum while below the level of nasofrontal angle, the incisions are through skin only and dissection at this area is blunt to avoid injury to the supratrochlear vessels.
6. Be sure there is adequate length, keeping in mind the fact that the flap must be rotated in loose fashion so as not to compromise the vascular supply.

Depicted is a nasal defect resulting from resection of a tumor; this type of reconstruction is equally well suited to a defect due to trauma.

A　Outline of the flap with associated blood supply and tumor of the nose to be resected. The upper extent of the midline incisions reaches the hairline. This portion of the flap is carried by sharp dissection down to the periosteum. From the nasofrontal angle, the incisions are carried only through the skin as outlined by the dotted lines. There is minimal interference with motor function of the forehead since little if any significant portion of the frontalis muscles is involved in the flap.

A¹　The flap is turned down to the nasofrontal angle with sharp dissection. From here down, meticulous blunt dissection is used to preserve the blood supply via the supratrochlear and dorsal nasal vessels. Interestingly enough, there are redundant skin and soft tissue in this area which facilitate rotation of the flap without tension. A patch of split thickness skin is sutured with 5-0 chromic catgut to the raw surface of the flap corresponding with the deep through and through defect in the nose.

B　Through and through defect of the nose.

C　The major portion of the donor site is closed by mobilization of the lateral skin margins. This may require rather extensive undermining of the skin. Inferiorly the donor defect is covered with a triangular section of split thickness skin; otherwise, mobilization of skin at this point will bring the eyebrows too far medially. When the flap is severed in about three weeks, the unused portion is returned to that portion of the donor site which had been covered with the split thickness skin graft.

D　Application of this flap to close a defect of the cheek just below the lower lid. The advantage of this type of reconstruction is ease of coverage with prevention of ectropion of the lower lid.

A modification of this flap is the island flap (Esser, 1917), in which the flap with its blood supply is tunneled under an intact bridge of skin at the glabella.

Plate 121   General Purpose Flaps

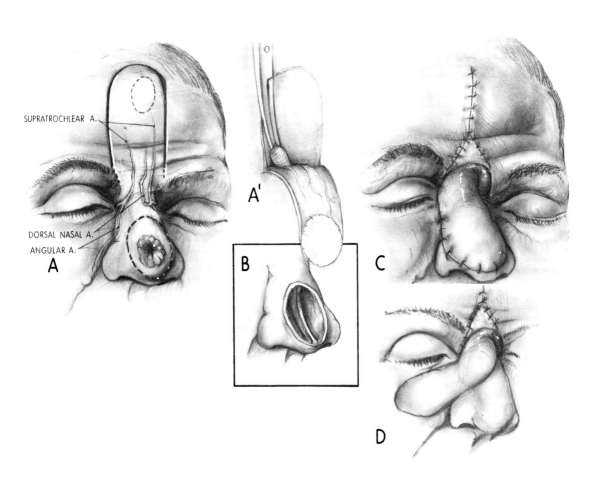

SUPRATROCHLEAR A.

DORSAL NASAL A.

ANGULAR A.

A

A'

B

C

D

FAT FLIP FLAP (After Millard, 1969)

Indication

To reduce bulging edema of transposed flaps.

Highpoints

1. Stage the procedure with one month interval, i.e., operate one border of flap at a time.
2. Excise skin scar along one edge.
3. Elevate skin and subcutaneous tissue of half of flap.
4. Dissect edematous and bulging fat in retrograde fashion as a second flap.
5. Elevate at a slightly more superficial plane surrounding adjacent skin juxtaposed to the flap.
6. Turn the fat flap back as far as possible and suture.
7. Skin closure is performed in a straight line if the closure follows a natural skin line; closure should be in multiple Z-plasties if it crosses a natural skin line.
8. Repeat the same technique on the other side of the flap about one month later.

A The skin scar is excised along one border of the flap.

B The skin and some subcutaneous tissue are elevated from both the flap and skin adjacent to the flap. The skin and subcutaneous tissue elevated from the adjacent area are slightly thinner than their counterparts from the flap. The fat flap is outlined with the dotted line. This includes the bulging edematous adipose tissue from the original flap.

C The fat flap is flipped over 180 degrees and sutured as far as possible across and under the elevated skin of the adjacent area. In this manner the bulging adipose tissue is transferred to the adjacent area which is depressed and wanting of adipose tissue.

D The final closure in cross section.

The skin closure is in a straight line approximating a natural crease. Where the skin closure crosses the natural lines, multiple Z-plasties are performed (see plates 18, 19 and 20).

Plate 122   General Purpose Flaps

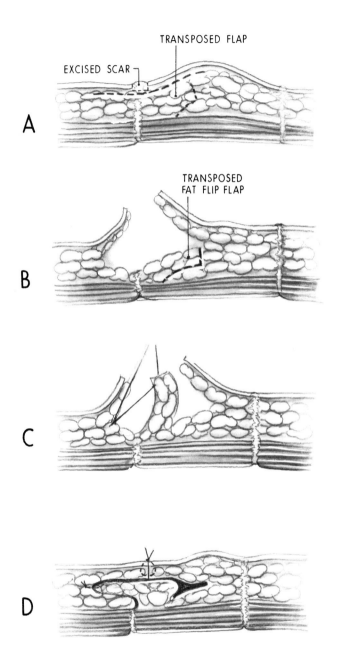

BIBLIOGRAPHY

Andrews, E. B.: Island flaps in facial reconstruction. Plast. Reconstr. Surg. *44*: 49–51, 1969.

Bakamjian, V. Y.: A two-stage method for pharyngoesophageal reconstruction with a primary pectoral skin flap. Plast. Reconstr. Surg. *36*:173–184, 1965.

Bakamjian, V. Y.: Total reconstruction of pharynx with medially based deltopectoral skin flap. New York J. Med. *68*:2771–2778, 1968.

Bakamjian, V. Y., Culf, N. K., and Bales, H. W.: Versatility of the deltopectoral flap in reconstructions following head and neck cancer surgery. Excerpta Medica International Congress, Series No. 174, Trans. Fourth International Congress of Plastic and Reconstructive Surgery, Rome, October 1967.

Chretien, P. B., Ketcham, A. S., Hoye, R. C., and Gertner, H. R.: Extended shoulder flap and its use in reconstruction of the defects of the head and neck. Amer. J. Surg. *118*:752–755, 1969.

Coleman, C. C., Jr.: Local flaps for reconstructions after head and neck tumor surgery. Plast. Reconstr. Surg. *42*:225–231, 1968.

Conley, J. J.: A one stage operation for the immediate reconstruction of the pharynx and cervical esophagus following radical resection. West. J. Surg. *63*: 344, 1955.

Conley, J. J.: One stage radical resection of cervical esophagus, larynx, pharynx, and neck with immediate reconstruction. Arch. Otolaryng. 58:546, 1963.

Conley, J. J.: The use of regional flaps in head and neck surgery. Ann. Otol. 69:1223, 1960.

Conway, H., Stark, R. B., and Joslin, D.: Cutaneous histamine reaction as a test of circulatory efficiency of tubed pedicles and flaps. Surg. Gynec. Obstet. 93:185, 1951.

Corso, P. F., Gerold, F. P., and Frazell, E. L.: The rapid closure of large salivary fistulas by an accelerated shoulder flap technic. Amer. J. Surg. *106*:691, 1963.

Cramer, L. M., and Culf, N. K.: Symposium on Cancer of Head and Neck. C. V. Mosby Company, 1969.

Davis, G. N., and Hoopes, J. E.: A new technique of delivery of the total forehead flap for intraoral reconstruction. Presentation at the Society of Head and Neck Surgeons Meeting, April 1970.

Dingman, R. O., Grabb, W. C., Oneal, R. M., and Ponitz, R. J.: Sternocleidomastoid muscle transplant to masseter area. Plast. Reconstr. Surg. *43*:5–12, 1969.

Edgerton, M. T., Jr.: Reconstruction of hypopharynx and the cervical esophagus after removal of cancer. Proceedings of the Fourth National Cancer Conference, p. 685, 1960.

Edgerton, M. T., and Snyder, G. B.: Combined intracranial-extracranial approach and use of the two-stage split flap technic for reconstruction with craniofacial malignancies. Amer. J. Surg. *110*:595–602, 1965.

Esser, J. F. S.: Studies in plastic surgery of the face. Ann. Surg. 65:297, 1917.

Farr, H. W., Jean-Gilles, B., and Die, A.: Cervical island skin flap repair of oral and pharyngeal defects in the composite operation for cancer. Amer. J. Surg. *118*:759–763, 1969.

Farrior, R. T.: Cancer of the head and neck. Primary and reconstructive surgery. Arch. Otolaryng. *71*:891–905, 1960.

Farrior, R. T.: Rehabilitation by skin grafting. Arch. Otolaryng. 83:120–134, 1966.

Gaisford, J. C.: Reconstruction of head and neck deformities. Surg. Clin. N. Amer. 47:295–322, 1967.

Haar, J.: Personal communication, 1970.

Hoopes, J. E., and Edgerton, M. L.: Immediate forehead flap repair in resection for oropharyngeal cancer. Amer. J. Surg. *112*:527, 1966.

Kazanjian, V. H.: The repair of nasal defects with the median forehead flap; primary closure of the forehead wound. Surg. Gynec. Obstet. 83:37, 1946.

Krizek, T. J., and Robson, M. C.: The split flap technique in head and neck reconstruction. Presentation at Society of Head and Neck Surgeons and American Society for Head and Neck Surgery, May 1973.

Loré, J. M., Jr., and Zingapan, E. G.: Deltopectoral flap. Arch. Otolaryng. 94:13–18, 1971.

McGregor, I. A.: The temporal flap in facial cancer: A method of repair. Third International Congress of Plastic Surgery, 1963.

Millard, D. R., Stokley, P. H., and Campbell, R. C.: The fat flip flap. Plast. Reconstr. Surg. *44*:202–204, 1969.

Milton, S. H.: Experimental studies on island flaps. 1. The surviving length. Plast. Reconstr. Surg. *48*:574–578, 1971.

Myers, M. B., and Cherry, G.: Differences in the delay phenomenon in the rabbit, rat, and pig. Plast. Reconstr. Surg. *47*: 73–78, 1971.

Narayanan, M.: Immediate reconstruction with bipolar scalp flap after excisions of huge cheek cancers. Plast. Reconstr. Surg. *46*:548–553, 1970.

Richardson, G. S., Hanna, D. C., and Gaisford, J. C.: Midline forehead flap nasal reconstructions in patients with low browlines. Plast. Reconstr. Surg. *49*: 130–133, 1972.

Schechter, G. L., Biller, H. F., and Ogura, J. H.: Revascularized skin flaps: A new concept in transfer of skin flaps. Laryngoscope *79*:1647–1665, 1969.

Sherlock, E. C., and Maddox, W. A.: The versatile deltopectoral skin flap in reconstruction about the head and neck. Amer. J. Surg. *118*:744–751, 1969.

Shumrick, D. A.: Reconstructive flaps in head and neck surgery. Otolaryng. Clin. N. Amer. pp. 685–702, October 1969.

Sisson, G. A., and Goldstein, J. C.: Flaps and grafts in head and neck surgery. Arch. Otolaryng. *92*:599–610, 1970.

Terz, J. J., and Lawrence, W., Jr.: Primary reconstruction of oropharyngeal surgical defects with a forehead flap. Surg. Gynec. Obstet. *129*:533–537, 1969.

Washio, H.: Retroauricular-temporal flap. Plast. Reconstr. Surg. *43*:162–166, 1969.

Wurlitzer, F., and Ballantyne, A. J.: Reconstruction of lower jaw area with a bipedicled deltopectoral flap and a ticonium prosthesis. Case report. Plast. Reconstr. Surg. *49*:220–223, 1972.

7. THE LIPS

PLANING OF LIP

Highpoints

1. The entire exposed vermilion of either the lower or upper lip or both may be excised for leukoplakia with immediate coverage using mucous membrane advanced from the inner aspect of the lip.
2. This operation may be combined with the shield type of excision (below) or the Abbe-Estlander operation (see plate 126).
3. Specimen must be labeled "right" and "left" for proper orientation of serial histologic study to rule out carcinoma.

A An incision is made through the mucosa about 0.3 to 0.5 cm beyond the extent of the leukoplakia.

B Following the vermilion border, or even including a small amount of skin if the leukoplakia has reached the cutaneous margin, a flap of mucosa is separated from the underlying muscle and excised.

C The remaining normal mucosa on the inner aspect of the lip is extensively undermined.

D Using 5-0 nylon, the advanced mucosa is approximated to the skin margin.

Complication

Some flattening of the natural contour of the lip.

SHIELD EXCISION OF LOWER LIP

Highpoints

1. Early carcinoma of lip less than 0.5 cm in diameter can be excised with adequate margins.
2. Up to one third of lower or upper lip may be excised – approximately 1.5 to 2.3 cm – and defect closed with simple approximation of edges. Larger defects require some type of reconstruction flaps.
3. Three-layer approximation: mucous membrane, muscle and skin.

A A "shield" type of incision is outlined with methylene blue. If the lesion is malignant, 1 cm of grossly normal tissue must be included on each side. The vermilion edges on both borders are marked by a needle dipped in the dye. This aids in an accurate approximation of the vermilion edges following the excision. The excision is made through and through skin, muscle and mucous membrane. Grasping the lip between index finger and thumb aids in the excision by stabilizing the lip and controlling hemorrhage. Only after the complete excision are the vessels clamped and tied.

B Layer closure is commenced by first approximating the mucosa with interrupted 4-0 or 5-0 nylon.

C The orbicularis oris muscle and other deep structures have been carefully approximated using 4-0 chromic catgut. The first skin suture of 5-0 nylon is placed through the dye marks on the vermilion borders.

D 5-0 nylon is used to complete the closure.

Plate 123   The Lips

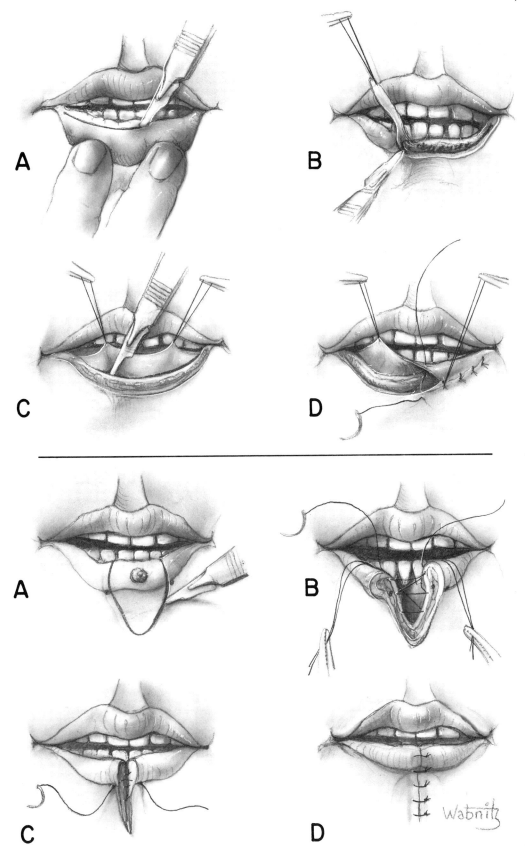

REPAIR OF LARGE VERMILION DEFECTS

Highpoints

1. Use mucous membrane and muscle pedicle flaps.
2. If donor site defect is large, dermal skin graft or free buccal mucous membrane serves as an excellent buccal inlay.
3. Flap and pedicles must be thick to preserve adequate blood supply.
4. Barton bandage necessary for cross oral pedicles.

A A traumatic defect involves the central portion of the lower vermilion. With both commissures evenly retracted a bipedicle mucous membrane–muscle flap is outlined on the upper lip. The outer or upper incision is made about 0.5 cm from the vermilion cutaneous border, splitting the entire lip and leaving enough attached at either side for an adequate blood supply. The incision is made 1 to 1.5 cm into the orbicularis oris muscle. Another inner parallel incision is made at least 1 to 1.5 cm from the first incision depending on the breadth of the defect in the lower lip. This likewise includes the muscle and is directed so that it meets the first incision deep in the muscle. The bipedicle flap thus mobilized contains the superior labial artery (A^1).

B The donor site can usually be closed by simple approximation. If this is not possible without distortion to the upper lip, especially the Cupid's bow, a free split thickness graft is inserted as depicted. The ragged edges of the defect are trimmed.

C The bipedicle flap is now rotated 90 degrees so that the inner edge of the flap is sewn to the skin margin of the defect and the outer edge of the flap sewn to the gingivobuccal margin of the defect. The pedicle is carefully tubed near its base and closed posteriorly so that there are no bare areas. A Barton bandage is applied. The pedicles are severed after two weeks.

D This defect is a partial loss of the lower vermilion. Reconstruction consists of the formation of a bipedicle tube of mucous membrane and muscle from the lower gingivobuccal sulcus, the donor site being covered with a dermal or free buccal mucous membrane graft.

E The bipedicle flap is elevated and tubed while the donor site is grafted.

F The next stage consists of transposing one end of the pedicle to the edge of the defect as shown by the direction of the arrow in step *E*.

G At the following stage, the defect is bared and the pedicle untubed. The tube edges are now sutured to the edges of the defect. A final stage may be necessary to correct any inequality with the opposite side of the lower lip.

Plate 124   The Lips

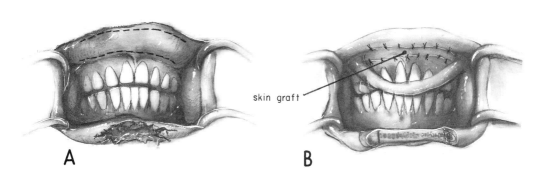

A

B

skin graft

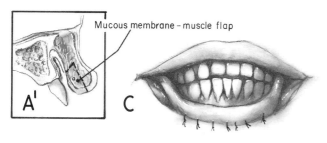

A'

Mucous membrane – muscle flap

C

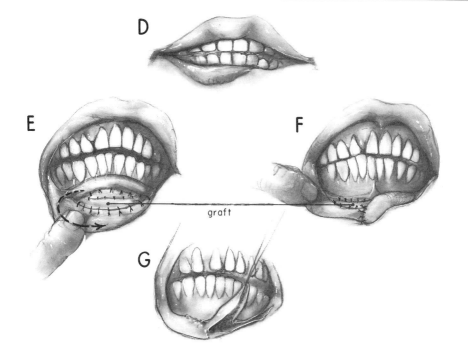

D

E

F

graft

G

CUPID'S BOW

Indication

When the upper lip is so deformed that the initial repair has resulted in a straight horizontal line that makes the reconstruction all the more obvious, restoration of a Cupid's bow is indicated (plate 135).

A   Triangular skin areas are outlined.

B   These areas are excised down to muscle which is superficially incised along the dotted lines at each side of the center of the bow. The mucosa of the lip is elevated from the muscle except in its midportion.

C   The completed restoration.

ELLIPTICAL EXCISION OF BENIGN LIP LESION

Indications

Small premalignant lesions and benign lesions.

D   An elliptical skin and mucosal incision is outlined.

E   The lesion with skin, mucosa and underlining muscle is excised. The muscle is approximated with one or more buried sutures of fine chromic catgut. The initial skin suture is placed at the vermilion border.

F   The completed closure.

DISTORTION OF MOUTH CORRECTED BY Z-PLASTY

G   A Z-type incision is made through and through the skin, muscle and mucous membrane (see plate 14).

H   The full thickness cheek flaps are swung as depicted. A three-layer closure is used.

The reverse Z-plasty can be used (Gerold, 1960) for a drooping commissure following section of the buccal division of the facial nerve.

EXCISION OF LARGE BENIGN LESIONS OF UPPER LIP WITH ROTATION FLAP

I   Skin incisions are made as outlined.

J   The flap is rotated and sutured in position. Extension of incision is made to allow closure of the donor site. The lateral skin margin is liberally undermined.

K   The completed closure. Buried sutures of fine chromic catgut or white silk are used subcutaneously.

Plate 125   The Lips

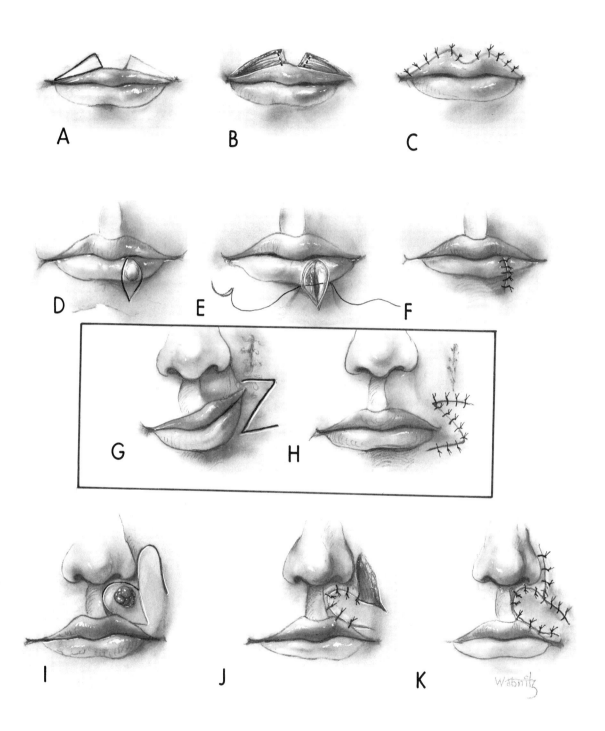

A

B

C

D

E

F

G

H

I

J

K

ABBE-ESTLANDER LIP OPERATION

Highpoints

1. One third to one half of upper or lower lip can be resected for carcinoma with immediate reconstruction.
2. Upper or lower lip defects following unsatisfactory cleft lip repair or trauma can be reconstructed.
3. Full thickness flap: skin, muscle, mucous membrane.
4. Preserve labial artery in flap pedicle.
5. Local anesthesia or general anesthesia.
6. With general anesthesia, extreme care during postoperative recovery phase regarding airway obstruction and disruption of suture lines.
7. Approximate vermilion borders.

A A shield type of incision is outlined in methylene blue (alcohol solution) with a minimum of 1 cm of grossly normal tissue on either side of the tumor. The vermilion border is marked at the point where the incisions cross with a needle dipped in the dye. This aids the approximation of the vermilion borders when suturing. Using calipers or other measuring device, a similar triangular area is outlined on the opposite lip, the length being equal to or slightly longer than that of the resected defect while the base or width is one half that of the defect. This achieves a proportionate shortening of upper and lower lips. The pedicle of the flap is usually medial and always contains the labial artery which must be carefully preserved. It is better to leave a larger pedicle — usually 5 to 8 mm — beyond the vermilion border than to risk injury to the artery. If the lesion is so located that the safety margin allows preservation of the natural commissure of the lips, this is preferable. Otherwise, the commissure is resected and reconstructed by a double Z-plasty or conversion of a **Y**-type incision to a **V** (see plate 128, steps *H, I, J* and *K*). The commissure can also be reconstructed by using the Gillies method (plate 127, steps *A, B, C* and *D*).

B The lesion with its borders is excised through and through. Using a clean knife, the flap is mobilized through and through except for the median pedicle.

C Using a stay suture, the flap is rotated.

D One suture of 5-0 nylon is placed through the needle marks of dye at the vermilion edges. It is left loose until a separate three layer closure is done with mucosa, muscle and skin. This closure is best begun along the medial margin of the pedicle. The muscle sutures are 4-0 chromic catgut; the mucosa suture is nylon or Dermalene.

E All the mucosal and muscle sutures are completed and the skin is approximated with 5-0 nylon.

F A crown-type suture approximates the lateral edges of the lips with the pedicle so that the otherwise exposed border of the pedicle is covered with mucosa of the lips.

G Approximation is complete. Feeding through a straw may be necessary. The pedicle is left intact for three to five weeks.

Plate 126   The Lips

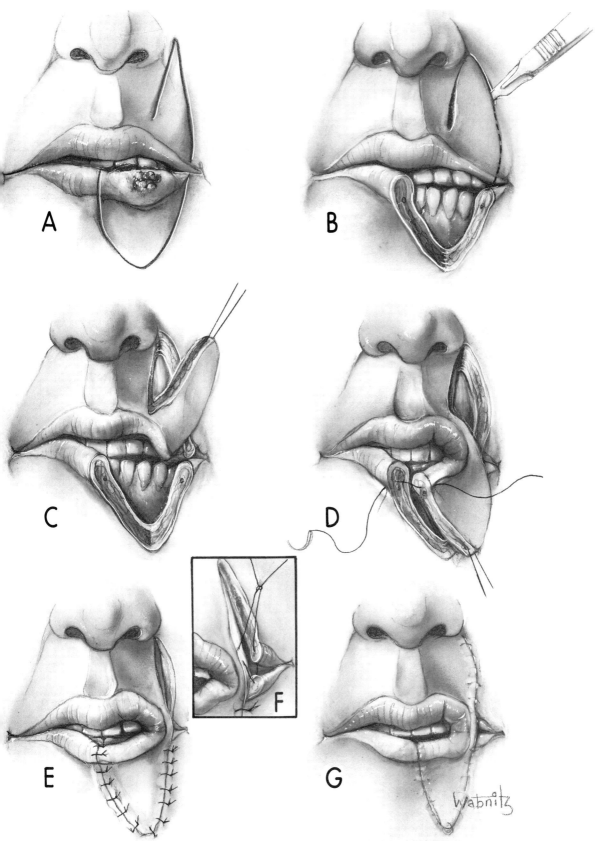

A

B

C

D

F

E

G

wabnitz

ABBE-ESTLANDER LIP OPERATION (*Continued*)

H　In three to five weeks the pedicle is transected (1–2) and reapproximation of the vermilion border accomplished by a modified Z-plasty. An incision (2–3) is made along the previous scar for a distance of 1 to 1.5 cm. A lateral extension (3–4) is made which is slightly longer.

I　The completed incisions.

J　Points 2 and 5 approximate one another, splitting the distance along the line 3–4. The vermilion edge is thus exactly realigned (1–6).

K　The completed reconstruction.

CORRECTION OF ROUNDED COMMISSURE OF LIPS (GILLIES)

Following major lip surgery in which the commissure has been either resected or displaced, the rounded corner may be corrected by the method of Gillies or that of May (plate 128, steps *H, I, J* and *K*).

Highpoints

The Gillies technique is as follows:
1. Excision of small triangle of skin.
2. Section of underlying muscle.
3. Advancement of mucous membrane.

A　A small triangle of skin is excised at the site of the new commissure. The vermilion of the lower lip is cut at an angle along the solid line.

B　The underlying muscle is cut slantwise at the site of the new commissure. The inside layer of mucous membrane is transected in a horizontal line leading to the new commissure.

C　The lower vermilion which was freed has been rotated into the new commissure forming a portion of the upper lip. It is sutured inside and outside. The buccal layer of mucous membrane of the lower lip is now freed with scissors or knife.

D　This mobilized mucous membrane is now approximated to the cutaneous border of the lower lip defect.

Plate 127   The Lips

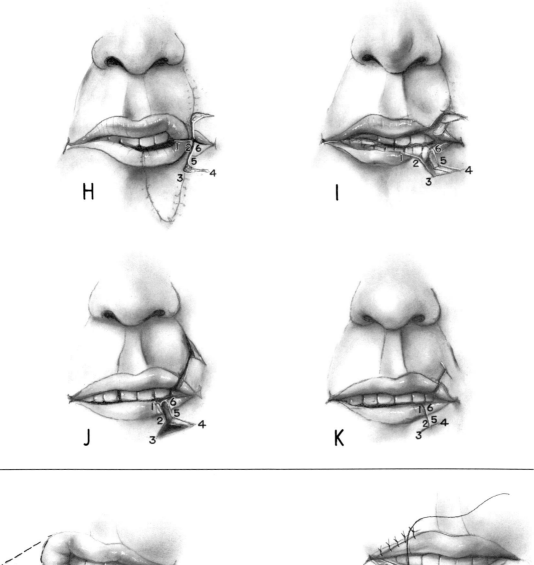

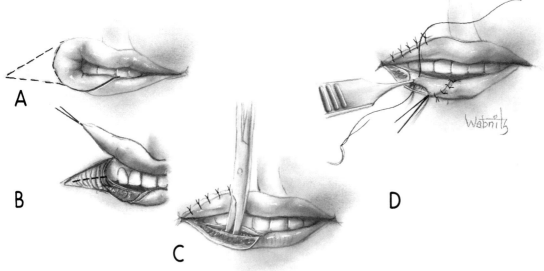

MODIFICATIONS OF ABBE-ESTLANDER LIP OPERATION

RECONSTRUCTION OF CENTER LOWER LIP DEFECT

A   Rotation of upper lip flap to close a center lower lip defect.

B   The commissure of the mouth is preserved. Operative details in plates 126 and 127.

C   When a crossed pedicle flap for center defects may not be tolerated by the patient or when general anesthesia is necessary, this type of transfer flap is used. During reaction from general anesthesia the patient may not be controllable and the usual crossed pedicle flap (steps A and B) is endangered.

    After the usual excision of the lesion, a lateral rectangular flap is advanced to close the center defect.

D   The resulting medial defect is closed with an upper lip flap which includes the commissure. The commissure can be preserved by following the technique in plates 126 and 127.

E   The completed closure.

RECONSTRUCTION OF UPPER LIP DEFECT

F   Defects in the upper lip are closed with a rotation flap from the lower lip.

G   A new commissure is formed by the pedicle from the rotated lower lip.

CORRECTION OF ROUNDED COMMISSURE OF LIPS (MAY, 1949)

Indication

    When the pedicle of a rotated lip flap forms the new commissure, the rounded corner is correctible.

H   A double Z-plasty (after May, 1949) is utilized to elongate and sharpen the commissure. This is done at least three to five weeks following the initial operation. Excision of a small triangle of skin may be required between flaps 4 and 2.

I   Flaps 1 and 3 are rotated outward, while flaps 2 and 4 are rotated inward—thus 2 and 4 are exchanged with 1 and 3.

J   Another method of correction for commissure deformity is conversion of a **Y**-type incision to a **V**. A **Y** incision is made as depicted. Some skin may require excision on the lateral borders.

K   Point 5 is then advanced to point 5'.

    For the Gillies method see plate 127, steps A, B, C and D.

Plate 128   The Lips

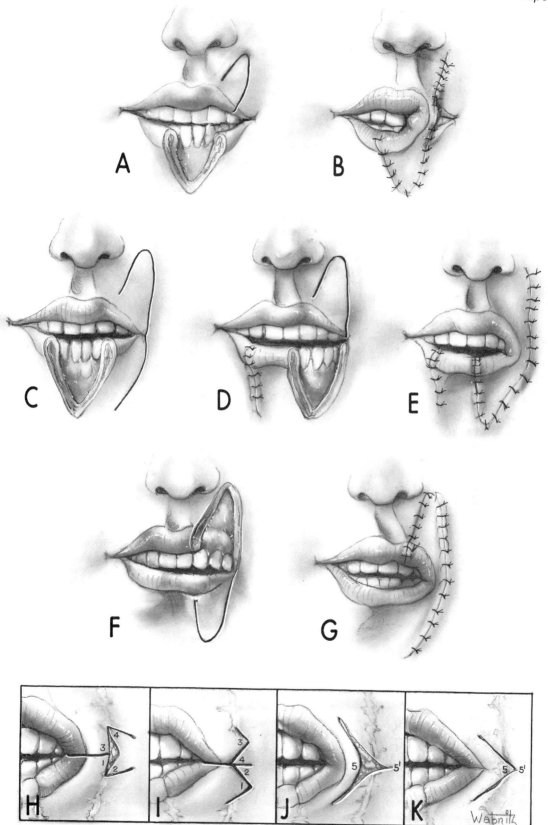

RECONSTRUCTION OF LARGE DEFECTS OF UPPER LIP

On the following five plates, different techniques are depicted for reconstruction of large full thickness defects of the upper lip. The first procedure is the use of the cheek flap (Paletta, 1954), with a tongue flap for inside mucous membrane lining (Bakamjian, 1971). The other flaps are the fan flaps, lateral flaps (Burow, Gillies), and forehead flaps. Each has its own advantages and disadvantages.

RECONSTRUCTION OF UPPER LIP WITH CHEEK FLAP
(After Paletta, 1954; Bakamjian, 1971)

Highpoints

1. Wide resection of tumor—this can include a portion of the base of the columella and floor of nose as well as full thickness of upper lip.
2. Medial border of cheek flap follows nasolabial fold leaving underlying muscles intact.
3. New vermilion and mucous membrane of reconstructed lip is formed by tongue flap.

A Malignant tumor involves major portion of upper lip. The cheek flap is outlined, its medial border following the nasolabial fold. Resection includes all layers of the upper lip and portion of columella and floor of the nose.

B A horizontal fishmouth incision is dotted along the tongue (Bakamjian). The cheek flap (Paletta) is already in position. The inferior tongue flap (1) will form the vermilion and lower portion of the reconstructed lip, while the upper tongue flap (2) will form the inner mucous membrane lining.

C The cheek flap fitted into the defect with tongue flap sutured in position. The cheek lateral to the flap site and portion of skin of cheek are undermined for closure of the donor site.

D Cross section depicts the position of tongue flaps.

E Close-up view of tongue flaps (1) and (2). A diamond-shaped area of tongue muscle may be excised at the time of the division of the tongue flaps to facilitate approximation of the tongue mucous membrane.

F
G The completed reconstruction.

This flap can be utilized to reconstruct the entire columella. The bare area on the contralateral side of the flap can be covered with a free skin graft if necessary.

Plate 129   The Lips

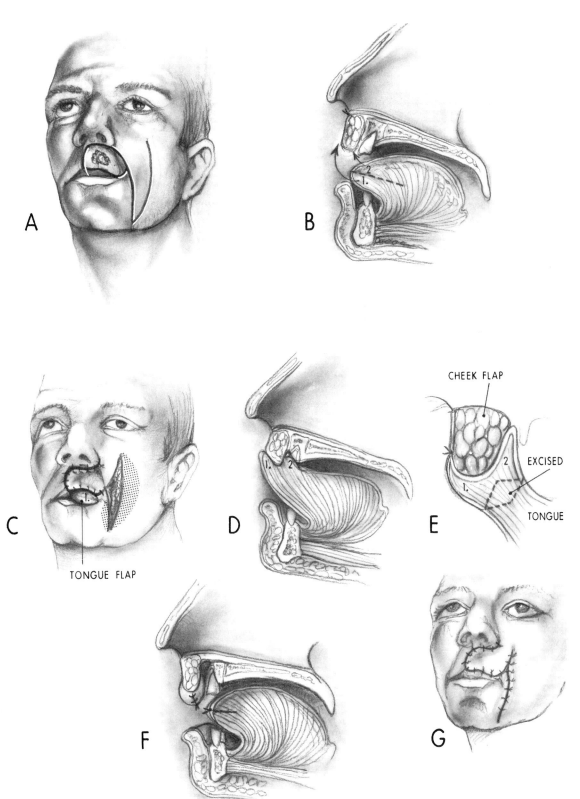

FAN FLAP RECONSTRUCTION FOR LARGE DEFECTS
OF UPPER LIP

Highpoints

1. Main blood supply is through the labial artery – same principle as an Abbe flap.
2. All incisions are through and through – into the oral cavity.

A Two thirds of the upper lip is excised or has been lost as a result of trauma. Skin incisions are made as outlined by the solid lines extending through all layers into the oral cavity. The distal extent of the incision (6) is 0.5 to 1.0 cm from the cutaneous-vermilion border to avoid injury to the labial artery. The lateral incision (7–8) is not made until the flap is rotated.

A¹ The mucous membrane is elevated from the inner aspect of a portion (1–2) of the
A² flap. This is advanced and sutured to the skin margin to form a new vermilion for the rotated flap.

B The flap is rotated into position.

C With the flap in position, the defect in the nasolabial region is closed in two or three layers. As this is done, the lateral incision (7–8) is made depending on the way the flap lies.

D Suturing the flap begins at the most advanced edge (2–3). A two- or three-layer approximation is made. Point 8 along the lateral border of the cheek is lost either by stretching or by trimming the corner.

E The completed reconstruction. The rounded commissure will require revision in three to five weeks (see plates 127 *A*, *B*, *C* and *D* and 128 *H*, *I*, *J* and *K*).

Complications

1. Involved procedure.
2. Results in excess scars in cheek.

Plate 130   The Lips

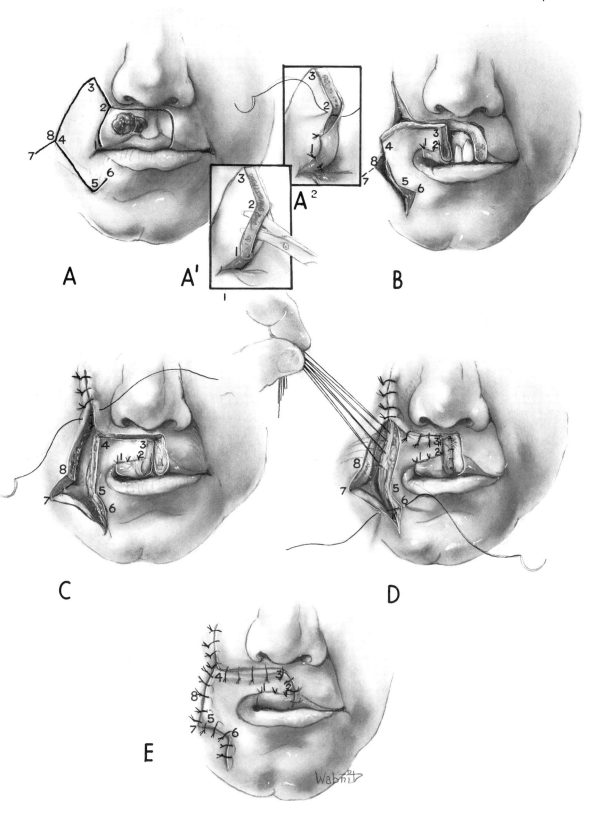

A

A'

A²

B

C

D

E

EXCISION AND REPAIR OF LARGE LESIONS OF UPPER LIP

In these drawings two types of operations are depicted. In the first operation the reconstruction is based on Burow's principle of excision of excess skin and muscle with straight horizontal advancement. In the second operation reconstruction is achieved by a fan flap as in the Abbe-Estlander procedure which utilizes the labial artery as the source of blood supply. Gillies has a modification of the fan flap which facilitates reconstruction of the skin of the columella when this is necessary. A significant drawback to both of these procedures is narrowing of the oral orifice. Paletta's technique may be preferred (plate 129).

BUROW'S TECHNIQUE

Highpoints

1. Full thickness excision of lesion and nasolabial crescents.
2. Adequate mobilization along gingivobuccal sulcus with preservation of rim of mucous membrane in gingiva.

A   An incision is made through and through the upper lip on both sides of the tumor with a horizontal connection at the base of the columella. Crescent-shaped arcs are outlined in the nasolabial areas to permit straight horizontal advancement of the sides of the defect.

B   The full thickness crescent-shaped areas and the tumor are excised.

C   Mobilization of the lateral flaps is achieved by liberal incisions on both sides of the upper gingivobuccal sulcus. Sufficient mucous membrane is left in the gingiva for suturing the advanced flap.

D   Three-layer closure is performed: mucous membrane, muscle and skin.

E   The mucous membrane closure is demonstrated. The rounded commissures may be corrected by following the technique of Gillies (plate 127, steps A, B, C and D) or May (plate 128, steps H, I, J and K).

GILLIES' TECHNIQUE

F   The major portion of the upper lip and skin of columella has been excised. Bilateral face flaps are made as follows. A point X is marked on the vermilion border at a distance from the commissure equal to approximately half the length of the defect of the upper lip. About 1.2 cm below and slightly lateral to this point, a through and through incision is made in the same direction away from the vermilion for a distance of about 2.0 cm. The labial artery, vital to this fan flap, is thus preserved. The incision is then carried in an easy sweep along the nasolabial fold to the lateral edge of the nose and then downward to the upper edge of the defect. The entire incision is through and through all layers. The gingivobuccal sulcus is also incised as in step C.

G   The mobilized lip flaps are rotated. Above point 2 on the lateral border of the lip flap, an incision (3–4) is made in the cheek flap to adapt the advanced cheek flap to the lip flap. Thus point 3 is approximated to point 1 and point 4 is approximated to point 2. Point 5 is rounded or lost as the cheek is advanced. Point 6 is used to reconstruct the columella.

H   The completed reconstruction.

Plate 131   The Lips

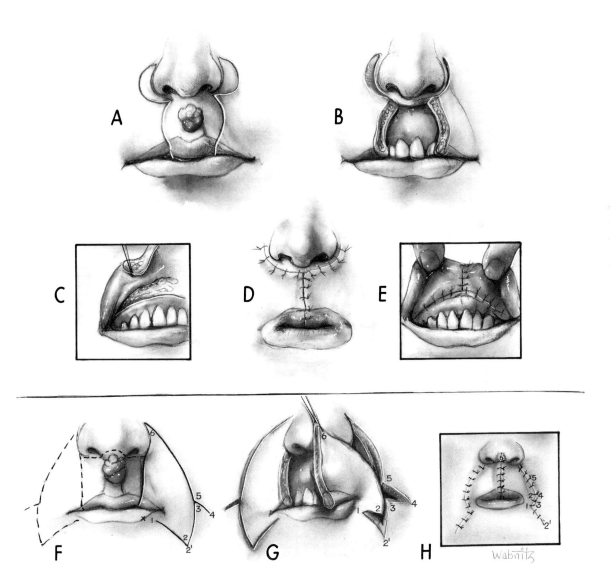

wabnitz

REPAIR OF LARGE DEFECTS OF UPPER LIP

Indications

    In the rare situation in which upper lip defect is due to patient neglect and poor or no treatment, when the defect is the result of tissue loss but mostly the result of retraction of the lip margins, an advancement with some of the fan flap principles is suitable. The associated cheek defect in this patient was covered with a forehead flap. The other complicating circumstance was the absence of well vascularized surrounding soft tissue as the result of radiation therapy. The fact that the lip margins were retracted cicatrix formation permitted this type of reconstruction with minimum narrowing of the oral orifice.

A   A very liberal incision is made in the gingivobuccal sulcus with mobilization of the lip and cheek beyond the nasolabial fold. Another incision is made in the nasolabial fold (1–2–3).

B   The incision in the nasolabial fold is then extended beneath the nares from point 4 to 5. This completely mobilizes the upper lip and cheek. A small triangle of tissue between 1–2–4 may require excision.

C   The upper lip flap is then advanced; the cheek is likewise advanced to close the defect in the nasolabial area. Three-layer closure is used if possible: mucosa, muscle and skin.

D   The lower lip is mobilized with a through and through incision following the fan flap technique (plate 130).

E   The inferior gingivobuccal sulcus is incised deeply, thus mobilizing the outer portion of the lower lip.

F   After the opposing ends of each flap are trimmed, a three-layer closure is mandatory.

G   The first layer is the mucosa, using nylon.

H   The second layer is muscle, using 3-0 chromic catgut.

I   The skin is approximated using fine nylon, the first suture being placed in the cutaneous-vermilion line.

The remaining cheek defect is reconstructed using a forehead flap (see plates 119 and 120).

Plate 132   The Lips

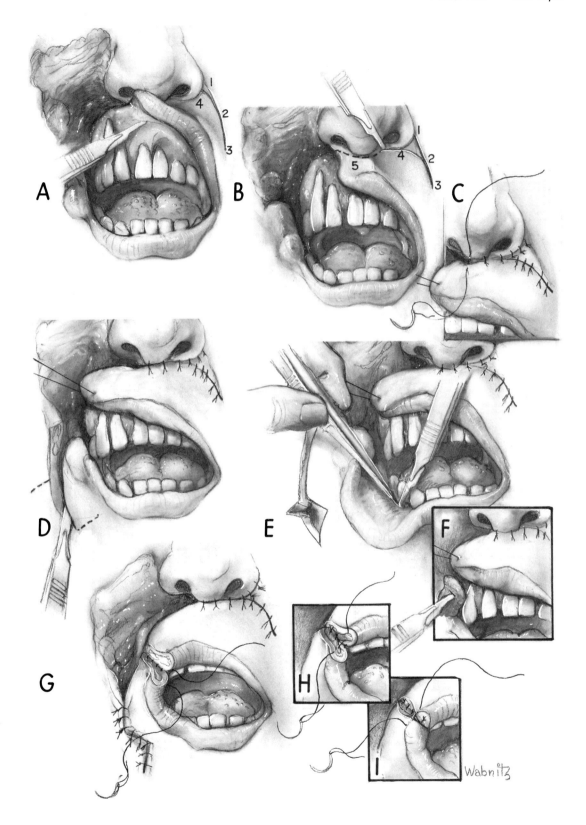

BITEMPORAL ("VISOR") FLAP FOR LARGE UPPER LIP AND CHEEK DEFECTS

Highpoints

1. No delay necessary.
2. If pedicles cannot be tubed, cover all bare areas with split thickness grafts.

A   After the hair is shaved, a bipedicle temporal flap is outlined including the major branches of the superficial temporal arteries in both pedicles. It is important to include a nonhair-bearing area for the lip turn-in portion of the flap. An alternate to this turn-in is a free split thickness skin or dermal graft. A tongue flap can also be used as mucous membrane lining (see plate 129). No delay is necessary and the bipedicle full thickness flap, including the galea, is immediately swung into position over the defect. This is particularly well suited to resections for cancer since the defect can be covered at the same operation. Another distinct advantage in resection of a malignant neoplasm is that local flaps are not used; hence spread of disease is detected more easily and not confused with the scars of local flaps.

Split thickness skin grafts are used to cover the donor site and the bare areas of the pedicles if tubing of the latter is not possible.

B   The underside of the central portion of the bipedicle flap is covered either with a nonhair-bearing turn-in fold from the flap itself or with a split thickness, dermal or buccal mucous membrane graft or a tongue flap or a combination of both. A horizontal row of sutures is placed along any remnant of the gingivobuccal mucous membrane. The lateral edges of the lip and cheek defect are approximated as well as possible to the bare undersurface of the bipedicle flap. This will require revision at a later stage.

C   The bipedicle flap in position with sutures along the upper edge of the flap to the upper edge of the cheek and lip defect. The dotted lines indicate the location of the turn-in fold or split thickness dermal graft or tongue flap which forms the inner covering of the upper lip.

D   The time of section of the pedicles will depend on the blood supply gained from the edges of the defect. Sectioning should be done in stages—one side at a time—and each side may be staged if necessary. The pedicles are then returned to the scalp, removing the split thickness grafts where necessary. The only scalp defect is in the center where it may be hidden by proper hair styling.

At a later stage, the vermilion of the upper lip can be restored by using cross lip grafts of vermilion from the lower lip. For restoration of a Cupid's bow see plate 125, steps *A*, *B* and *C*. If a forehead defect exists caused by the use of a non-hair-bearing turn-in portion, this can be covered by rotation flaps from the scalp and forehead in place of split thickness skin grafts.

Plate 133   The Lips

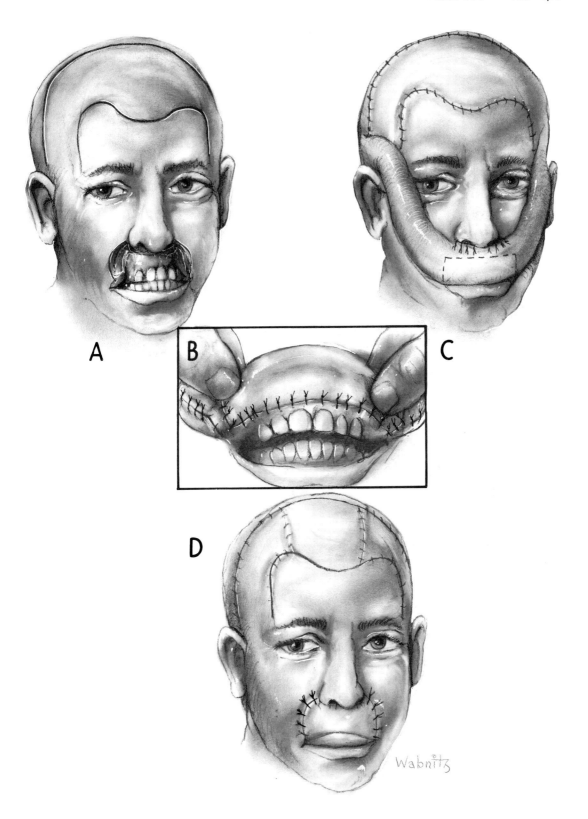

A

B

C

D

Wabnitz

RESECTION OF LOWER LIP WITH BERNARD RECONSTRUCTION

Highpoints

1. Resect adequate margins, especially down to chin.
2. Preserve external maxillary arteries.
3. If neck dissection is necessary, perform as second stage (Martin et al., 1941).
4. Virtually entire lower lip can be excised.
5. Preserve mucous membrane in lateral triangular cheek flaps — this forms vermilion for reconstructed lower lip.
6. Preserve some mucous membrane in gingivobuccal sulcus for suturing lateral cheek flaps.
7. Tailoring of excess skin and muscle is performed as last stages of operation.

A A rectangular full thickness excision of the lower lip and entire chin is performed. A narrow rim of gingivobuccal mucous membrane (A) is preserved on the alveolar ridge. This serves as suture sites for the lateral cheek flaps. With a suitable dye, two lateral nasolabial triangles are outlined. The base of each triangle is slanted slightly upward and each base is equal to half of the length of the excised lower lip. The median border of the triangle follows the nasolabial fold as closely as possible so that with its closure a more natural fold will result. The skin and muscle (1) of these nasolabial triangles are now excised carefully, preserving the underlying mucous membrane (2 in A, B and C). This mucous membrane (2) is now mobilized, preserving its base. A small triangle of skin (X) is excised as the mucous membrane flap (2) is tailored to form the new lower lip vermilion. The two triangles (Y) below the chin margin are not outlined or excised until the cheek flaps are mobilized.

B It may be necessary to excise some muscle and subcutaneous tissue from the lateral area of this triangle where the cheek is thick. On the right side of the patient, the mucous membrane flap is already sutured.

C The cheek flap has been mobilized along the mandible as far lateral as the masseter muscle, taking care not to injure the external maxillary artery which is the principal blood supply to the cheek flap. The anterior margin of the masseter muscle may be freed if additional mobilization is necessary. The closure is begun by approximation of the mucous membrane of the cheek flap to the mucous membrane of the gingivobuccal sulcus left attached to the lower alveolar ridge. These sutures are placed to facilitate the median advancement of the cheek flap. Before all these sutures are tied, the mucous membranes of the edges of the nasolabial triangle are closed. As the cheek flaps are advanced, the two triangles below the chin (Y in step A) are excised to adapt the midline closure in a satisfactory manner. Three-layer closure is used wherever possible.

Plate 134   The Lips

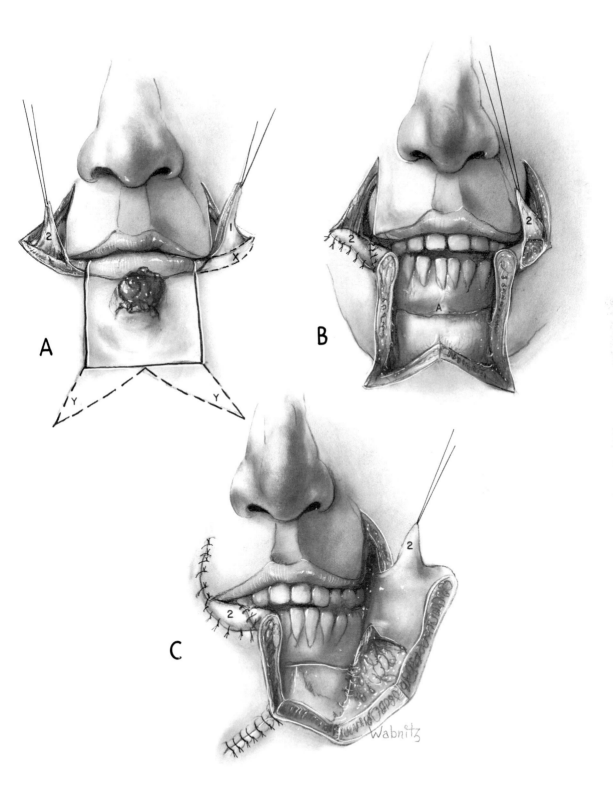

A

B

C

Wabnitz

CLEFT LIP REPAIR

To properly understand the objectives in cleft lip repair not only must the deformity be evaluated but also its relationship to the normal anatomy.

Normal Anatomy (After Millard, 1968)

A   Anterior view—the labeled structures and their relationships are the normal landmarks important in cleft lip repair.

B   Lateral view—depicted is the protruding lower two thirds to three fourths of the upper lip known as the "pout" which likewise is important in the cleft lip repair.

Types of Cleft Lip Deformities

    a. Incomplete.
    b. Complete.
    c. Unilateral.
    d. Bilateral.
    e. Median (extremely rare).

Just about any combination of the above types is possible. In addition, varying degrees of each deformity are possible. Varying types of the cleft palate are likewise possible. In general, simultaneous repair of a cleft lip combined with cleft palate is not performed for a number of reasons: optimal time is different and there are increased morbidity and mortality due to possible airway problems and blood loss.

Basic Deformities of Cleft Lip

1. Vertical shortness or narrowing of the lip on the side of the cleft.
2. Cleft alveolus (complete or incomplete).
3. Maxillary deformity and distortion.
4. Nasal deformities:
    a. Alar nasi distortion—flattened, flared, collapsed, recessed or widened at its base.
    b. Columella deformities—shortened, inadequate or twisted to the noncleft side.
    c. Attenuation (thinning) of any of the lower nasal cartilage.
    d. Deviated septum in either the vertical or horizontal plane, or both.
5. Cupid's bow for the most part exists but is distorted on the median portion of the cleft.

Basic Objectives of Repair

1. Recognize, identify and preserve normal landmarks and as much tissue as possible.
2. Realign these normal landmarks into their normal position both from the anterior aspect and the lateral aspect.
    Specifically—
    a. Widen cleft lip in its vertical diameter.
    b. Preserve philtrum, Cupid's bow, the "pout" and the mucocutaneous junction.
    c. Correct the distortion of the alar base and columella with undermining and mobilization rather than any cartilage incision.
    d. May require orthodontic correction for deformed alveolus.

Do NOT in General

    a. Perform any nasal tip modification concomitantly with cleft lip repair.
    b. Damage or excise any nasal cartilage.
    c. Perform simultaneous cleft palate repair.
    d. Excise any normal landmarks.
    e. Use straight line scar except in the minimal cleft lip.

(Text continued on opposite page.)

Plate 135   The Lips

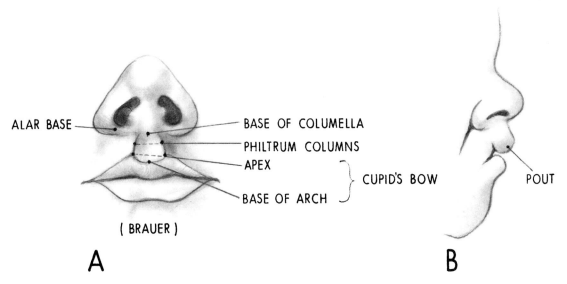

ALAR BASE

BASE OF COLUMELLA

PHILTRUM COLUMNS

APEX

CUPID'S BOW

BASE OF ARCH

POUT

(BRAUER)

A   B

There are exceptions to these dicta depending on the procedure utilized as well as the skill and experience of the surgeon. As the child grows, nasal tip, alar cartilage and nasal septal surgery can be performed at a later time. More than ever is the surgeon's oath of *primum non nocere* applicable—when not sure seek help.

Optimal Age for Operation

There is considerable difference of opinion regarding the optimum time of operation. Although the repair can be done on the first day of life, the earliest age that is reasonable is 10 to 14 days after birth, provided that the infant has started to gain weight and is otherwise normal, especially in blood count. The rule of "over 10" is a good guide—over 10 weeks old, over 10 lb in weight and over 10 gm of hemoglobin. Three months of age is felt by others as the most opportune time.

Remember that other anomalies may exist. A complete physical examination and chest x-ray are mandatory.

With marked deformity of the prelabium and premaxilla (the central portion of the upper alveolar ridge and maxilla from which the upper incisors arise) combined with alveolar cleft, the repair should not be delayed beyond three months since the deformity will become aggravated with growth. The cleft lip repair will tend to realign the premaxilla and aid in closure of the alveolar defect. Earlier repair at the age of 10 to 14 days in these extreme cases may be preferred. With bilateral cleft lip and when the premaxilla is asymmetrically distorted, a staged repair of the cleft lip will tend to realign the premaxilla. For example, if the premaxilla is to the right of the midline, the cleft lip on the left side is repaired first, thus pulling the premaxilla to the left and center. Then the right-sided cleft is repaired. Under no circumstances is any portion of the premaxilla or prelabium excised except for some excess of the vermilion as determined during the final steps of the operative procedure.

Anesthesia

General endotracheal anesthesia is preferred with the endotracheal tube brought out through the mouth across the midportion of the lower lip. Care must be taken that no tension be placed on the upper lip or the commissures. The author does not usually use any local anesthesia and never infiltrates epinephrine with a local anesthetic agent under any circumstances since it is felt that it is the epinephrine that may result in cardiac irregularities.

(Text continued on page 322.)

321

CLEFT LIP REPAIR (*Continued*)

Classification of Types of Repair of Unilateral Cleft Lip

It was once felt that the surgeon should become familiar with one basic type of repair, make that choice and then adapt it to all forms of cleft lip deformities. This concept still has some merit but the mere fact that there are so many techniques and modifications thereof is ample proof that the perfect all-around method is yet to be proven. Hence a knowledge of several techniques is advantageous. Musgrave has recommended certain techniques for certain deformities based on his experience of utilizing five types of repair. Some of his recommendations will be outlined; others will be modified.

It is somewhat difficult to classify the types of repair. Yet there appear to be several general categories with some common characteristics.

Cleft Lip Repair

Type of Operation	Indication or Advantage	Disadvantages
I STRAIGHT LINE		
Rose-Thompson (with Z-plasty on inner aspect of lip)	Only minimal incomplete cleft	Contracture of straight scar; incomplete Cupid's bow
II BROKEN LINE		
1. *Triangular flap* (type of Z-plasty)		
a. Tennison (Marcks, Randall, Hagerty)	Moderately sized complete and severe incomplete cleft	Philtrum distortion; tension of lower portion of lip; excess tissue loss; complex measurements
b. Millard (rotation-advancement)	Minimal and moderately sized incomplete (recent modification for large sized) cleft	Some difficulties in severe incomplete and complete
c. Mirault (Blair-Brown-McDowell)	Relatively easy procedure	Loss Cupid's bow; tight and flattened lip; nasal distortion
d. Jayapathy-Huffman-Lierle	True mathematical Z-plasty	May distort philtrum
2. *Rectangular or Quadrilateral Flap* Hagedorn, LeMesurier, Steffensen (May's modification of Axhausen)	Wide and severe, incomplete and complete cleft	Distortion of Cupid's bow may occur; excessive vertical width of lip

TRIANGULAR FLAP CLEFT LIP REPAIR
Tennison Technique (after Hagerty, 1958)

Highpoints (After Brauer)

1. Z incision on lateral border of cleft which is thus unfolded.
2. Reverse ∟ (**J**) incision on medial border of cleft which is thus lengthened and opened to receive the triangular flap of the **Z** from the lateral border.
3. Final closure is virtually the shape of a **Z**.

The geometric calculations have been carefully outlined by Hagerty, Randall and Jayapathy with Huffman and Lierle. Hagerty (1958) plan is described.

(Text continued on opposite page.)

Plate 136   *The Lips*

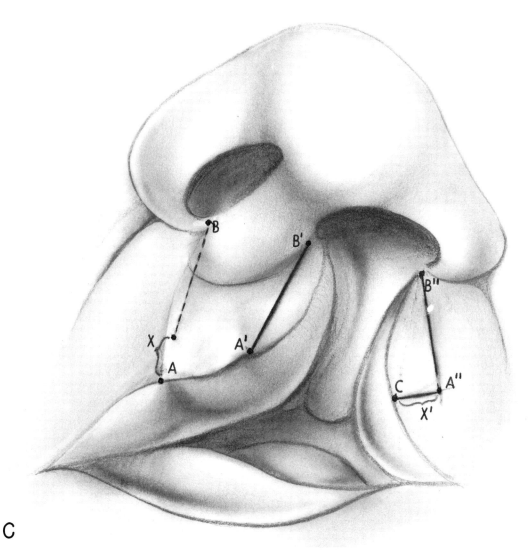

C

C   Line A–B extends from the apex of Cupid's bow to the base of the columella on the
normal side, whereas line A¹–B¹ is the same line on the cleft side (except for length).
(If the apex of Cupid's bow on the cleft side is not discernible, it is calculated by being
equidistant from the midline of the arch of Cupid's bow to the apex on the normal
side.)

Point B″ is located at the alar base so that when approximated to B′ it will shape the
naris on the cleft side similar to the naris on the normal side. Point C is located on
the mucocutaneous border on the lateral side of the cleft where the vermilion begins
to narrow.

A compass is set with a distance equal to line A′−B′. Its pivot leg is then placed at point
B″. A small arc is scribed in the vicinity of A″. The compass is now set with a distance
equal to length X (length X=X′=(A−B)−(A′−B′) equals a vertical gain to be achieved on
the cleft side; distance X′ will form the base of an isosceles triangle with its pivot leg set
at point C. A small arc is scribed to intersect the first arc scribed from point B″. Where
the two arcs intersect is point A″. (A small **V** wedge may have to be excised just inferior to
point B″ in extreme cases to avoid rotation of the triangular flap off the lip.)

D An imaginary dotted line is now drawn from the midportion of the base of the columella (*1*) to the midportion of the arch of Cupid's bow (*2*). Another imaginary dotted line is drawn at right angles to this former line (1–2) to meet point A'. At a point (*3*) which is equidistant from point 2 to where the two above imaginary lines intersect (4), a solid line is drawn (A'–3). This is the incision which opens the lateral side of the cleft—its length is equal to the sides of the isosceles triangle (base distance C–A'' = X', plate 136). The isosceles triangle is then constructed using a compass. The apex of this triangle is point 3'.

The shaded area represents the tissue to be excised which some surgeons feel is too much tissue to be discarded.

Plate 137   The Lips

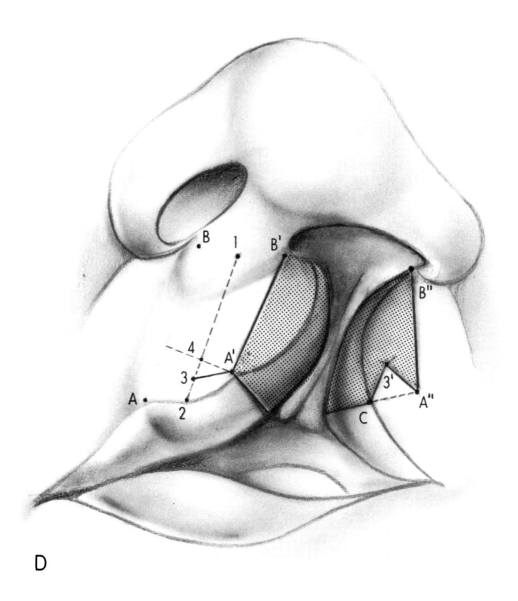

D

TRIANGULAR FLAP CLEFT LIP REPAIR (*Continued*)

E Full thickness incisions are now made on the medial side of the cleft extending from B' to A' and thence to 3. The excess lip is trimmed as in the shaded area in step *D*. Another full thickness incision is made on the lateral side of the cleft from point B'' to A'' to 3' and thence to C. The excess lip is trimmed as in the shaded area in step *D*. Mobilization of the alar base and cheek is then performed sufficiently to realign the naris on the cleft side to match as closely as possible the normal naris. Approximation is in three layers.

F The completed repair.

G Repair of deformity of the naris is best delayed to a much later stage. One such correction is depicted along the rim. Other naris modifications are described in plate 80. Plate 125, steps *A*, *B* and *C*, describes a modification referable to Cupid's bow. Plates 78 and 79 describe techniques utilized in severe nasal deformities following cleft lip repair.

Plate 138   The Lips

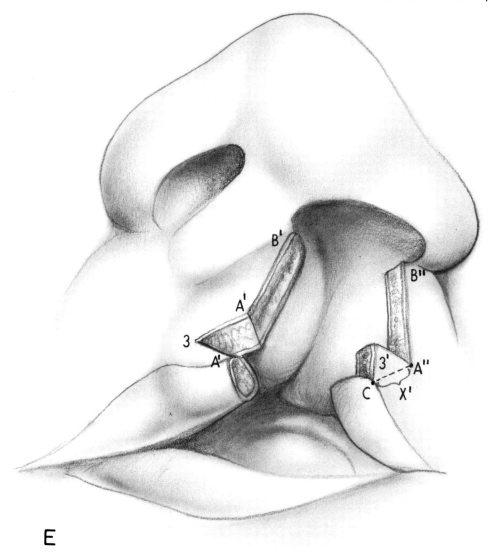

E

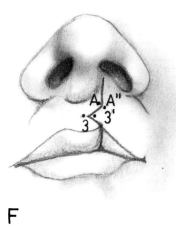

F

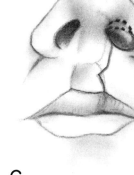

G

RECTANGULAR OR QUADRILATERAL FLAP CLEFT LIP REPAIR
(After Axhausen, 1941; Hagedorn, 1884; LeMesurier, 1952; May, 1949)

The following cleft lip repair has been found helpful in wide unilateral cleft lip with cleft alveolus and marked distortion of the lip. It is basically a "cut as you go" method founded on the quadrilateral flap technique. With marked deformity of the prelabium and premaxilla (the central portion of the upper alveolar ridge and maxilla from which the upper incisors arise) combined with alveolar cleft, the repair should not be delayed beyond three months since the deformity will become aggravated with growth. The cleft lip repair will tend to realign the premaxilla and aid in closure of the alveolar defect. Earlier repair at the age of 10 to 14 days in the extreme cases may be preferred.

Highpoints

1. Avoid a straight vertical scar.
2. Adequate mobilization of both sides of lip along the gingivobuccal sulcus with advancement of sides of lip toward cleft.
3. Liberal undermining of the ala nasi and cheek on the same side as the cleft.
4. Three-layer closure: mucous membrane, muscle and skin.
5. Accurate alignment of the vermilion borders with outward bulge to form a puckered upper lip at Cupid's bow (plate 135).
6. Avoid injury to cartilage or bone.

A An initial measurement is made (with the columella deformity pushed toward the midline) on the medial side from the base of the columella (A) at the tip of the median vermilion border to the apex of Cupid's bow (B). Point A' is at the tip of the lateral vermilion border. Distance $A–D–C–B$ = distance $A^1–D^1–C^1–B^1$. Three or 4 mm ($B–C = B^1–C^1$ = minor distance) is subtracted from this initial distance (usually 11 or 12 mm) yielding 8 mm ($A–D = A^1–D^1$ = major distance). Hence $(A–D) + (B–C) = (A^1–D^1) + (B^1–C^1)$ = vertical width of the normal side and in turn equals the desired vertical width of the cleft side. Points D, B and B^1 are located on the mucocutaneous line. C is 3 to 4 mm directly above B, while C^1 is 3 to 4 mm on a line at right angles to the mucocutaneous junction. Incisions are not made along lines D–C and D^1–C^1 until the close of the operation, since mobilization and rotation of the alar base may change some of the initial measurements. Refer to step *M* for the orientation of points.

B Reconstruction of the floor of the nose anteriorly is begun with a median turnout flap of mucous membrane from the edge of the alveolar cleft. Care is taken not to tear this flap nor to injure the underlying bone or cartilage. This flap should not extend beyond the point at which the premaxilla meets the vomer.

 A lateral turn-out of mucous membrane flap is then developed, starting at the edge of the alveolar process and thence upward into the nose.

C The median and lateral turn-out flaps have been approximated with interrupted 5-0 or 6-0 chromic catgut. Mobilization of the lateral portion of the lip is begun by an incision in the gingivobuccal sulcus leaving sufficient mucous membrane on the alveolar ridge for placement of sutures to advance the lip. This incision begins at the tip of the lip near the ala nasi and extends well along the canine fossa. This incision must not be too close to the cartilage and rim; otherwise, the nares will collapse. If made too far posteriorly the nares will be too bulky.

D Using a small curved blunt scissors, the cheek is mobilized up to within several millimeters of the inferior orbital rim, taking care not to injure the infraorbital nerve. The lip, cheek and ala nasi are thus freed as one unit.

E
F A similar gingivobuccal incision is made on the opposite side extending well beyond the midline. If there is columella displacement, this incision is extended deeper to free the columella. Small curved scissors are used. Care must be taken to avoid injury to the cartilage and anterior nasal spine.

(Text continued on opposite page.)

Plate 139   The Lips

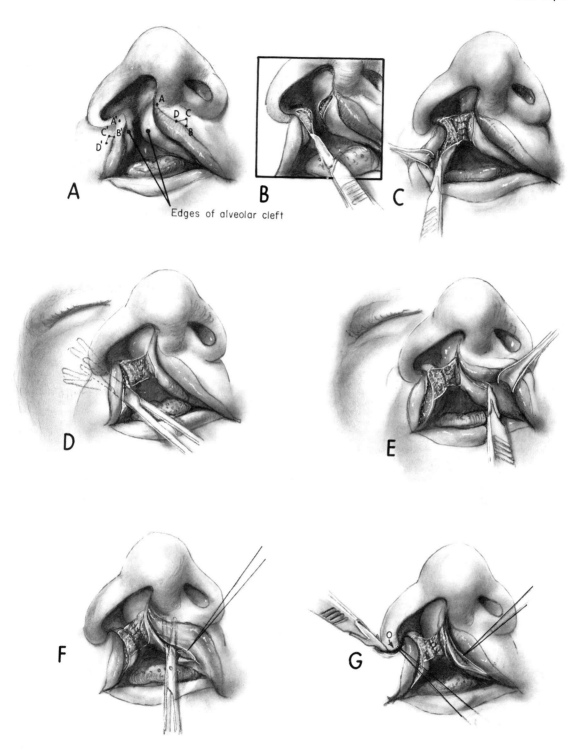

Edges of alveolar cleft

G   With marked deformity of the ala nasi, an incision is made along the edge of the ala. This facilitates approximation of the laterally displaced ala (point O) to the columella, thus narrowing the naris and forming a more normal floor of the naris. The alar flap (O) is better too short than too long.

H   To facilitate the approximation of the alar flap to the base of the columella, the median vermilion incision is begun at point A. The tip of the alar flap is sutured to the tuberculum of the columella.

I
J   Suturing of the alar flap is completed, its inner edge approximated to the presenting edge of the reconstructed floor of the nose (the median and lateral turn-out flaps) and its outer edge to the remaining bare area at the base of the columella.

A through and through incision is now made commencing at point A^1 (see step A), which is at the superior tip of the mucocutaneous junction on the lateral side of the cleft. This incision is best temporarily stopped at C^1 while the incision on the medial side is extended. The length of this incision from point A^1 depends on the initial measurement of the vertical width of the lip on the normal side — the wider the lip required, the longer the incision.

K   The median vermilion flap incision is carried along to point D on the mucocutaneous line and thence toward point C (see step A). It is best to delay completion of the incision until further evaluation of the vertical width of the lip is made.

L   The flaps are now crisscrossed and the width of the repaired lip compared with the normal side. If the vertical width of the lip is too narrow, both incisions are extended. The medial lip flap is now advanced (arrow) toward the cleft and fixed with 4-0 chromic catgut sutures through the edge of mucous membrane which was left along the alveolar ridge.

The lateral lip flap is advanced and sutured in a similar fashion.

M   The upper portion of the lateral lip flap (A^1) is now sutured to the floor of the naris reaching the columella (A). The excess portions of the vermilion skin flap are now excised after a careful evaluation following the crisscross maneuver depicted in *L*. Puckering of the lip should be achieved. The first layer of fine chromic catgut sutures is placed in the mucous membrane with knots tied on the mucous membrane surface. At least three muscle sutures of 5-0 or 4-0 chromic catgut are used for the second layer. Before the third layer is sutured, the skin edges are elevated slightly to facilitate some eversion of the skin closure. Skin approximation uses 5-0 nylon. The vermilion borders must be painstakingly aligned in perfect fashion.

N   The completed closure. A collodion strip gauze dressing is placed over the repair extending well out on the cheeks. The elbows are immobilized.

If asymmetry of the axis of the nares or nasal tip exists, repair should be deferred until about the age of five years. Time and soft tissue pulled from the initial repair will tend to reshape the bony framework and those changes should be allowed to occur before nasal tip surgery is performed.

Complications and Drawbacks

1. Portion of Cupid's bow may be lost.
2. Incision across philtrum column on cleft side.
3. Tension across lip repair if inadequate cheek mobilization.

Plate 140   The Lips

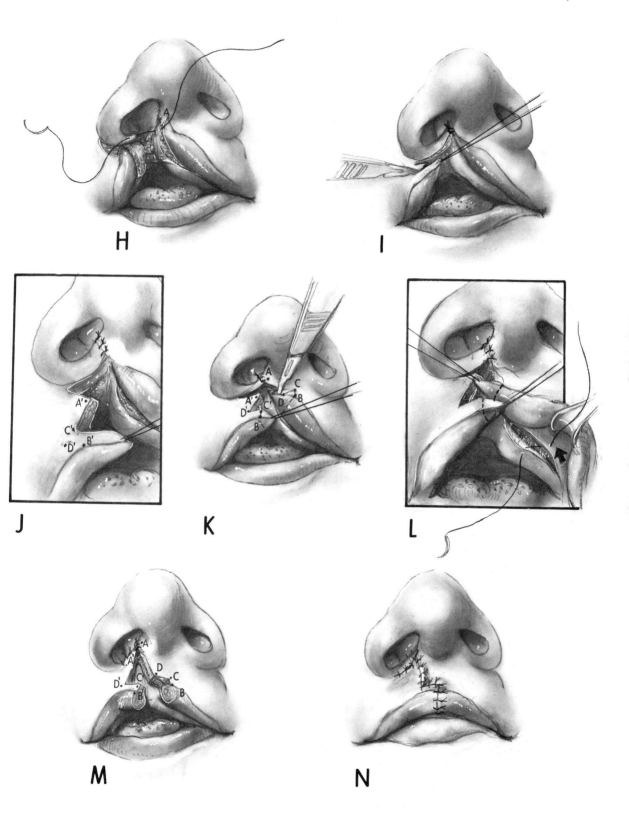

H

I

J

K

L

M

N

ROTATION-ADVANCEMENT CLEFT LIP REPAIR (Millard, 1964)

Indication

Although Millard emphasizes the adaptations and modifications of this technique for all types of cleft lip deformity, the consensus of opinion at this point in time directs its use primarily to the moderate cleft lip deformity.

Highpoints

1. The rotation-advancement technique is basically a double Z-plasty closure.
2. No measurements are used. "Cut as you go."
3. Rotation (downward) of Cupid's bow into a normal position with its preservation.
4. Advancement (medially) of the upper portion of the lateral border of the cleft with correction of alar flare and improvement in distal septal.
5. Preserve as much muscle and mucosa as possible by making an incision of flap A on the bias and by carefully stripping the vermilion on the lateral flap.

A   An incision is made starting at the medial edge of the cleft lip in a plane which is almost at a right angle to the cutaneous vermilion junction, intersecting this junction at the potential height of Cupid's bow on the cleft side (point 1). This through and through incision is carried upward following the reciprocal curvature and position of the philtrum on the normal side until it reaches the region of the base of the columella. Here the incision curves under the base of the columella and extends toward the normal side as far as is necessary to rotate and drop the Cupid's bow (flap A) into a normal horizontal plane. A small cutback incision (point 2) may facilitate this rotation. To preserve as much muscle and mucosa on this flap as possible, the incision is placed on the bias from the outside in. Thus two flaps are formed—A and C. Flap A is Cupid's bow and philtrum; flap C will become the nostril sill.

B   A fine hook exerts upward traction on the roof of the alar nasi on the cleft side. This results in a bare area on the medial side approximating the extent of lengthening to be achieved at the columella. Flap C is thus raised and approximated to itself to aid in the maintenance of this lengthening. The number of sutures depends on the desired lengthening.

C   Flap B is now developed, taking care to preserve a small flap just above and contiguous with the cutaneous vermilion border—the "white skin roll" (point 3). This small flap interdigitates with a reciprocal cutout in flap A. When developing flap B, the vermilion is only shaved from the underlying muscle, thus preserving as much muscle and mucosa as feasible. The line of shave starts at a point on the lateral edge of the cleft in a plane at a right angle to the cutaneous vermilion junction. This point is located where the vermilion commences to narrow and where the resulting preserved length of the lateral element when sutured to the medial element (flap A) will result in a normal balanced upper lip. The length of the tip of flap B depends on the width of the cleft and can be extended into the vestibule skin as necessary.

D   Flap B is now advanced medially to reach the apex of the defect resulting from the rotation of flap A. Flap C is advanced laterally but not the entire distance toward the apex of the defect, resulting from the advancement of flap B. The apex of this defect is closed by one or two sutures reapproximating the base of the alae nasi as depicted.

    The dotted line depicts the crescent-shaped portion of the drooping roof (web) of the alae nasi which is excised.

E   To facilitate an upward advancement of the alar nasi after the excision of the alae nasi web as depicted in step *D*, a short relaxing incision (point 4) is made.

F   One suture is placed to close the gap, thus increasing the length and relaxing the inner flap—a **V–Y** gain. The closure is thus completed.

G   The completed repair.

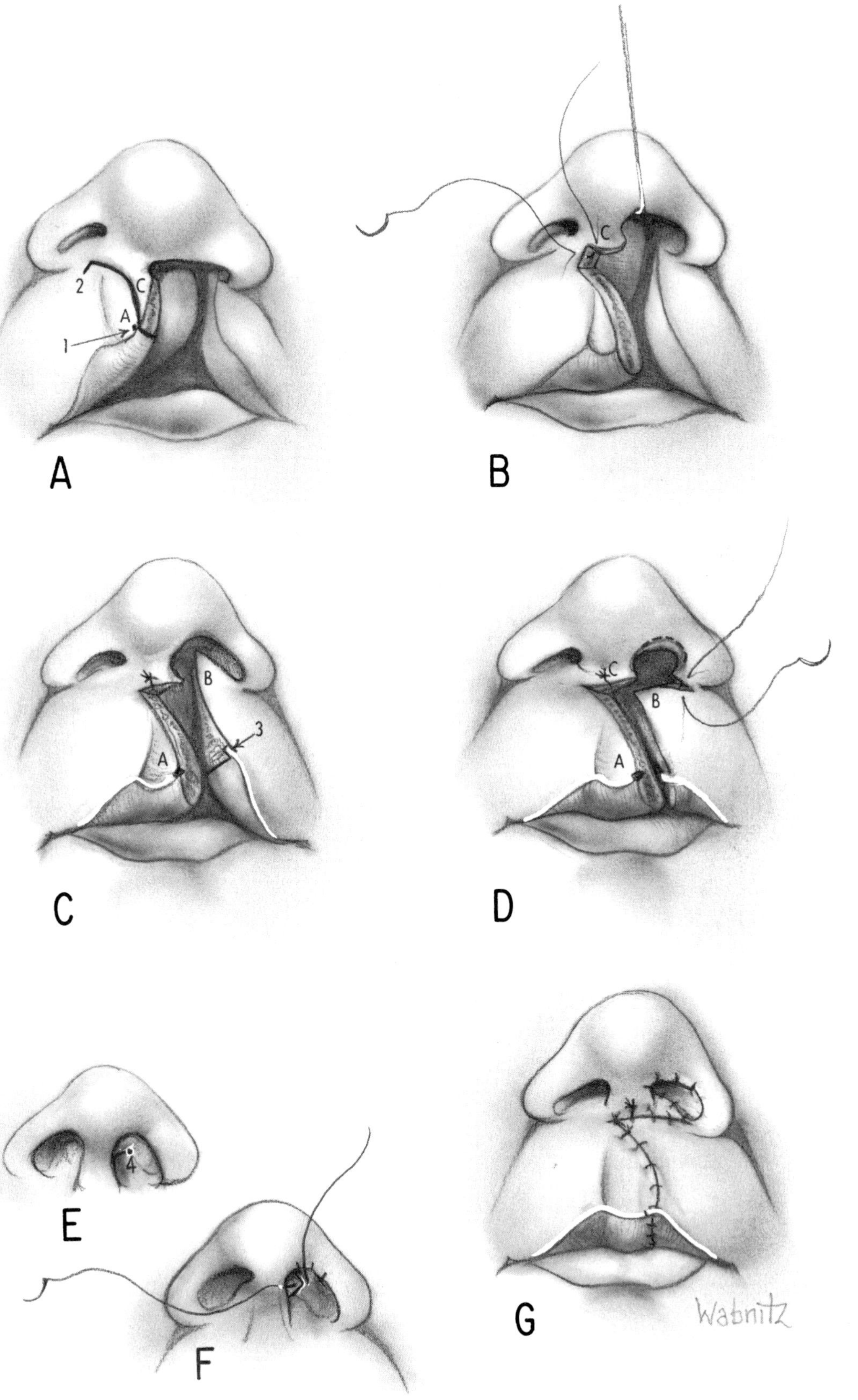

Plate 141   The Lips

A

B

C

D

E

F

G

Wabnitz

BILATERAL CLEFT LIP REPAIR

Highpoints

1. Vermilion of prelabium is preserved and used as oral lining for center portion of reconstruction.
2. Three-layer closure: mucous membrane, muscle and skin.
3. Small relaxing incisions for the alae nasi.

A   Incisions along the vermilion edges are made as outlined by the dotted lines (after Brown and McDowell, 1947).

B   Flaps indicated by **X** and **Y** are mobilized.

C   The vermilion of the prelabium **Z** is incised along its exterior border. The interior border is preserved. The vermilion of the prelabium is thus hinged and turned downward and inward. Relaxing incisions are made at the base of the alae nasi along the dotted lines.

D   The lateral lip flaps are approximated to the central portion of the lip in three layers: mucous membrane, muscle and skin.

E   The lateral flaps X and Y are trimmed and interposed across the prelabium. The vermilion of the prelabium **Z** is sutured to the lower edge of the reconstructed upper lip, forming an intraoral lining.

F   The completed restoration.

With bilateral cleft lip and when the premaxilla is asymmetrically distorted, a staged repair of the cleft lip will tend to realign the premaxilla. For example, if the premaxilla is to the right of the midline, the cleft lip on the left side is repaired first, thus pulling the premaxilla to the left and center. Then the right-sided cleft is repaired. Under no circumstances is any portion of the premaxilla or prelabium excised except for some excess of the vermilion as determined during the final steps of the operative procedure.

Plate 142   The Lips

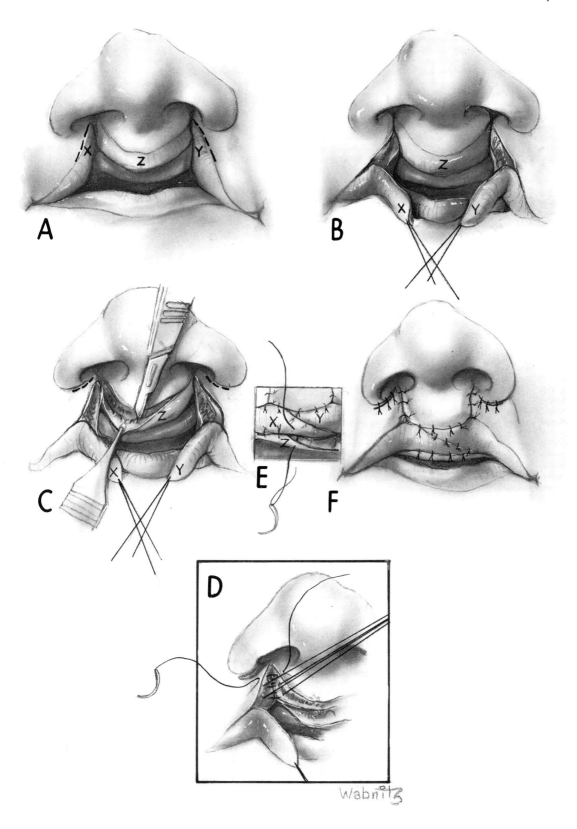

A

B

C

E

F

D

Wabnitz

BIBLIOGRAPHY

Abbe, R.: A new plastic operation for the relief of deformity due to double hare-lip. The classic reprint. Plast. Reconstr. Surg. 42:481–483, 1968.

Ashley, F. L., McConnell, D. V., Machida, R., Sterling, H. E., Galloway, D., and Grazer, F.: Carcinoma of the lip. A comparison of five year results after irradiation and surgical therapy. Amer. J. Surg. 110:549–551, 1965.

Axhausen, G.: Technik und Ergebnisse der Lippenplastik. Georg Thieme, Leipzig, 1941.

Bakamjian, V. Y.: Personal communication, 1971.

Berkeley, W. T.: Correction of secondary cleft-lip nasal deformities. Plast. Reconstr. Surg. 44:234–241, 1969.

Bernard, C.: Cancer de la Lèvre inférieur opéré par un procédé nouveau. Bull. Soc. Chirurgie Paris 3:357, 1853.

Bernstein, L.: Secondary reconstructive procedures for cleft lip and nose. Trans. Amer. Acad. Ophthal. Otolaryng. January-February 1967.

Bowers, D. G., Jr.: Double cross-lip flaps for lower lip reconstruction. Plast. Reconstr. Surg. 47:209–214, 1971.

Brauer, R. O.: A comparison of the Tennison and Le Mesurier lip repairs. Plast. Reconstr. Surg. 23:249–259, 1959.

Brown, J. B., McDowell, F., and Byars, L. T.: Double clefts of the lip. Surg. Gynec. Obstet. 85:20, 1947.

Craig, R. D. P.: The management of complete clefts of the lip and palate. Brit. J. Surg. 54:923–931, 1967.

Dingman, R. O., and Grabb, W. C.: A rational program for surgical management of bilateral cleft lip and cleft palate. Plast. Reconstr. Surg. 47:239–242, 1971.

Estlander, J. A.: Méthode d'autoplastic de la joue ou d'une lèvre par un lambeau emprunte à l'autre lèvre. Rev. Mém. Méd. Chir. 1:344, 1877.

Filatoff, W.: Plastic a tige ronde. Westnik Oftalmol. Avril Mai, 1917.

Fishman, L. S., and Stark, D. B.: The maxillary arch prior to surgical closure of a cleft lip. Plast. Reconstr. Surg. 42:572–576, 1968.

Gage, A. A., Koepf, S., Wehrle, D., and Emmings, F.: Cryotherapy for cancer of the lip and oral cavity. Cancer 18:1646–1651, 1965.

Georgiade, N. G.: Improved technique for one-stage repair of bilateral cleft lip. Plast. Reconstr. Surg. 48:318–324, 1971.

Gerold, F.: Personal communication, 1960.

Guerrero-Santos, J.: Use of a tongue flap in secondary correction of cleft lips. Plast. Reconstr. Surg. 44:368–371, 1969.

Hagerty, R. F.: Unilateral cleft lip repair. Surg. Gynec. Obstet. 106:119–122, 1958.

Jayapathy, B., Huffman, W. C., and Lierle, D. M.: The Z-plastic procedure—Some mathematic considerations and application to cleft lip. Plast. Reconstr. Surg. 26:203–208, 1960.

Jesse, R. H.: Extensive cancer of the lip. Arch. Surg. 94:509–516, 1967.

Kernahan, D. A.: The striped Y—A symbolic classification for cleft lip and palate. Plast. Reconstr. Surg. 47:469–470, 1971.

Kiehn, C. L., DesPrez, J. D., and Brown, F.: Maxillary osteotomy for late correction of occlusion and appearance in cleft lip and palate patients. Plast. Reconstr. Surg. 42:203–207, 1968.

Kluzák, R.: Transplantation of rib growth cartilage. Experimental study and possible use in primary cleft lip repairs. Plast. Reconstr. Surg. 49:61–69, 1972.

Le Mesurier, A. B.: The treatment of complete unilateral harelips. Surg. Gynec. Obstet. 95:17–27, 1952.

Maisels, D. O.: Chronic lip fissures. Brit. J. Derm. 81:621–622, 1969.

Marcks, K. M., Trevaski, A. E., and daCosta, A.: Further observations in cleft lip repair. Plast. Reconstr. Surg. 12:392, 1953.

May, H.: Plastic and Reconstructive Surgery. 3rd ed. Philadelphia, F. A. Davis Company, 1971.

Martin, H. E., MacComb, W. S., and Blady, J. V.: Cancer of the lip. Ann. Surg. 114:226, 1941.

McCabe, P. A.: A coding procedure for classification of cleft lip and cleft palate. Cleft Palate J. 3:383–391, 1966.

McConnel, F. M. S., Zellweger, H., and Lawrence, R. A.: Labial pits—Cleft lip and/or palate syndrome. Arch. Otolaryng. *91*:407–411, 1970.

Millard, D. R.: A radical rotation in single harelip. Amer. J. Surg. *95*:318–322, 1958.

Millard, D. R.: Closure of bilateral cleft lip and elongation of columella by two operations in infancy. Plast. Reconstr. Surg. *47*:324–331, 1971.

Millard, D. R.: Extensions of the rotation-advancement principle for wide unilateral cleft lips. Plast. Reconstr. Surg. *42*:535–544, 1968.

Millard, D. R.: Refinements in rotation-advancement cleft lip technique. Plast. Reconstr. Surg. *33*:26–38, 1964.

Paletta, F. X.: Cancer of the lip. From symposium on cancer of the head and neck. *In* Gaisford, J. C. (ed.): Total Treatment and Reconstructive Rehabilitation. Vol. II. St. Louis, C. V. Mosby Company, 1969.

Paletta, F. X.: Early and late repair of facial defects following treatment of malignancy. Plast. Reconstr. Surg. *13*:95–108, 1954.

Randall, P.: A triangular flap operation for the primary repair of unilateral clefts of the lip. Plast. Reconstr. Surg. *23*:331–347, 1959.

Saemann, O.: Die Transplantations – Methode der Herrn. Prof. Dr. Burow. Dtsch. Klin. *20*:221, 1853.

Steffensen, W. H.: A method for repair of the unilateral cleft lip. Plast. Reconstr. Surg. *4*:144, 1949.

Steffensen, W. H.: Further experience with the rectangular flap operation for cleft lip repair. Plast. Reconstr. Surg. *11*:49, 1953.

Tennison, C. W.: The repair of unilateral cleft lip by the stencil method. Plast. Reconstr. Surg. *9*:115, 1952.

Thompson, J. E.: An artistic and mathematically accurate method of repairing the defect in cases of harelip. Surg. Gynec. Obstet. *14*:498–505, 1912.

Uchida, J.-I.: A new approach to the correction of cleft lip nasal deformities. Plast. Reconstr. Surg. *47*:454–458, 1971.

Villoria, J. M. F.: A new method of elongation of the corner of the mouth. Plast. Reconstr. Surg. *49*:52–55, 1972.

von Bruns, V.: Das Handbuch d. praktisch Chir. Tübingen, Lauppsche Buchhandlung, 1859.

Wynn, S. K.: Primary nostril reconstruction in complete cleft lips. The round nostril technique. Plast. Reconstr. Surg. *49*:56–60, 1972.

8. PERIORBITAL REGION

Many of the principles outlined are from Mustardé, 1969.

ANATOMY

A   Anatomy of the eye and its relationship to the bony orbit.

B   Additional anatomy is depicted on plates 157, steps *B* and *B'*, 158, steps *D* and *G*, and 52.

Plate 143   Periorbital Region

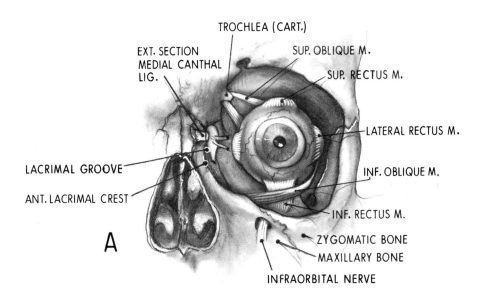

TROCHLEA (CART.)

EXT. SECTION
MEDIAL CANTHAL
LIG.

SUP. OBLIQUE M.

SUP. RECTUS M.

LATERAL RECTUS M.

LACRIMAL GROOVE

ANT. LACRIMAL CREST

INF. OBLIQUE M.

INF. RECTUS M.

ZYGOMATIC BONE

MAXILLARY BONE

INFRAORBITAL NERVE

A

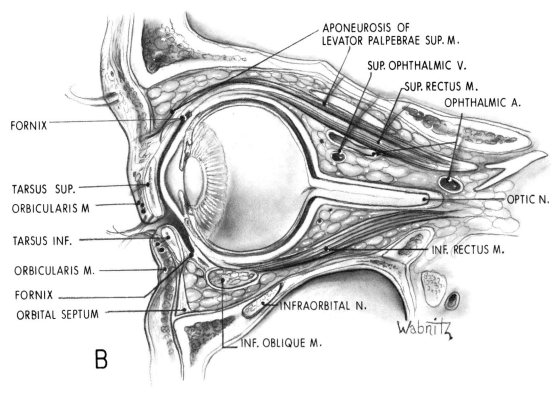

APONEUROSIS OF
LEVATOR PALPEBRAE SUP. M.

SUP. OPHTHALMIC V.

SUP. RECTUS M.

OPHTHALMIC A.

FORNIX

TARSUS SUP.

ORBICULARIS M

TARSUS INF.

ORBICULARIS M.

FORNIX

ORBITAL SEPTUM

OPTIC N.

INF. RECTUS M.

INFRAORBITAL N.

INF. OBLIQUE M.

Wabnitz

B

WOUNDS OF THE CONJUNCTIVA

A
 a. Laceration at right angle (1) to the fornix requires repair. Meticulously placed 6-0 catgut sutures are used for repair; otherwise, scar contractures will occur.

 b. Lacerations parallel (2) to the line of the fornix usually require no suturing.

 c. Lacerations of the palpebral (lid) conjunctiva are repaired with 6-0 nylon pull-out sutures (3) in steps *B* and *C*. Such lacerations more often than not involve the entire lid. No knots are permissible on exposed conjunctiva to prevent corneal damage. Replacement of missing conjunctiva can be accomplished with conjunctiva from the opposite eye or from the fornices. This has drawbacks; hence, usually a mucosal graft from the inner aspect of the lips, cheek or nasal septum is preferred. Never use split thickness skin. A free foreskin graft (prepuce) (Smith, 1965) can be used to replace bulbar conjunctiva (over the sclera) for large defects. Lip and cheek mucosa are abundant but tend to contract 50 to 60 per cent. Nasal mucosa is best and is obtained ideally by dissecting the mucous membrane from the underlying perichondrium—a different plane than in the submucous resection operation (plates 64 and 65). If the perichondrium is removed, there is no harm except that the graft is somewhat thick and tends to contract. If only the mucous membrane is excised, then the donor site re-epithelializes well by being covered with antibiotic ointment. If the perichondrium is removed with the mucous membrane, it is best to cover the bare cartilage with a split thickness epidermal or dermal graft.

REPAIR OF LID LACERATIONS

B
C
 A three-layer closure is performed: conjunctiva with continuous 6-0 nylon pullout sutures (3) which splint the edges of the tarsus together (the ends of this pullout suture are secured with tape as depicted)—a small portion of the tarsal plate is included in this suture; orbicularis oculi muscle with only one or two 5-0 catgut sutures (5); and the skin with 5-0 or 6-0 silk or nylon. If nylon is used, the ends should be either very short or very long to avoid injuring the cornea. A small suture (4) of 6-0 silk is utilized to approximate the lid margins exactly at the gray line. This suture is left long—2.5 cm or longer—to prevent a turning-in, thus avoiding injury to the cornea.

MANAGEMENT OF DISRUPTION OF THE CANALICULI
(See plate 158 *G*)

D
 Depicted is a "near-far, far-near" type of suture (Smith, 1965) for approximation of lid margins. This aids in the prevention of notching of the lid margins.

Plate 144   Periorbital Region

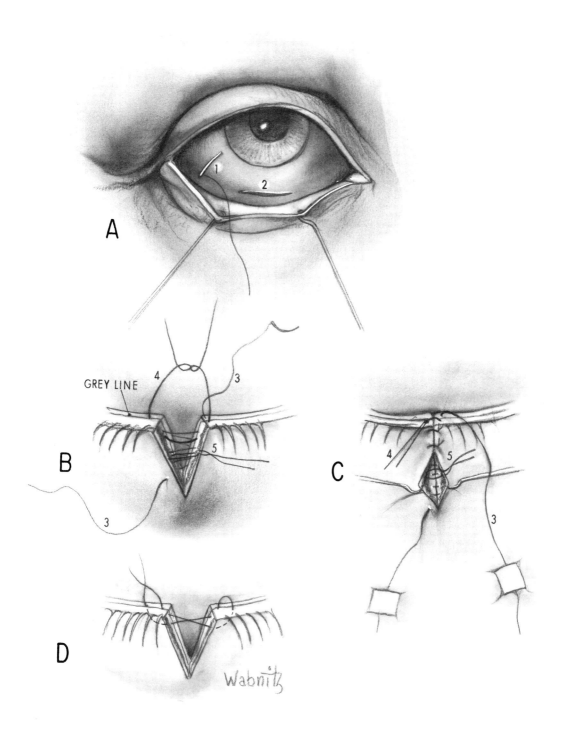

GREY LINE

Wabnitz

A

B

C

D

RECONSTRUCTION OF LIDS

Basic Principles

These principles can be applied to tissue loss and severe scars resulting from trauma.

a. The *upper lid* is more important than the *lower* lid since significant defect in the upper lid, especially in the midline, will eventually lead to a corneal ulceration and *loss of vision*. Hence, do not use the upper lid to reconstruct the lower lid except possibly for the use of a small amount of redundant skin of the upper lid. The lower lid may be used to reconstruct the upper lid.

b. Twenty-five per cent (up to 30 per cent in the elderly) of the *vertical* lid (full thickness) defect can be closed by primarily approximating the edges if both canthal areas are uninvolved. If the defect is greater, additional length can be achieved by a lateral cantholysis. Hence a 25 per cent defect requires no grafting technique. This is the principle of "quarters."

c. Horizontal lid defects are separate problems and, if of any size, require transposed tissue or rotated flaps (plate 155, steps D and E; plate 160, steps E and F).

d. Use a three-layer closure, except in situations in which the conjunctiva loss is small and less than the skin and muscle loss. In such cases the conjunctival layer can be omitted (steps C^2 and C^3).

Alternate and additional concepts:

a. Some surgeons (McCoy; Smith) feel that portions of the full thickness layers of the upper lid can be safely utilized to reconstruct the lower lid using the rotated (switch) or pedicle flap technique. This would be the reverse situation as depicted in plate 151. With *larger* flaps from the upper to the lower lid or vice versa, a "sharing" procedure is utilized (Hughes, 1954; Kolner; Cutler-Beard, plate 152). The important principle in any modification of this technique is that the lid margin of the donor lid is *not* transected or violated (plate 152). Smith points out that this feature is the reason why Mustardé and other surgeons have abandoned this method—it is actually a failure of application of surgical technique rather than a failure of the basic method itself.

b. When there is only skin loss of the lids, free graft from the opposite lid (opposite side if necessary) or from the postauricular region or a thick split graft (freehand) is used.

c. When utilizing the Fricke upper lid flap (plate 155, steps D and E) McCoy emphasizes that the entire length of the skin of the upper lid should be used to avoid disparity when closing the donor site.

d. Both these surgeons (McCoy and Smith) avoid the Mustardé technique of a lateral cheek flap (plate 148) to reconstruct the lower lid. The lateral cheek flap may result in a downward pull on the reconstructed lower lid. To aid in the prevention of this problem, refer to plate 148 which demonstrates that the lateral side of the excised triangle is longer and more oblique than the medial side.

e. When excising skin of the lower lid, Smith emphasizes the importance of having patients open their mouths widely to evaluate the downward traction on the lower lid in order to prevent ectropion.

f. Wheeler advises in repairing lid defects that the layer closure of the inner and outer incisions should not be directly in the same plane (halving technique). This is more theoretical than practical.

RECONSTRUCTION OF LOWER LID

Plates 146, 147 and 148 depict in outline fashion the basic principles of lower lid reconstruction for vertical defects following the "quarter" rule of Mustardé. Details of technique for large lower lid defects are depicted on plate 148.

A   Vertical lid defect.

B   Horizontal lid defect (requires transposed tissue or rotated flaps). Refer to plate 155, steps D and E and plate 160, steps E and F.

(Text continued on opposite page.)

Plate 145   Periorbital Region

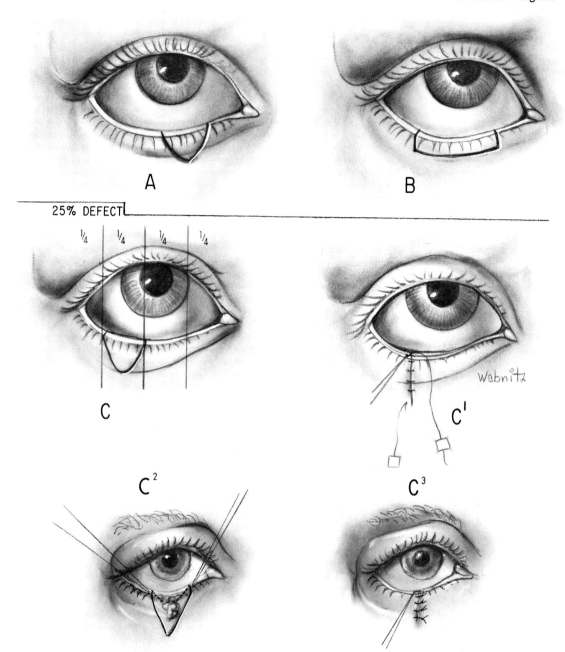

25% DEFECT

A

B

C

C¹

C²

C³

Wabnitz

Reconstruction of lower lid with 25 per cent defect

C   *Vertical Defect.* For suturing details refer to plate 144, steps *B*, *C* and *D*.
C¹ Twenty-five per cent defect—primary closure when both canthal areas are intact. (In elderly patients up to 30 per cent of the lid may sometimes be resected and a primary simple closure performed.)

C² If a lesion is superficial, an excision of somewhat less of the palpebral conjunctiva (Fox, 1958) can be performed along the dotted lines. In such circumstances, suture approximation of the conjunctiva is not necessary (Martin, 1957), provided the fornix is not violated. The use of stay sutures on the lid margin is of great aid in the initial incision of the lesion.

C³ The completed closure.

*Reconstruction of Lower Lid with 25 per cent defect
at Lateral Canthus*

D
D¹
D²

Twenty-five per cent defect at lateral canthal region. This usually requires a lateral canthoplasty (D¹). Either the inferior or superior crus or both crura of the lateral canthal ligaments are transected. A *medial* canthoplasty is *not* used because of possible injury to lacrimal apparatus.

Reconstruction of Lower Lid with 30 per cent defect

E
E¹

Thirty per cent defect.
A lateral cantholysis is again usually necessary except in the elderly, in which there is more tissue laxity.

Plate 146   *Periorbital Region*

25% DEFECT AT LATERAL CANTHUS

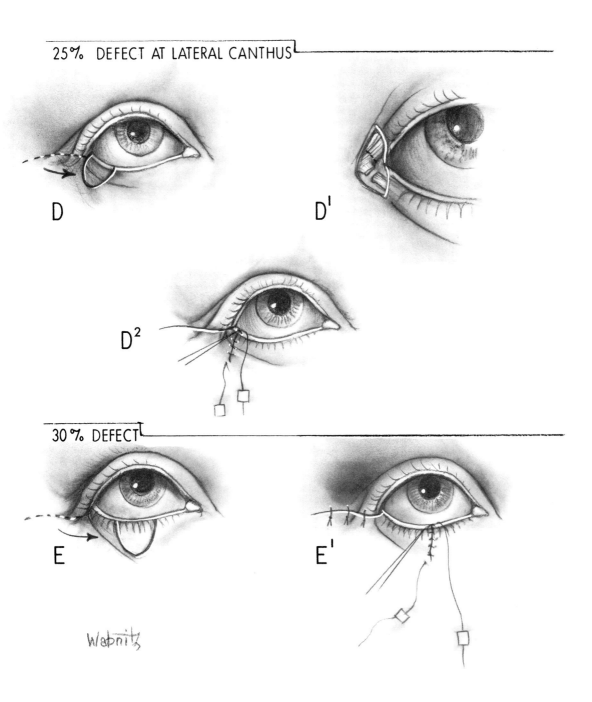

D

D'

D²

30% DEFECT

E

E'

Wabnitz

Reconstruction of Lower Lid with 30 to 50 per cent defect

F Thirty to 50 per cent defect.

F¹ A lateral cantholysis plus an advanced cheek flap is required for closure. Lining of the flap can be obtained from some redundant conjunctiva at the lateral canthal region. Note that the lateral side of the excised triangle is longer and more oblique than the medial side to prevent inferior contracture of the reconstructed lid. This principle is applicable to the procedure in steps G and H. Details of technique are on the following plate.

Reconstruction of Lower Lid with 50 to 75 per cent defect

G Fifty to 75 per cent loss.

G¹ A lateral cantholysis plus a larger rotated cheek flap with cutback (1) incision is required for closure. The lining of this flap will require a free septal mucous membrane graft (X). Be sure the mucosal surface is identified and distinguished from the raw undersurface when suturing the graft in place. 6-0 nylon pullout sutures are used. Details of technique are on the following plate.

Reconstruction of Lower Lid with 100 per cent defect

H One hundred per cent loss of lower lid.

H¹ A lateral cantholysis plus a somewhat larger rotated cheek flap with cutback incision is required for closure. The lining of this flap will require a free septal cartilage and mucous membrane graft (X). Details of technique are on the following plate.

Paletta (1973) has demonstrated the use of an extended nasofacial flap (see plates 81 and 83), superiorly based to reconstruct lower lid defects.

Plate 147   Periorbital Region

30%–50% DEFECT

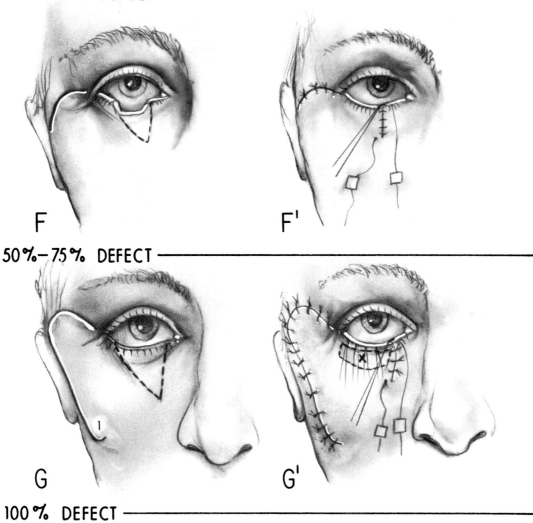

F

F'

50%–75% DEFECT

G

G'

100% DEFECT

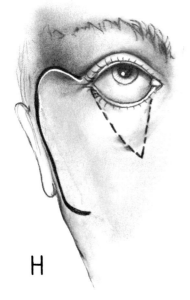

H

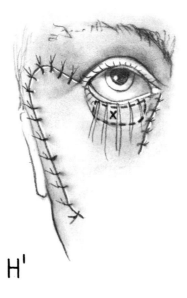

H'

RESECTION OF LARGE BASAL CELL CARCINOMA OF LOWER LID WITH RECONSTRUCTION USING LATERAL CHEEK FLAP
(After Mustardé, 1969)

Highpoints

1. Full thickness resection.
2. Immediate reconstruction with lateral cheek flap.
3. Total release of cheek flap in front of ear with right angle back cut at distal end of incision of cheek flap when two thirds or more of lower lid is resected.
4. Lower lid resection includes an elongated inverted triangle or "shield" below the tumor to ensure proper advancement of cheek flap.
5. The sides of this triangle or shield are unequal in length and direction: the medial side is shorter and vertical; the lateral side is longer and slanted obliquely downward and medially. This is done to prevent downward pull of reconstructed lower lid.
6. The cheek flap is extended slightly upward at the lateral canthus and the release extends 1 cm below the apex of the excised triangle.
7. The deep portion of the cheek flap is sutured to the orbital rim, especially at the lateral canthus to prevent downward tension on reconstructed lid.
8. Lining of the newly reconstructed lid is ideally achieved by utilizing a free mucosal chondral graft from the nasal septum.
9. Do not injure lacrimal punctus and canaliculus if this is compatible with adequate resection of the primary tumor; otherwise, resect these areas. Troublesome epiphora may or may not occur and this can be corrected later if need be by the utilization of a conjunctival flap (plate 156, step C).
10. Margins of tumor must be adequately identified—sutures or staining with silver nitrate—for frozen sections.
11. Refer to page 344 for alternate and additional concepts.

A　Depicted is a tumor requiring resection of almost the entire lower lid, sparing the canaliculus. The area of resection with a large cheek flap and back cut (1) is outlined.

A¹　Schematic outline of procedure emphasizing five important features of the incision for the cheek flap.
1. The medial incision of the excised triangle is almost vertical; the lateral incision is longer and oblique.
2. Adequate undermining below and especially lateral to the apex of the excised triangle.
3. Cutback (1) incision is made just below the lobule of the ear.
4. A vertical relaxing incision on the cheek flap may be necessary with an excision of small triangles (2) to increase the length of the cheek flap. The cheek flap consists of skin and subcutaneous tissue but *not* the parotid fascia. The facial nerve and its branches are thus spared.
5. The portion of the incision forming the cheek flap is curved slightly upward toward the level of the brow (3).

B　The tumor is excised with a full thickness resection and a free graft consisting of septal cartilage, and attached mucosa is sutured in place as a replacement for the tarsus and conjunctiva. One or two continuous 6-0 nylon pullout sutures (4) are utilized. *No* knots are tied on the conjunctival surface. To increase support inferiorly 5-0 or 6-0 catgut sutures may be necessary.

C　The inner subcutaneous tissue of the rotated cheek flap is sutured (5) to the periosteum of the infraorbital portion of the maxilla to prevent downward pull on the newly reconstructed lower lid. Similar sutures (6) are also used to support the flap at the lateral canthal region by fixing the sutures superiorly along the lateral orbital margin.

D　Long 5-0 silk sutures are used to approximate the cheek flap to the mucocartilage

(Text continued on opposite page.)

Plate 148   Periorbital Region

75% – 90%   DEFECT

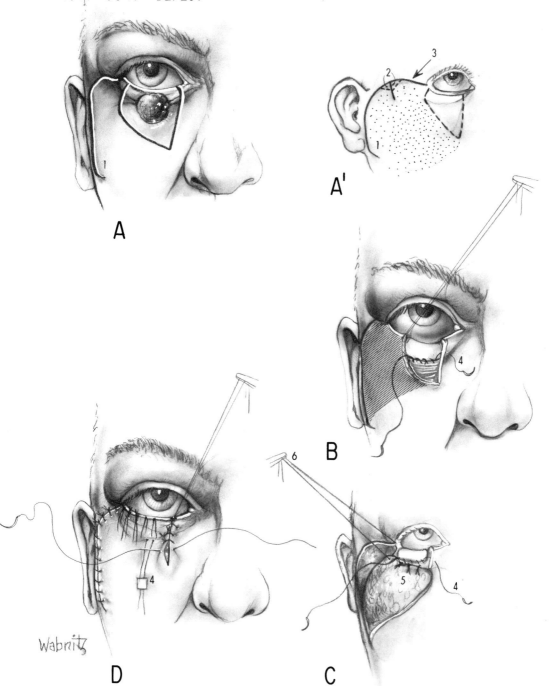

graft. For the remainder of the skin closure 5-0 nylon is used. The pullout sutures securing the septal graft are depicted (4).

Complications

1. Nylon pullout sutures may break, so take care in removing them.
2. Downward droop of new lid – perform lateral canthoplasty.
3. Fold and edema of rotated cheek flap.
4. Failure of nasal graft, especially the cartilage.

351

Highpoints

1. Upper lid reconstruction is most important in order to protect the cornea.
2. Upper lid reconstruction must encompass the following characteristics:
   a. Ability to cover and protect the cornea during sleep.
   b. Ability to elevate if at all possible, hence it must have some neuromuscular function.
   c. Must be lined with smooth mucous membrane to protect cornea.
   d. Must be rigid enough to maintain its shape and curvature in order to protect the cornea.
3. Lower lid or portion thereof best suited for reconstruction whenever possible.
4. Use all layers of lower lid.
5. Preserve vascular supply to rotated lower lid — pedicle in smaller flaps 5 mm wide and in the larger flaps 6 mm wide.
6. Suture tarsal plate of rotated lower lid to remaining portion of levator palpebrae superioris muscle or its aponeurosis (plate 151, step *L*).
7. As with lower lid, the principle of quarters is applicable (page 344).
   a. Defect of up to one quarter (25 per cent) is accomplished by direct closure (no rotated flap from lower lid necessary).
   b. Defect greater than one quarter and up to two quarters is reconstructed by up to one quarter lower lid flap with direct closure of donor site of lower lid.
   c. Defect of greater than two quarters and up to three quarters is reconstructed by a lower lid flap up to two quarters of its length with a rotation of the lateral cheek flap to close the donor site of the lower lid.
   d. Defect of greater than three quarters to total loss is reconstructed by a lower lid flap up to three quarters of its length preserving the medial quarter of the lower lid, thus avoiding any injury to the punctum and lacrimal apparatus.
8. The vascular hinge for lower lid flaps a, b and c under #7 are placed laterally, whereas flap d under #7 is placed medially.
9. Avoid kinking of vascular supply in pedicle when flap is rotated.
10. Refer to basic principles of lid reconstruction (page 344).

Reconstruction of Upper Lid with 25 per cent defect

A Twenty-five per cent defect repair is depicted. The lids are divided into quarters for clarity. Direct three-layer closure is performed following the technique on plate 144, steps *B*, *C* and *D*. If the defect is only slightly greater than 25 per cent of the lid, several additional millimeters can be gained by a lateral cantholysis (canthotony) in the elderly patient (plate 146, step *D*[1]). In a younger patient, it is best to rotate a flap from the lower lid.

A[1] The completed closure. The 6-0 nylon conjunctival suture (1) and the gray line fine silk suture (2) are depicted.
Refer to plate 152 for an alternate technique.

Reconstruction of Upper Lid with 30 to 50 per cent defect

B Thirty to 50 per cent defect repair is depicted by rotation of the lower lid flap measuring in width *one half* of the upper lid defect and *equal* in height (vertical) to the upper lid defect.

Using fine hooks, the upper lid defect is reduced 25 per cent. The original defect (dotted lines) is thus reduced to the solid lines. The defect is equal to distance X–Y, which is equal to distance X′–Y′ of the lower lid flap. The midpoint of this defect then locates the point (1) on the lower lid where the vascular pedicle is planned. When the

(Text continued on page 354.)

Plate 149   Periorbital Region

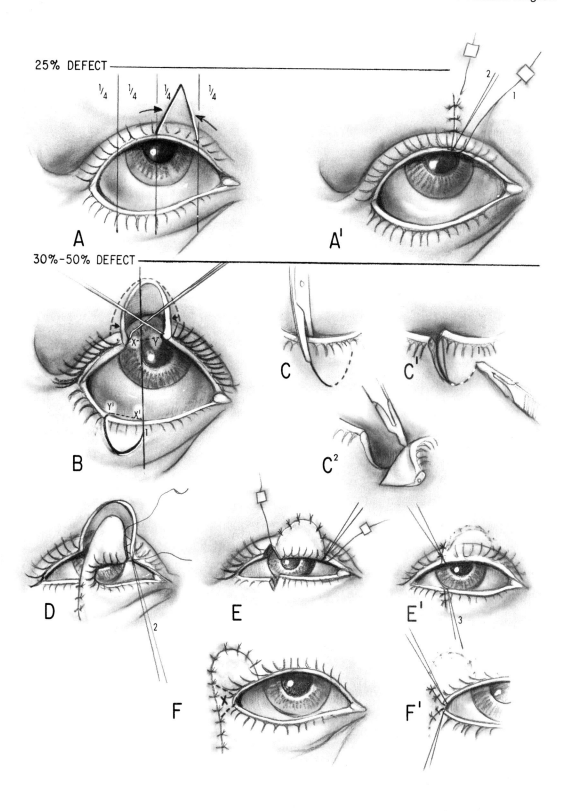

25% DEFECT

30%-50% DEFECT

A

A'

B

C

C'

C²

D

E

E'

F

F'

Reconstruction of Upper Lid with 30 to 50 per cent defect (Continued)

resulting upper lid defect is less than 6 mm in width (using the fine hooks), the lower lid flap width for practical purposes should not be less than 6 mm, since a rotation of a lower lid flap less than 6 mm is too minute.

C   The lower lid flap is outlined and rotated from the *lateral* portion of the lower lid by first using scissors through the lid margin (along the solid line) and then by using a knife (along dotted line, steps C^1 and C^2) up to within 5 mm of the lid margin where the pedicle (1) is located, thus carefully preserving the vascular arcade. The knife cut is made away from the pedicle. This vascular arcade is actually 3 mm from the free border of the lid margin (Whitnall), and hence if meticulous pains are taken, some additional relaxation of the rotated flap can be achieved by incising the skin and conjunctiva another millimeter or so.

D   The flap is rotated and sutured in place using a standard three-layer closure. Depicted is placement of the conjunctival 6-0 nylon pullout suture. One suture (2) is placed in the gray line of the lid margin at the medial border of the defect. When there is not more than a 50 per cent defect of the upper lid, it is not necessary to suture the levator palpebrae superioris to the flap, since there is sufficient attachment to the remaining upper lid. However, if practical, such attachment can be done with 5-0 chromic catgut.

If additional relaxation is deemed necessary, a lateral cantholysis (plate 146, step D^1) is performed.

Sutures are placed in such a fashion as not to kink the vascular pedicle. These sutures are removed on the fifth postoperative day, except for the margin gray line suture (2) which is removed two days later.

E
E¹   The vascular pedicle is transected in two to three weeks, and the lid margins tailored by an excision of small triangles to facilitate good realignment of the lid margins. A near-far, far-near suture may be placed along the gray line to prevent notching (plate 144, step *D*). This suture is left long (3).

F
F¹   If the defect is at the lateral canthus, the procedure is modified in that a single triangle (X) from the pedicle can be excised at the lateral canthus to form a sharper lateral canthus and to lengthen the palpebral fissure.

Plate 149 Repeated   Periorbital Region

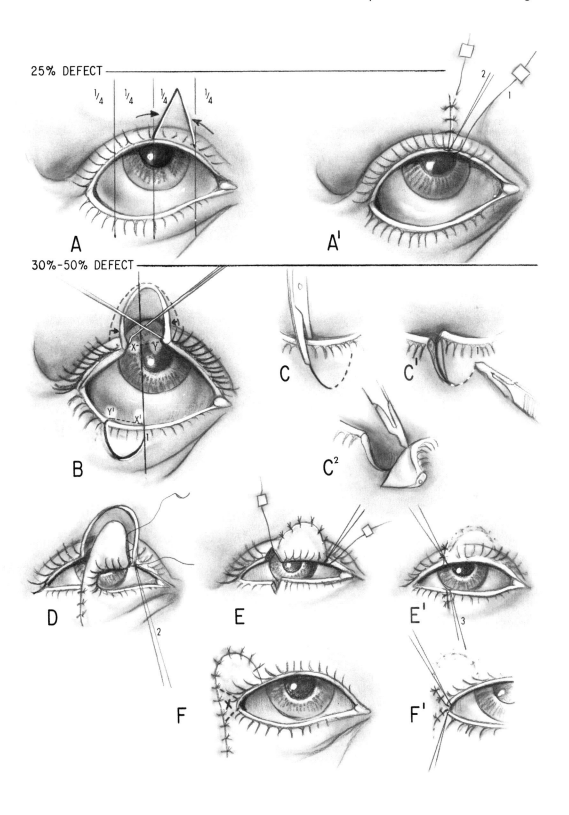

25% DEFECT

¹/₄ ¹/₄ ¹/₄ ¹/₄

A

A'

2
1

30%-50% DEFECT

B

X Y

Y' X'

1

C

C'

C²

D

2

E

E'

3

F

X

F'

Reconstruction of Upper Lid with 50 to 60 per cent defect
(After Mustardé, 1969)

This group is divided into two techniques:
1. Fifty to 60 per cent defect—closed with pedicle of flap based and swung laterally.
2. Sixty to 75 per cent defect—closed with pedicle of flap based and swung medially.

Laterally Based Flap

G   A defect somewhat greater than two quarters is depicted. Fine hooks simply put normal tension on the cut edges but do *not* attempt to decrease the defect by a quarter. Hence, quite a different mathematical plan is used to calculate the position and width of the flap from the lower lid as compared with the smaller defects. This is first done by marking the corresponding width of the defect on the edge of the lower lid with a dye (points 1 and 2). Then this marked defect is reduced by a distance equal to one quarter the entire length of the lower lid, the subtraction being done on the *lateral* side of the marked defect. This is the distance between points 2 and 3. Point 3 then becomes the location of the pedicle of the lower lid flap which is to be rotated from the lateral portion of the lower lid. This obviates injury to the lacrimal apparatus.

H   The flap is outlined. Distance 3–4 is equal to distance 1–3 in step G. Point 4 on the lateral portion of the lower lid flap is to be transposed to point 4' on the medial edge of the upper lid defect.

I   Rotation of flap. In order to close the donor site, an advanced lateral cheek flap will usually be necessary (except on the elderly when more lax skin is present). Refer to plates 147 and 148.

I^1   The closure is the standard three-layer approximation (plate 144). Transection of the pedicle is performed at two and one half weeks (plate 149, steps *D*, *E* and *E*^{1}). The nylon pullout conjunctive sutures (5) are taped to the skin.

Reconstruction of Upper Lid with 60 to 75 per cent defect

Medially Based Flap (Close to 75 Per Cent Defect)

When the defect in the upper lid is close to 75 per cent loss, a medially based flap is necessary since there is not sufficient length laterally for a rotated lower lid flap.

J   Defect and calculation of the flap are depicted. The calculation is the same as in step G but it is obvious that there is not sufficient length laterally; hence, it is rotated from the medial side. Distance 3–4 is the width of the flap after one quarter length of the lid has been subtracted (distance 2–3). Point 4 on the medial portion of the lower lid flap is to be transposed to point 4' on the lateral edge of the upper lid defect. Caution must be taken not to involve that portion of the lower lid flap with the canaliculus. At times the outline of the flap must be shifted slightly laterally to preserve this vital apparatus.

K   The flap is outlined and elevated medially and the remaining portion of the lower lid with the vascular pedicle is advanced *medially* by a zygomatic and cheek relaxing incision as shown in plates 147 and 148. This closes the defect of the donor site.

    In no case is the canaliculus included in the flap.

K^1   The closure is depicted. A standard three-layer closure is performed as described in plate 144, steps *B*, *C* and *D*. The muscle layer closure must be carefully performed to restore motor function to the transposed flap. It may be necessary to suture the muscle or the connective tissue of the flap to the aponeurosis of the palpebrae superioris muscle (plate 151, step *L*).

    The conjunctival pullout sutures (5) are taped to the skin.

    Transection of the pedicle is performed at two and one half weeks following the technique depicted on plate 149, steps *D*, *E* and *E*^{1}.

Plate 150   Periorbital Region

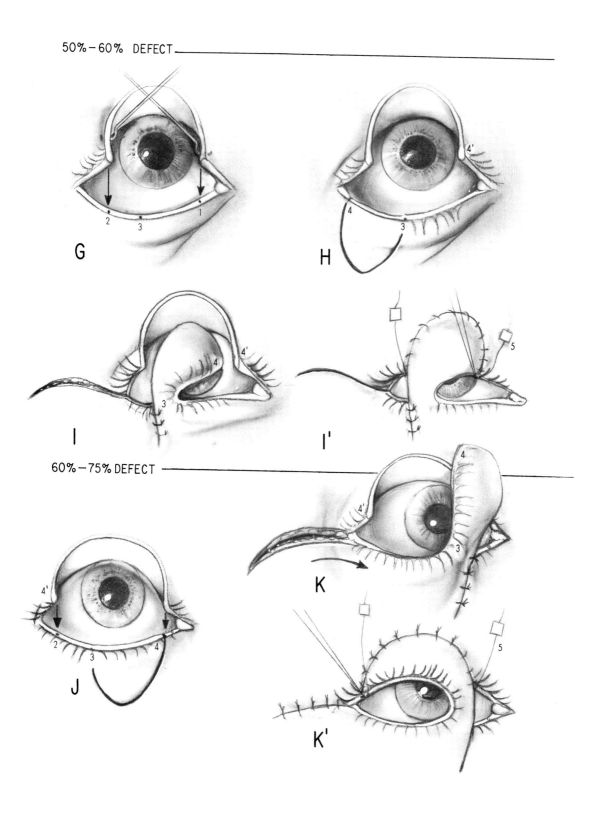

50%–60% DEFECT

G

H

I

I'

60%–75% DEFECT

J

K

K'

The lower lid flap in this size defect must always be rotated from the medial side, preserving, however, the medial quarter of the lower lid, thus preventing injury to the canaliculus. Hence, no more than a maximum of three quarters of the lower lid is utilized. No calculations are necessary with total defect since the pedicle is always located at the lateral edge of the lower lid.

Since the flap is large, the width of the pedicle should be larger—6 mm rather than 5 mm as in the smaller flaps. The tarsus requires transection and this will carry the incision farther, leaving only about 4 mm on the inner side of the pedicle.

The flap must be sutured to the palpebrae superioris muscle.

L Depicted is total loss of the upper lid with an outline of the lower lid flap. Point 2 on the medial side of the lower lid is transposed to point 2^1 on the lateral side of the upper lid defect. The stippled area on the cheek represents a triangle of skin to be excised to facilitate the advancement and closure of the lower lid defect. Note that the medial side of this triangle is shorter than the lateral side of the triangle. This aids in the prevention of scar contracture and drooping of the reconstructed lower lid. Additional details of this phase are on plate 147, steps *F* and *G*, and plate 148.

The cut edge (X) of the remaining portion of the palpebrae superioris muscle is tagged with two or three fine silk sutures for later approximation to the rotated lower lid flap. A vertical relaxing incision (3) on the cheek flap may be necessary with excision of small triangles (4) to increase the length of the cheek flap.

M The full thickness flap is elevated and the relaxing incision is made with an elevation of the cheek flap down to but not including the underlying muscles. Injury to the branches of the facial nerve is avoided.

The flap with pedicle is advanced and rotated into the defect. Care is taken not to kink the vascular pedicle; it is better to leave a bit of a gap on the edges surrounding the pedicle. Any resulting small defect is corrected at the second stage when the pedicle is divided in two and one half weeks. Septal cartilage with mucosa (Y) is utilized to line the reconstructed donor site and sutured in place using 6-0 nylon pullout sutures.

The rotated lower lid flap is first sutured by approximation of conjunctiva of the lid flap to the stump of conjunctiva of the upper fornix. If the sutures are clear of the cornea 6-0 chromic catgut is used; otherwise, a 6-0 nylon pullout suture is utilized to prevent ulceration of the cornea. The next layer is the approximation of the previously tagged stump of the palpebrae superioris muscle to the connective tissue of the lower lid flap using 6-0 chromic catgut. The third layer is the skin closure, taking care to avoid injury to the vascular pedicle.

N The completed closure.

O
O¹ The pedicle is sectioned in two and one half weeks excising two small triangles of lid margin to produce a smooth curved lid margin. This is performed under local anesthesia. The lid margins are approximated with 6-0 silk sutures, the ends being left long. A near-far, far-near suture can be used on the margins to prevent notching (plate 144, step *D*).

Plate 151   Periorbital Region

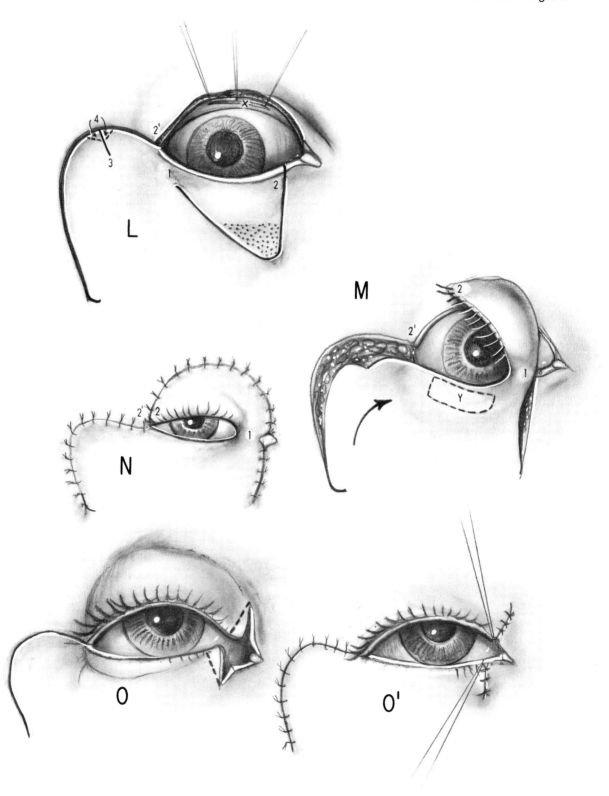

BRIDGE FLAP REPAIR OF LARGE UPPER LID DEFECTS, CUTLER-BEARD TECHNIQUE (After Smith and Obear, 1967; Fox, 1964)

There is a difference of opinion regarding the reconstruction of upper lid defects. Esser's technique (plates 149 and 150) has some drawbacks in that the rotation flaps from the lower lid for large defects necessitates a rather formidable procedure to reconstruct the lower lid which may in turn cause drooping of the reconstructed lower lid and shortening of the length of both lids.

The various techniques are:
1. Composite grafts.
2. Temporal and forehead pedicle flaps.
3. Lower lid flaps.
   a. Bridge flap of Cutler-Beard technique.
   b. Tarsal sharing flap of Hughes technique.
   c. Rotation flap of Esser.

Highpoints

1. Full thickness flap from lower lid and portion of cheek.
2. Keep lower lid margin with marginal artery intact—a width of 3 to 4 mm.
3. Two stages—up to two months between stages—the patient must be informed that the eye will be sutured closed for this period of time.
4. Lash graft may be performed as third stage.
5. Protect cornea with scleral contact lens during all but the final steps of stage 1.
6. Width of flap equals horizontal width of upper lid defect prior to resection.
7. Suture transected edge of levator palpebrae superioris muscle to orbicularis oculi muscle and orbital septum at the superior edge of the flap.

A   A scleral contact lens has been inserted to protect the cornea. The width of the area to be resected is measured. This will determine the width of the bridge flap.

Resection of full thickness of the upper lid is then performed with adequate margins. Stay sutures are used both on the corners of the resected specimen and on the corners of the remaining lid. The area resected includes the tarsus or part thereof depending on adequate ablative surgery.

B   The lower lid flap is scribed, preserving 3 to 4 mm of the lower lid margin which preserves the lid contour with the marginal artery. The horizontal width of the flap is determined from the preresection measurements of the upper lid defect since after resection the remaining edges of the upper lid retract.

B¹   Cross section at the same stage as step *B*.

C   The lower lid flap has been mobilized as a full thickness flap. The skin, orbicularis oculi muscle and orbital septum are cut with a knife, while the underlying conjunctiva is cut with a scissors. The skin extending down to the cheek is mobilized to prevent undue tension on the final suture lines. The arrow depicts the course of the flap under the lower lid margin (the bridge flap). Stay sutures or fine skin hooks on the flap facilitate this maneuver. The scleral contact lens is then removed just prior to approximation of the flap which consists of:
   a. Suturing the conjunctiva layers of the upper lid defect and the conjunctiva of the flap with 6-0 chromic catgut with knots buried (not contacting the cornea).
   b. Suturing the remnant of the levator to the orbicularis oculi muscle and orbital septum of the flap with interrupted buried 6-0 silk. This facilitates relatively normal function of the levator to the flap.

(Text continued on page 362.)

Plate 152   Periorbital Region

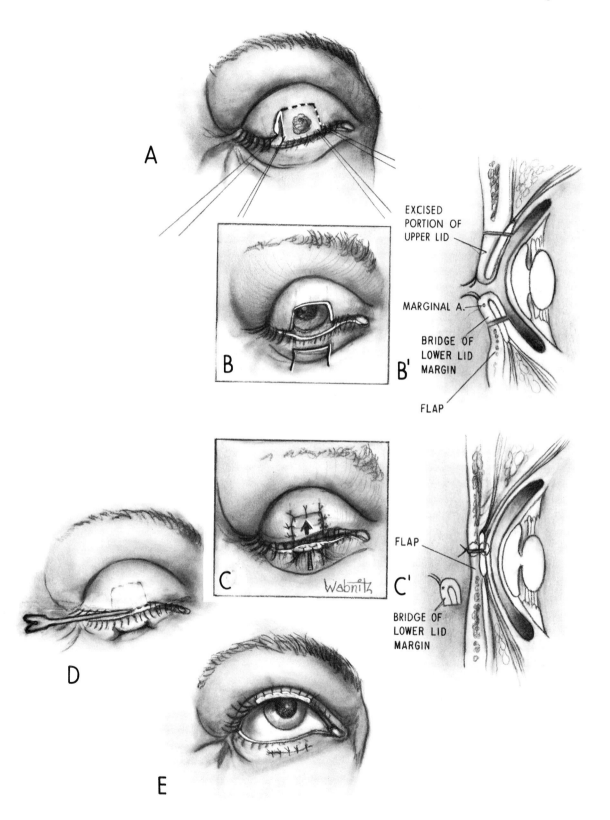

EXCISED
PORTION OF
UPPER LID

MARGINAL A.

BRIDGE OF
LOWER LID
MARGIN

FLAP

A

B

B'

C

Wabnitz

C'

FLAP

BRIDGE OF
LOWER LID
MARGIN

D

E

    c. Suturing the medial and lateral borders of the remaining upper lid to the flap with two 4-0 silk mattress sutures without vertical tension.

    d. Suturing the skin edges with interrupted or continuous 6-0 silk sutures.

    e. Suturing the lower lid vertical incision with 6-0 silk after all tension is relieved by an additional release incision if necessary.

    No sutures are placed in the preserved lower lid margin.

    Skin sutures are removed in six days.

    Mattress sutures are removed in 10 days.

C¹   Cross section at the same stage as step C.

D   The flap is transected over a groove director as depicted about 1 to 2 mm below the normal lid margin to allow for some postoperative retraction of the transposed flap. The conjunctiva of the flap is sutured to the skin of the flap with interrupted 6-0 plain catgut sutures or a 6-0 nylon pullout suture forming the upper lid margin.

E   The remaining stump of the base of the flap is repositioned into the donor site. Its edge is then sutured to the freshened inferior edge of the margin of the lower lid. The remaining skin edges and conjunctiva are approximated in two layers following the excision of any redundant skin.

An eye lash graft to the upper lid margin (see plate 155, step *F*) can be performed six weeks after the first stage (two weeks before transection of the flap) or after the second stage.

Plate 152 Repeated   Periorbital Region

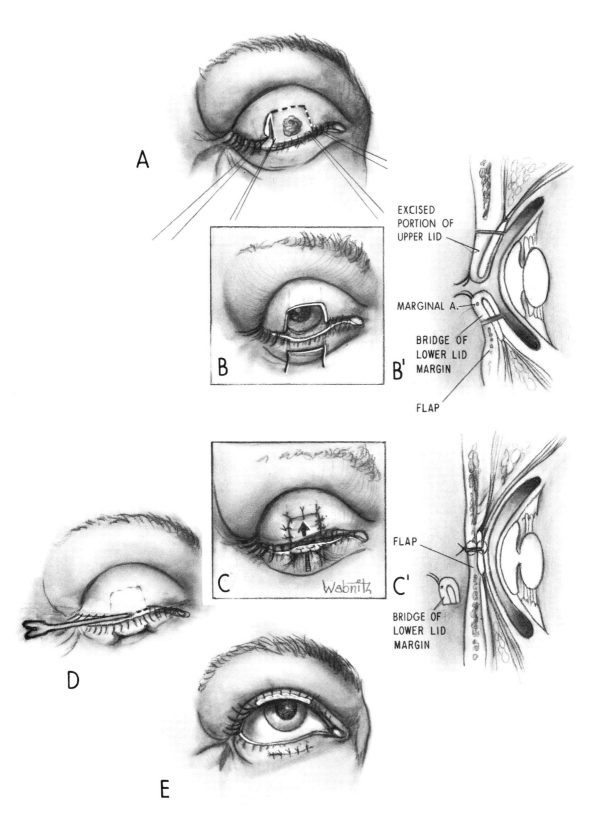

A

B

B'

EXCISED
PORTION OF
UPPER LID

MARGINAL A.

BRIDGE OF
LOWER LID
MARGIN

FLAP

C

Wabnitz

C'

FLAP

BRIDGE OF
LOWER LID
MARGIN

D

E

Highpoints

1. Retain as much of upper lid as possible (compatible with good tumor surgery) since this structure is most important to protect the cornea and subsequent vision. The new upper lid must protect the cornea during sleep and ideally be able to elevate while awake.
2. Protect globe.
3. Resect entire lacrimal apparatus.
4. Cheek flap highpoints (refer to page 350).
5. Septal mucosa graft for upper lid and septal cartilage and mucosal graft for lower lid.
6. Adequate forehead and scalp flap.
7. Adequate margins (at least 1.5 cm) around tumor and resect underlying periosteum and perichondrium—check margins with frozen sections with *careful labeling*. This is most important since gross evaluation can be misleading.
8. Once bone is invaded with basal cell carcinoma, radical resection of the osseous structure is often necessary with enucleation. Locally, invasive basal cell carcinoma is *extremely* lethal. Gross extension of disease is no criterion for microscopic extension.

A   Outline of incisions for resection, and forehead, scalp and cheek flaps for reconstruction. The basic principle is the retention of as much of the upper lid as possible to protect the cornea without compromising adequate resection.

A^1 An alternate plan would be to rotate the remaining lower lid (3) to replace the defect
A^2 in the upper lid (refer plate 151). Only 75 per cent replacement is necessary (Mustardé). Depicted is a Fricke supraorbital flap (2) to reconstruct the lateral portion of total loss of the upper lid. This flap is lined with septal mucosa. A rotated cheek flap is used for the lower lid (refer to plates 147 and 148).

B   A forehead-scalp flap with a back cut (4) is elevated to reconstruct the medial portion of the upper lid. This is lined with septal mucosa. Cartilage is optional since the flap is quite thick and stiff. The cheek flap is elevated also with a back cut (5) in the fashion described on plate 148. The only modification is the mobilization of the conjunctiva on the lower lid with an incision laterally along the fornix to permit lateral advancement of the entire remnant of the lower lid.

C   The lined area on the upper lid indicates the location of the septal mucosal graft, while the lined area on the lower lid indicates the septal cartilage and mucosal graft. These grafts are secured in position by 6-0 nylon pullout sutures or 5-0 catgut sutures. Long 5-0 or 6-0 silk sutures are placed along the lid margins. A split thickness epidermal graft (X) covers the nasal defect. This could also be covered with further mobilization and a larger scalp flap (plate 90). If there is undue tension with primary closure of the scalp defect, the defect can be closed with a split thickness epidermis graft (Y).

    Reconstruction of a lacrimal apparatus may be necessary if epiphora occurs. This can utilize the basic principle of a dacryocystorhinostomy by construction of an outlet into the nasal cavity (refer to plate 159) or a conjunctival flap (plate 156, step C).

Plate 153   Periorbital Region

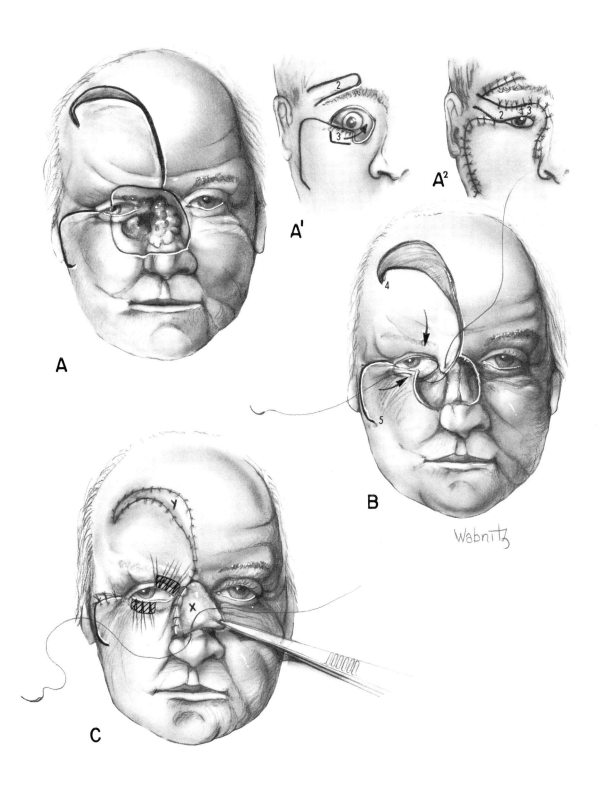

A

A'

A²

B

Wabnitz

C

EXCISION OF SUPERFICIAL BASAL CARCINOMA
IN REGION OF LATERAL CANTHUS OF LOWER LID

Although the lesion depicted could be excised by the method described in plate 146, step *D*, since the lesion is superficial, full thickness resection of the lid is not necessary.

A Excision of lesion including a portion of the underlying orbicularis oculi muscle. Outline of skin flap (Fricke, 1829) from upper lid. This is permissible since the lid margin is not disturbed and there is redundant skin present and no deformity of the upper lid will result (refer to page 344 for details in regard to principles of lid reconstruction).

B Rotation of flap. Approximation with 5-0 silk or nylon.

C Completed procedure.

D Depicted is a superficial basal carcinoma below the lateral canthal region. Excision is performed including a portion of the underlying muscle. The incision for the small flap is at or slightly above the level of the lateral canthus.

E The flap advanced. It is important that no downward pull is placed on the lower lid. If necessary, a subcutaneous suture is placed through the flap into the margin of the orbit to prevent tension on the lower lid.

F The completed procedure.

Plate 154   Periorbital Region

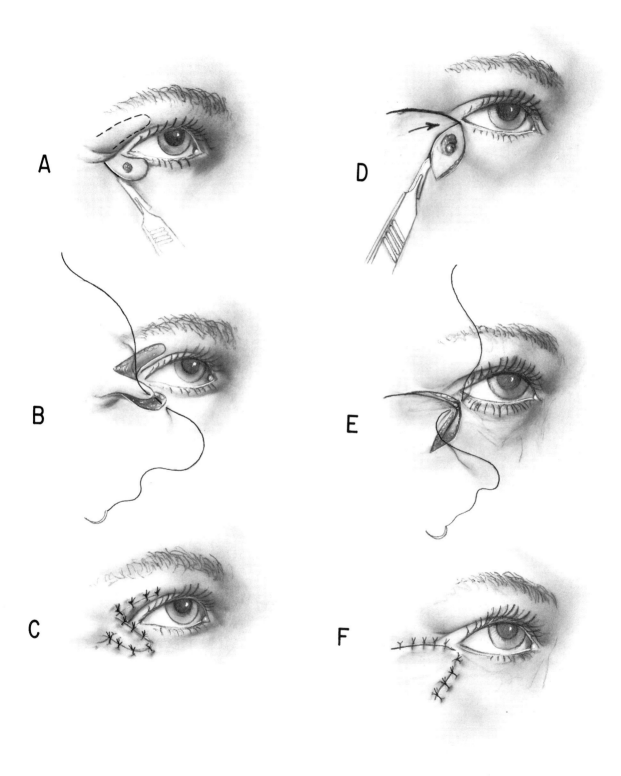

A

B

C

D

E

F

EXCISION OF BENIGN LESION OF UPPER LID

When simple approximation of skin edges following resection of a lesion near the medial canthus would distort the medial canthus, an advanced skin flap from the more central portion of the lid may be indicated.

A The line of excision with lateral extension for advanced flap is depicted.

B The skin flap is advanced. A relaxing incision (dotted line) may be necessary to avoid a dog-ear.

C The completed closure.

RECONSTRUCTION OF SUPERFICIAL HORIZONTAL DEFECT OF PORTION OF LOWER LID (Fricke, Upper Lid Flap)

D Depicted is a long horizontal defect of the skin of the lower lid. The dotted line outlines an upper lid skin flap which is to be rotated nondelayed to close the defect. Since there is usually considerable redundant skin of the upper lid, this is quite feasible, especially in the elderly. Some surgeons emphasize that the upper lid skin flap should extend virtually the entire distance of the upper lid to avoid any uneven contractures which may occur with only a 50 per cent length flap. Care must be taken not to injure the deeper structures of the upper lid, e.g., the underlying muscle and tarsus, nor the most important lid margin. This must not be violated under any circumstances.

E The flap in place. Depending on the extent of the defect at the lateral canthus, the base of the flap "x" can be returned to the donor area at a second stage. Sutures must be carefully placed to avoid injury to the globe. Edema of the lower lid margin can occur if this margin is too wide.

When there is a narrow horizontal defect of the free margin of the lower lid, a bipedicle flap of skin from the upper lid appears preferred as is depicted in plate 160, steps E and F. The conjunctiva of the remaining portion of the lower lid is freely mobilized to the lower fornix, excised and sutured to the inner portion of the bipedicle flap to form the inner lining. Although this procedure is simple, the surgeon must be aware that the skin flap may curl on itself and later on droop after the pedicles are returned to the upper lid. It might be fortuitous to leave the pedicles attached for a prolonged period of time. (Fricke's supraorbital flap is described on plate 153, Step A[1].)

(Text continued on page 370.)

Plate 155   Periorbital Region

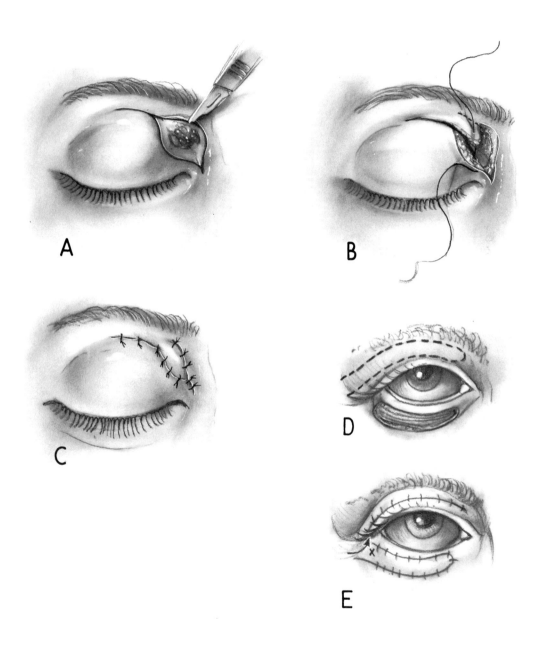

A

B

C

D

E

EYELASH RECONSTRUCTION

There is some difference of opinion regarding the advisability of eyelash replacement for the lower lid; yet, there is less question as to the advisability of upper eyelashes.

Several methods are described, especially regarding the donor site, e.g., eyebrow, temporal region or postauricular region.

Highpoints

1. Evaluate proper direction of hair and maintain this direction in graft.
2. Do not injure hair follicles—these are *upward obliquely* and hence an incision deep to skin must follow this angle.
3. Trim excess adipose tissue from graft.
4. Avoid donor site which may become bald later.

F Depicted is the temporal region donor site with the incision placed in a relatively horizontal plane. The hairs thus will be in the same plane when transferred to the lid margin. Two or three rows of hairs are excised.

F¹ The hair follicles extend upward in an oblique direction and care must be taken that the incision (dotted line) for the graft follows this same angle; otherwise, the follicles will be injured.

G The free graft (about 2 mm in width) consisting of two or three rows of hairs with follicles. Although some adipose tissue is necessarily excised when the graft is removed, as much of this fat is trimmed with fine scissors as is possible. The rounded black protuberances of the follicles must be preserved.

H An incision parallel and slightly outside or distal (1.0 to 2.0 mm) to the free lid margin is made deep enough to accommodate the free graft. Care must be taken that the direction of the hair is in the correct plane. Sutures through both lid edges and the graft are carefully placed without injury to the globe.

The original hairs may fall out with new growth in about three weeks. These hairs will require a periodic trimming.

Complications

1. Failure of graft—repeat.
2. Scarring with inturning of new lashes against the cornea; such hair will require removal by electrolysis.

EYEBROW RECONSTRUCTION

Reconstruction of the absent eyebrow can be usually achieved following a technique similar to that used for the grafting of an eyelash, except that the graft is wider and through and through sutures are not used. The wider the graft, however, the greater the possibility of failure. Hence, an island flap of hair-bearing scalp can be used based on a branch of the superficial temporal artery and vein. Avoid donor site which may become bald later.

Plate 155 Continued   *Periorbital Region*

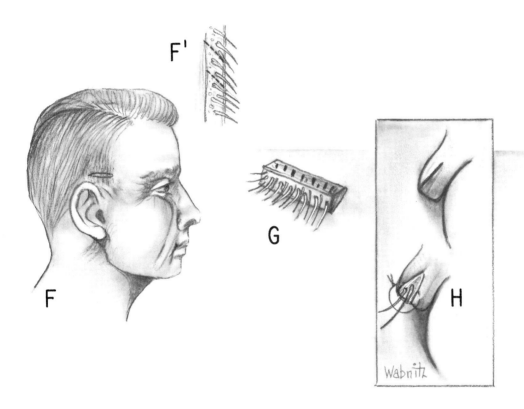

F'

G

F

H

Wabnitz

EXCISION OF LESIONS AT THE MEDIAL CANTHUS

When the loss of tissue is at the medial canthal region, a lateral cantholysis usually will not afford enough relaxation, and a free full thickness graft or transposed flap will be necessary. If the defect is superficial and the canaliculi are preserved, a free graft is utilized (plate 86, steps *E*, *F* and *G*). However, if the defect is full thickness with loss of the canaliculi but yet quite small, the defect is closed in three layers as depicted in plate 144, steps *B* and *C*. The tarsus is sutured to the medial end of the stump of the canthal ligament or to the periosteum. A lateral canthoplasty may be necessary to gain an additional length for one or both lids (refer to plate 146, step *D¹*). Either the superior or inferior crus or both crura of the lateral canthal ligament are transected. When the defect is larger, a transposed flap is necessary.

A For a moderate defect, the glabella flap is utilized resorting to the **V–Y** principle. The flap is full thickness and must not include the brow. Only a few millimeters' defect of the lids can be reconstructed with this flap.

A¹ The **V** flap is lowered and the donor site is closed in **Y** fashion. A three-layer closure is utilized in which the lids approximate the flap, attempting to suture conjunctiva to conjunctiva.

For a larger defect a midline forehead flap is necessary (refer to plate 121).

B A modification of the forehead flap with base at the contralateral side of the nose is
B¹ depicted. The dotted line represents the discarded tip of the flap. This flap is performed in one stage while the flap on plate 121 requires a second stage to transect and return the pedicle. The disadvantages of the contralaterally based flap are the horizontal scars plus the fact that the brows may well meet one another in the midline. Mucous membrane lining is usually necessary and this is obtained from the nasal septum as described on plates 147 and 148. Be sure to suture the inner side of the flap to the periosteum where it dips into the canthal region to produce a concavity.

C A somewhat distressing problem may arise regarding tearing associated with the loss of the canaliculi — epiphora. To reconstruct a suitable duct at the initial operation is a matter of judgment, since some patients do not develop epiphora. Depicted is Mustardé's method for construction of a new duct. A flap of conjunctiva along the inferior fornix is rotated medially and sutured to the remaining lacrimal sac if present or into the nasal cavity utilizing principles of a dacryocystorhinostomy (refer to plate 159).

Other surgeons have indicated that skin defects in this region may require no covering, allowing the defect to close by granulations and secondary intention. This entails a rather protracted course. Another method of handling such lesions is by radiotherapy or using the technique of Mohs' paste.

Plate 156   Periorbital Region

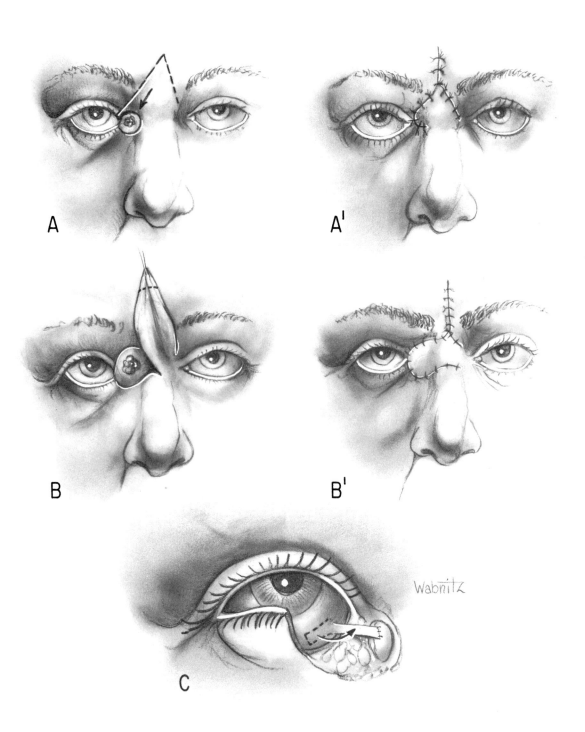

A

A'

B

B'

C

Wabnitz

MEDIAL CANTHOPLASTY AND REPAIR OF RELATED INJURIES

Highpoints

1. Disruption of the medial canthal ligament may be associated with other local deformities:
   a. Naso-orbital fracture.
   b. Injury to the nasolacrimal apparatus: puncta, canaliculi, lacrimal sac and naso-lacrimal duct.
   c. May be bilateral.
2. If such injuries are present, all should be corrected concomitantly including a dacryocystorhinostomy (refer to plate 159), if indicated.
3. More seriously, intracranial injuries may be present, and if so, these take precedence over any repair in the region of medial canthus.
4. Protect cornea during operation.

A Typical deformity in the left medial canthal region characterized by displacement of the medial canthus primarily laterally and slightly downward and forward. The canthus itself is rounded and blunted and may be partially obscured by redundant tissue of the lids. Distances a and b are the normal relationships, whereas distance b^1 is longer than b and a^1 is shorter than a. Although this deformity may be entirely and solely due to rupture of the medial canthal ligament, fracture of the medial wall of the orbital can also contribute to this clinical picture. X-ray films are performed, and if indicated, laminograms.

   If the trauma is some weeks or months old and associated with persistent swelling at the medial canthal region, especially below the level of the medial canthal ligament, injury to the lacrimal apparatus has occurred with the probable formation of a mucocele of the lacrimal sac. A dacryocystorhinostomy (plate 159) would be indicated. In either event all such associated deformities must be corrected concomitantly. The procedure described in the following illustration depicts only repair of the medial canthal ligament and reduction and fixation of fresh naso-orbital fractures.

B Surgical anatomy of the medial canthal (pàlpebral) ligament and associated lacrimal
B^1 apparatus. B^1 is a coronal section through the medial canthal ligament. The medial canthal ligament splits into a thicker anterior section and a much thinner posterior section, thus enveloping the lacrimal sac. Horner's muscle lies just deep to the posterior section of the medial canthal ligament. The anterior section is attached to the anterior lacrimal crest behind the plane of the cornea; the posterior section along with Horner's muscle is attached to the posterior lacrimal crest. In the illustration (B), the anterior section of the ligament has been ruptured in its midportion. However, other variations of disruption of the ligament can occur. The disruption may be more laterally at a point just over the proximal portions of the canaliculi. Here the ligament is thinner. Repair in this situation must approximate the upper and lower origins of the ligament from the upper and lower lids. Another type of disruption of the ligament may involve an avulsion of a portion of the underlying bone with a small fragment of bone attached to the medial end of the ligament. This affords an excellent point for the through and through wire suture to be described. Laterally, the ligament is attached to the medial angles of the two tarsal plates. Medially it arises from the frontal process of the maxilla in front of the lacrimal groove.

Plate 157   *Periorbital Region*

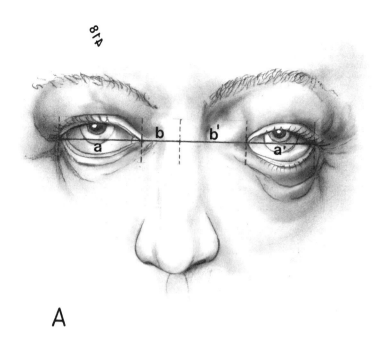

A

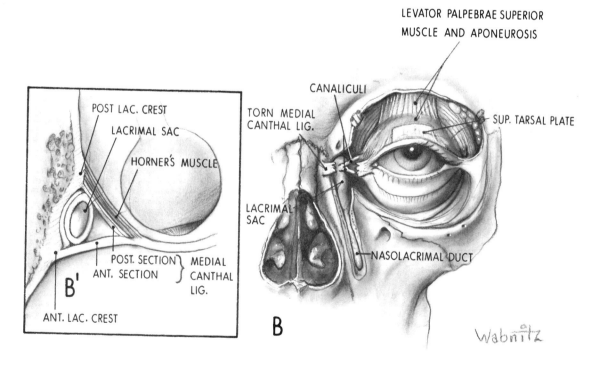

LEVATOR PALPEBRAE SUPERIOR
MUSCLE AND APONEUROSIS

CANALICULI

TORN MEDIAL
CANTHAL LIG.

SUP. TARSAL PLATE

POST LAC. CREST

LACRIMAL SAC

HORNER'S MUSCLE

LACRIMAL
SAC

POST. SECTION
ANT. SECTION } MEDIAL
CANTHAL
LIG.

NASOLACRIMAL DUCT

B'

ANT. LAC. CREST

B

Wabnitz

MEDIAL CANTHOPLASTY AND REPAIR OF RELATED INJURIES
(*Continued*)

C   A small curved incision is made on the side of the nose anterior to the medial canthus, avoiding the skin of the eyelid. Care must be taken not to injure the cornea of each globe during the operation. The lids can be temporarily sutured together. With a small periosteal elevator, the bone is exposed at the selected site for fixation of the ruptured ligament. A similar incision is then made on the opposite side of the nose. Two drill holes about 5 mm apart are made in the medial wall of the orbit through the exposed bone bilaterally. A small dental bur or drill is utilized. No. 32 wire attached to the bur or drill is then pulled through the holes, first above and then through the ligament and through the holes below.

D   Insert drawing depicts detail of wire suture through ruptured ligament.

E   The wire is tightened on the contralateral side and carefully twisted. The cut twisted end is then buried in one of the drill holes. When scarring prevents complete approximation, the attachment of the orbital septum (plate 143) to the periosteum along the orbital rim is incised. Section of the lateral canthal ligament (plate 146, step D^1) and the tarso-orbital fascia may likewise be necessary.

F   If an associated deformed fracture of the naso-orbital compound is present and no intracranial complications exist, through and through wires similar to those used to repair the medial canthal can be utilized if necessary. These are placed slightly more anteriorly and they pass through the skin and acrylic plates or Silastic guards on either side of the nose. Care must be exercised so that no excess pressure is applied on the acrylic plates or Silastic guards that might cause skin necrosis.

G   If there is injury to the canaliculi, repair should be done immediately since secondary repair is extremely difficult. Basically, this entails passing a plastic tube 1 mm in diameter through the lumen of the canaliculus and approximating the ends with two or three 6-0 or 7-0 catgut sutures. The tubing, acting as a stent, is sutured to the lower lid with fine silk sutures and left in place two weeks. Dilatations are usually necessary following removal of the tubing. An operation microscope may be necessary to locate the distal end of the canaliculus. The microscope may also aid in the suturing of the severed ends. If the distal severed end cannot be located with the microscope, methylene blue can be instilled in the other canaliculus if intact. This will usually extrude through the distal severed end of the injured canaliculus.

An alternate technique for reconstruction of the medial canthal ligament has been described by M. K. Wang using a triangular skin flap as a substitute for the torn ligament. This technique has specific use when sufficient length of the torn medial canthal ligament is absent or cannot be identified.

If there is associated depressed fracture of the glabella resulting from a previous injury, a concomitant bone graft is performed (Smith, 1965).

When obstruction of the nasolacrimal duct is present, a concomitant dacryocystorhinostomy is performed (refer to plate 159).

Plate 158   *Periorbital Region*

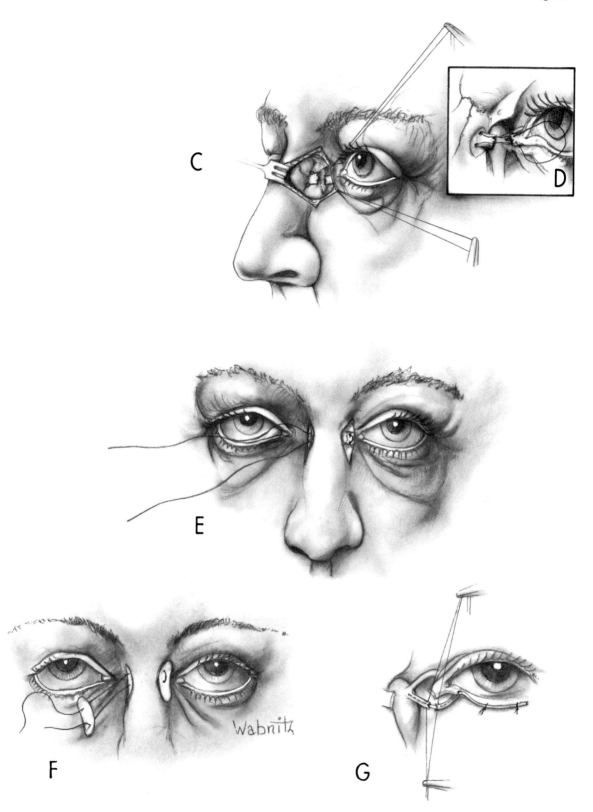

C

D

E

F

Wabnitz

G

DACRYOCYSTORHINOSTOMY (After L. Q. Pang, 1971)

Indications

Obstruction of the nasolacrimal sac with or without dacryocystitis.

Highpoints

1. Canaliculi must be patent; otherwise, they require reconstruction (refer to previous plates and plate 156, step *C*).
2. Any nasal or ethmoid sinus disease must be corrected.
3. Anesthesia—local (Pang) or general.
4. Place skin incision 3 mm medial to the medial canthus to avoid the angular vessels.
5. Do not transect the medial canthal ligament if feasible—if lacerated or torn this requires repair at the same sitting. Refer to previous plates.
6. Place vertical incision in lacrimal sac between the middle and posterior thirds, thus forming a longer (or wider) anterior mucosal flap (step *D*).
7. Do not injure the canaliculi—at times catheterization may be helpful to identify canaliculi and lacrimal sac if severe scarring is present.
8. Refer to plates 143 and 157 for anatomic relationships of lacrimal sac.

A   Lateral view of the bony framework forming the lacrimal fossa. The lateral portion of the maxilla has been omitted for the sake of clarity. Dotted lines indicate bone removal to form a new drainage route from the lacrimal sac into the nose. The bone removed includes the entire lacrimal fossa and a portion of thick anterior lacrimal crest. If need be, the posterior extent can be enlarged by reaching the posterior margin of the lacrimal bone and even up to the lamina papyracea of the ethmoid.

B   A vertical 2 to 2.5 cm long skin incision has been made commencing 2 to 3 mm superior to the medial canthal ligament and 3 mm medial to the medial canthus. This tends to avoid the angular vessels. The muscle fibers of the orbicularis oculi muscle are split. The medial canthal ligament is identified and preserved. Retraction or at times transection of this ligament is necessary. It must be repaired in any event. Using sharp dissection, the fascia attaching the lacrimal sac to the anterior lacrimal crest is transected along the dotted line. Care must be taken not to tear the sac. It is then completely mobilized from its bed by removing the periosteum with the sac.

C   Using a small trephine saw, an opening is made in the anteroinferior portion of the lacrimal fossa and anterior lacrimal crest. Care is taken not to injure the underlying nasal mucosa. The opening is then enlarged with Kerrison forceps to the shape of an oval—up to 15 mm long and 12 mm wide.

D   At this point a cotton-tipped nasal applicator (dotted lines) is inserted into the nasal cavity up to the region of the trephine opening. If the nasal mucosa bulges into the opening, all is clear; otherwise, some interposing ethmoid cells will require removal. For the sake of clarity, the medial canthal ligament is omitted.

A vertical incision is made in the lacrimal sac in a plane between the middle and posterior thirds. This results in an anterior flap (1) which is longer (or wider) in the horizontal plane than the posterior flap (2). This is most important since the distance between the posterior flaps of the sac and nasal mucosa is shorter than the distance between the anterior flaps. A similarly placed vertical incision is then made in the nasal mucosa using the cotton-tipped applicator as support to steady the nasal mucosa.

Short horizontal incisions are made at each end of the vertical incisions. This aids in the reflection of the flaps.

If necessary, because of lacerations and severe scarring, the flaps may be varied and even placed in a horizontal plane.

E   The posterior flaps are then approximated with three 6-0 or 5-0 chromic catgut sutures. The anterior flaps are then sutured in similar fashion. For the sake of clarity, the medial canthal ligament is omitted. If repair of this ligament is performed, the drill holes are made and sutures are placed (refer to previous plates, steps *D* and *E*) but not secured until approximation of the flaps is completed.

 (Text continued on opposite page.)

Plate 159   Periorbital Region

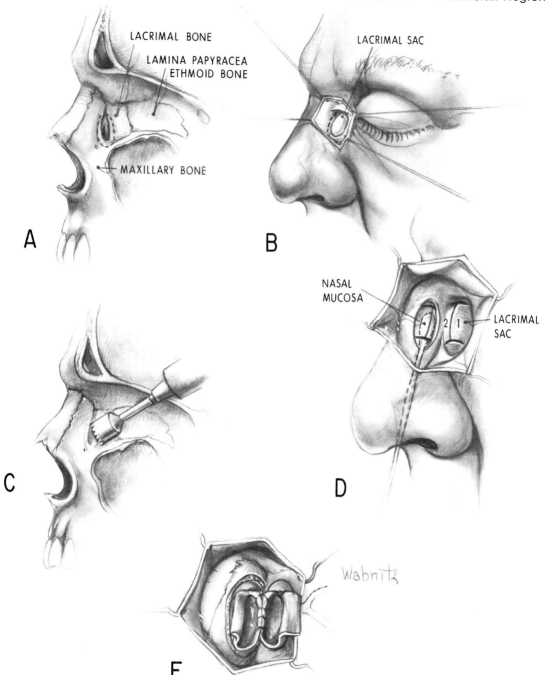

A

LACRIMAL BONE

LAMINA PAPYRACEA
ETHMOID BONE

MAXILLARY BONE

B

LACRIMAL SAC

C

D

NASAL
MUCOSA

LACRIMAL
SAC

E

Wabnitz

Some surgeons insert a fine plastic tube through the canaliculus and thence into the nose. If the reconstruction has gone smoothly, this seems superfluous.

Postoperative Care

1. Do *not* blow nose.
2. Decongestants.
3. Antibiotics are optional.

Complications

Stenosis due to cicatrization requires revision.

An alternate technique is described by Iliff, 1971.

CORRECTION OF SCAR CONTRACTURE OF THE LIDS AND ECTROPION

A   Scar contracture of the lower lid. The *entire* scar must be excised. A Z-plasty is outlined with wide undermining of the surrounding skin as in the stippled areas.

B   The Z-plasty completed.

      If the scar is exceedingly large, a transposed flap may be necessary from the mid-forehead (refer to plate 121) or an advanced lateral cheek flap (plates 147 and 148).

C   Scar contracture of upper lid with ectropion. A Z-plasty is outlined with an additional area of scar excised.

D   The completed Z-plasty with a full thickness graft (3) inserted in the large defect. If the defect is small, a simple closure is feasible. Pullout 5-0 nylon sutures through the tarsoconjunctival layer can be used to aid in the approximation of the flaps of the Z-plasty.

      For severe ectropion of the lower lid secondary to scarring and tissue loss, a bipedicle flap (Tripier) from the upper lid may be of help.

E   A section of skin from the upper lid with some underlying fibers of the orbicularis oculi muscle is mobilized. A bipedicle flap of skin and muscle is thus developed. A temporary tarsorrhaphy is performed (plate 162, steps *F* and *G*).

F   The flap is swung into the defect and approximated with 5-0 nylon sutures. Both pedicles are tubed. The donor site is closed by simple approximation. Sponge rubber roll is sutured over the flap to help prevent curling or bulging of the flap. The pedicles may be left intact for months to act as suspensory slings for the lower lid, or they may be transected and returned to the ends of the donor site.

Plate 160   Periorbital Region

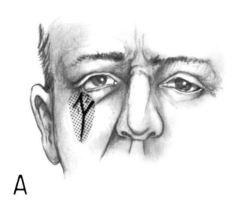

A

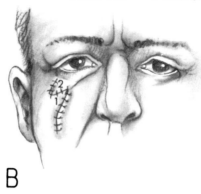

B

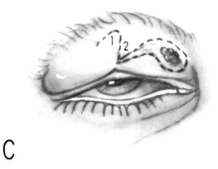

C

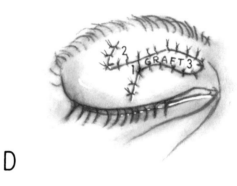

D

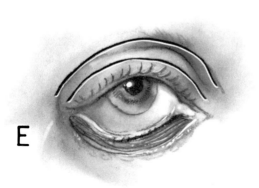

E

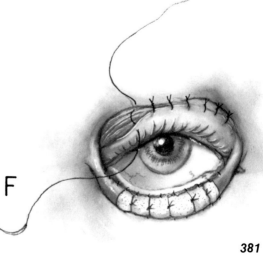

F

TARSORRHAPHY

Indications

To protect cornea.

LATERAL PERMANENT TARSORRHAPHY OR CANTHORRHAPHY

This type of intermargin adhesion is particularly adaptable for paralytic ectropion and drooping of the lower lid which is of a permanent nature. It is used in deformities associated with facial nerve paralysis involving the orbicularis oculi muscle and minor deformities secondary to lower lid surgery.

Highpoints

1. The upper lid is made to support the lower lid.
2. Preserve most of the upper tarsal plate.

A   The lids are drawn together to the desired position and the lid margins are marked with a suitable dye. This point is usually 6 to 8 mm from the commissure of the lateral canthus.

B   The lids are split along the gray line with a knife, using fine hooks on the lids as traction points. An incision is carried through the canthus for 2 mm (point X). The lids are then separated into two layers for a distance of 3 mm (point Y), starting at the dye marks.

C   On the lower lid the skin and underlying orbicularis oculi muscle are excised, while on the upper lid the conjunctiva and a small portion of the tarsus are excised as per dotted lines.

D   Using a 6-0 nylon mattress suture, the two bare areas are approximated with a guard of Silastic or cotton over the skin.

E   A long 5-0 silk suture is placed at the point in which the two lids meet. In 10 days the nylon suture is removed, and in another three or four days the silk suture is removed.

TEMPORARY TARSORRHAPHY (Weeks)

This procedure is utilized when there is facial nerve paralysis following facial nerve surgery or parotid surgery when return of function is expected.

Highpoints

1. Correct alignment of upper and lower lids.
2. Excise small longitudinal area (6 to 8 mm) of mucocutaneous intermarginal tissue to form a bare area.
3. Incise base of each bare area to open wounds.

F   After the lids have been approximated and the exact opposing sites for the tarsorrhaphy have been marked with the point of a knife, 6 to 8 mm mucocutaneous rectangular areas are excised, leaving a thin strip of epithelium on both ciliary and conjunctival edges of the lid margins. The cilia are thus not injured and normal lid contour is preserved.

A longitudinal incision 2 mm deep is made in the base of each bare area. When the lid edges are approximated, this incision facilitates flaring of the wounds with more surface area for healing. Through and through horizontal mattress sutures of 4-0 silk guarded with small polyethylene tube booties are inserted and tied snugly.

G   The completed tarsorrhaphy. The sutures are left in place for eight to 10 days, or longer. With return of function, the lids are then separated by a simple incision of the scar tissue.

Plate 161   Periorbital Region

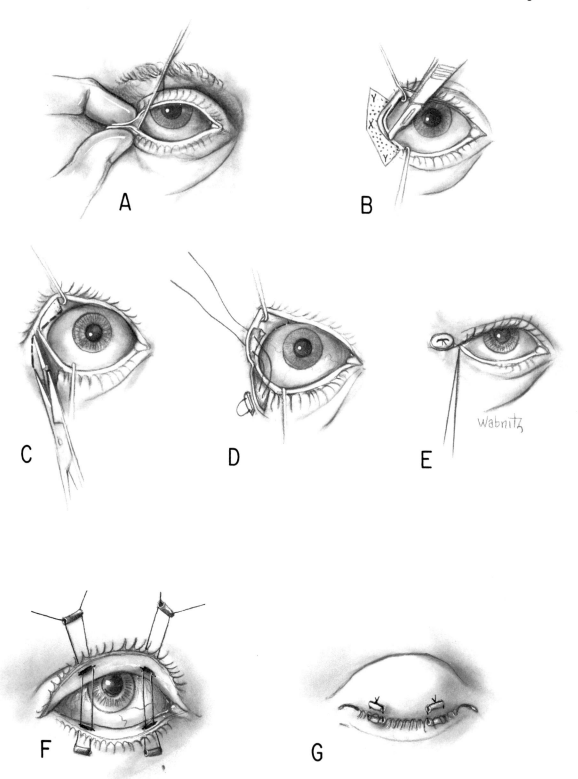

A

B

C

D

E

wabnitz

F

G

GRAFT FOR DEFECT OF INFRAORBITAL RIM

Highpoints

1. Incision in lower lid is made as close to eyelashes as possible.
2. Cartilage graft should have some perichondrium left attached. Silastic can also be utilized.
3. Avoid pressure on infraorbital nerve.

A An incision is made through the lower lid just below the lashes. This location of the incision prevents postoperative edema of the lower lid which would occur if the incision were lower; however, this incision may result in ectropion.

B Following a temporary tarsorrhaphy, the orbicularis oculi muscle is exposed and split parallel to its fibers. The defect in the infraorbital rim is exposed.

C Scar tissue around the infraorbital nerve is carefully freed and excised. The edges of the bony defect are cleaned and freshened. Using a small drill point, a hole is placed at an angle in the edge of the defect for a distance of 0.5 to 1.0 cm. It does not pass through the bone.

D Another drill hole is placed in the anterior aspect of the zygoma at such an angle as to
D^1 reach the blind end of the first hole. This is achieved by inserting a straight needle into the first hole to help locate the blind end. The two holes are connected.

E With the same type of drill holes placed in the medial edge of the defect in the maxilla, a section of costal cartilage (plate 22) previously shaped is now sewn into position, using fine tantalum braided wire. An adequate notch is cut to avoid pressure on the infraorbital nerve. It is important to preserve a section of perichondrium on the cartilage. This aids in its "take." Silastic (silicone rubber) cut from a suitable block can also be utilized.

F The cartilage graft in place. The skin is approximated with fine silk, the ends being left long to avoid injury to the cornea. The tarsorrhaphy may be opened immediately or left until the skin sutures are removed.

Complications

1. Absorption of cartilage.
2. Ectropion.

Plate 162   Periorbital Region

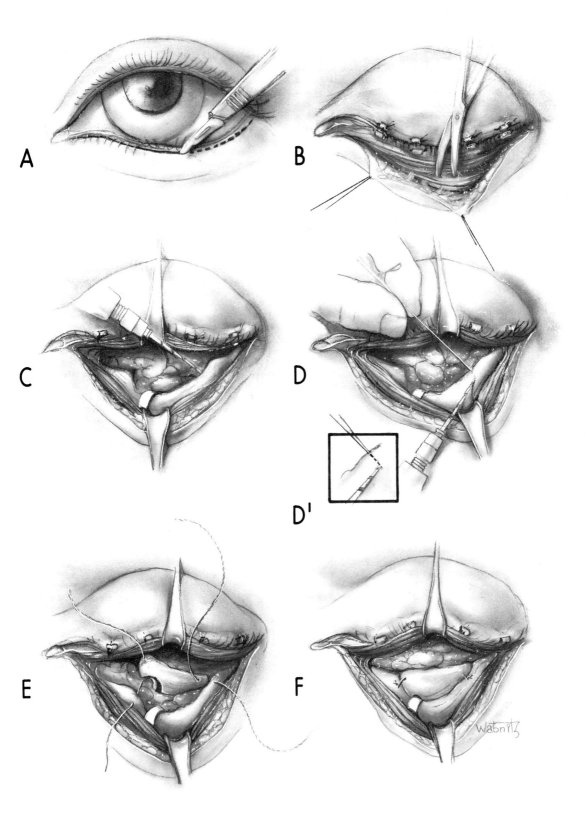

DECOMPRESSION OF THE ORBIT FOR EXOPHTHALMOS
(After Walsh, Ogura and Pratt, 1971)

Progressive exophthalmos (malignant) is usually associated with Graves' disease—toxic goiter. Following a subtotal thyroidectomy, the exophthalmos, either unilateral or bilateral, may become stationary or progress. Total thyroidectomy (Perzik, 1963) has been shown to be the more effective procedure to halt or even cause regression of the exophthalmos. If the exophthalmos becomes progressive, corneal ulceration, edema of the eyelid and of the conjunctiva, epiphora, diplopia and finally loss of vision can occur. The cosmetic deformity alone is an indication for an operation to decompress the orbital contents.

Several procedures have been described:
1. Removal of lateral wall of orbit (Kronlein; Swift).
2. Removal of roof of orbit, allowing the orbital contents to herniate into the anterior cranial fossa (Naffziger).
3. Removal of floor of the orbit, allowing the orbital contents to herniate into the antrum (Hirsch, 1950).
4. Removal of medial wall of the orbit, allowing the orbital contents to herniate into a cavity formed by removal of the ethmoid sinus cells and floor of the frontal sinus (Sewall, 1936).
5. Removal of floor and medial wall of orbit—a combination of #3 and #4 (Walsh and Ogura, 1957).

Depending on the degree of exophthalmos, either the Hirsh procedure or the Walsh-Ogura procedure appears to be the most adaptable.

The Walsh-Ogura technique is depicted.

A The areas excised are shown via a Caldwell-Luc operation (plates 28 and 29). The opening into the antrum is made as large as possible so that adequate visualization of the ethmoid labyrinth and roof of antrum is possible.

B Using various types of forceps, a complete ethmoidectomy is performed up to the anterior wall of the sphenoid sinus. (This approach is similar to the transantral ethmoidal sphenoidal hypophysectomy.) A mastoid curet or osteotome may be necessary to excise thicker portions of bone. If possible, leave the anterior and posterior ethmoid arteries intact. The lamina papyracea is thus also excised.

C Using Kerrison forceps, the floor of the antrum is removed, preserving at this stage the superior layer of periosteum; otherwise, premature herniation of orbital fat will obstruct vision. The infraorbital nerve should likewise be saved as well as, if feasible, a narrow strip of bone to support the nerve. The bone lateral to the nerve is also excised as far as the heavier bone of the zygoma. The foramina of the optic nerve must not be violated.

D After all the bone is removed, the periosteum of the floor of the orbit is incised in several locations to allow the orbital contents to herniate into the antrum.

A large nasoantral window is then made. The antrum may be packed with strip gauze impregnated with an antibiotic ointment for 24 hours.

The incision in the canine fossa is closed with 4-0 continuous nylon.

Complications

1. Intraorbital hemorrhage.
2. Damage to the optic nerve.
3. Subcutaneous emphysema.
4. Diplopia.

Plate 163   Periorbital Region

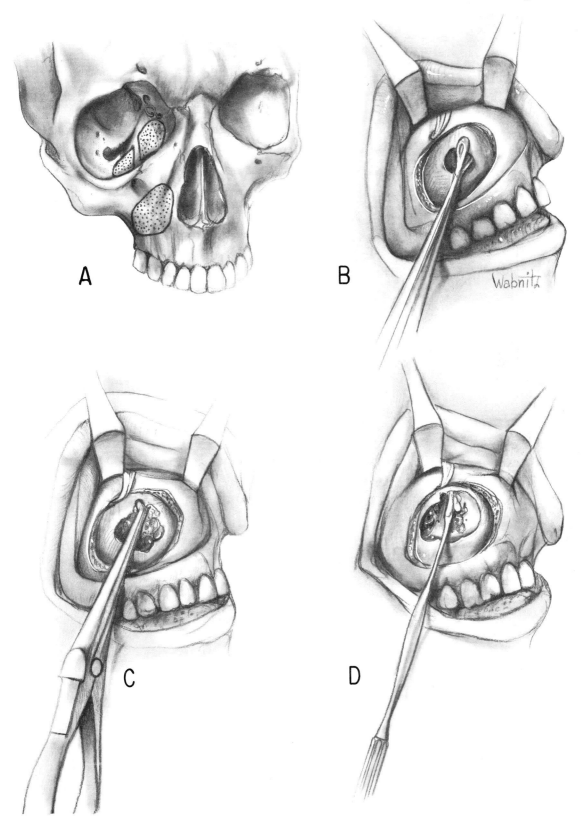

BIBLIOGRAPHY

Aiello, L. M., and Myers, E. N.: Blow-out fracture of the orbital floor. Arch. Otolaryng. *82*:638–648, 1965.

Cutler, N. L., and Beard, C.: A method for partial and total upper lid reconstruction. Amer. J. Ophthal. *39*:1–7, 1955.

Esser, J. F. S.: Ueber eine gestielte Ueberpflanzung eines senkrecht angelegten Keils aus dem oberen Augenlid in das gleichseitige Unterlid oder umgekehrt. Klin. Mbl. Augenheilk. *63*:379–381, 1919.

Fox, S. A. (ed.): Affections of the lids. *In* International Ophthalmology Clinics. Vol. 4. Boston, Little, Brown and Company, 1964.

Fox, S. A.: Ophthalmic Plastic Surgery. 2d ed. New York, Grune & Stratton, Inc., 1958.

Fricke, J. C. G.: Die Bildung neuer Augenlider (Blepharo plastik) nach Zerstorungen und dedurch hervorgebrachten Auswartswendungen derselben. Hamburg, Perthes & Basser, 1829.

Hughes, W. L.: Reconstructive Surgery of the Eyelids. 2nd ed. St. Louis, C. V. Mosby Company, 1954.

Iliff, C. E.: A simplified dacryocystorhinostomy: 1954 to 1970. Trans. Amer. Acad. Ophthal. Otolaryng. *75*:821–828, 1971.

Lewis, J. R., Jr.: The Z-blepharoplasty. Plast. Reconstr. Surg. *44*:331–335, 1969.

Musgrave, R. H., Smith, B., Wang, M. K.-H., Horton, C. E., and McCoy, F. J.: Panel Discussion. Surgical Management of Tumors and Deformities of the Eyelids. 57th Annual Clinical Congress, American College of Surgeons, Atlantic City, 1971.

Mustardé, J. C.: Repair and Reconstruction in the Orbital Region. Edinburgh, E & S Livingstone Ltd., 1966.

Neuman, Z., and Giladi, A.: Plea for a radical approach in so-called keratoacanthoma of the eyelid. Plast. Reconstr. Surg. *47*:231–233, 1971.

Ogura, J. H., and Pratt, L. L.: Transantral decompression for malignant exophthalmos. Otolaryng. Clin. N. Amer. *4*:193–203, 1971.

Pang, L. Q.: Dacryocystorhinostomy: A technique under local anesthesia. Instruction section. Trans. Amer. Acad. Ophthal. Otolaryng. Meeting, Las Vegas, 1971.

Perzik, S. L.: Total thyroidectomy. Amer. J. Surg. *106*:744, 1963.

Smith, B., and Obear, M. F.: Bridge flap technique for reconstruction of large upper lid defects. Trans. Amer. Acad. Ophthal. Otolaryng. *71*:897–901, 1967.

Smith, J. P.: Progressive exophthalmos: Case presentations — Preliminary report of new surgical technique used in treatment. Laryngoscope *75*:1160–1172, 1965.

Snow, J. W., and Johnson, H. C.: One-stage reconstruction of the lacrimal apparatus. Plast. Reconstr. Surg. *48*:453–456, 1971.

Symposium: Cosmetic blepharoplasty. Trans. Amer. Acad. Ophthal. Otolaryng. *73*:1141–1164, 1969.

Walsh, T. E., and Ogura, J. H.: Transantral orbital decompression for malignant exophthalmos. Laryngoscope *67*:544, 1957.

9. THE EAR

OTOPLASTY

Types of Operation

There are a number of various techniques described to correct the protruding auricle with the absence of the antihelix. Two different techniques will be described which have a significant variation. The first method completely incises the cartilage, whereas the second method rolls the cartilage and to a large extent depends on suturing for the correction. The criticism of the first method is often a rather sharp edge to the antihelix; in the second method, the sutures can fail.

Occasionally this deformity is associated with extremely thin cartilage which is so flexible that additional sutures are necessary to correct the deformity.

CARTILAGE INCISION TECHNIQUE (After Luckett, 1910)

Highpoints

1. Depend on complete incision of cartilage rather than sutures to correct deformity.
2. Extreme care with dressings.
3. Do not operate before age of three years.
4. Extend incision superiorly and inferiorly.

A The ear is pushed back against the mastoid to its normal position. This forms a fold in the ear cartilage which becomes the new antihelix. A straight cutting edge needle is then inserted from front to back at multiple sites along this new antihelix. As the needle is withdrawn, its tip is colored with an alcohol solution of suitable dye. This maneuver stains the posterior surface of the ear cartilage indicating the line of incision to be made later in the cartilage (refer to plate 165 for normal anatomy).

B An ellipse of skin is excised in the posterior auricular sulcus, the major portion of the excised skin being from the auricle itself. Depending on the degree of the deformity, the width of skin excised may be from 0.5 to 1.5 cm.

C A posterior auricular skin flap has been developed, leaving the perichondrium intact. This flap is freed 4 to 6 mm beyond the dye marks, thus allowing sufficient space to place the cartilage sutures. The incision in the cartilage is made along the dye marks, taking care that the perichondrium and skin on the anterior surface are not incised. This is most important since both perichondrium and skin act as a hinge. If the index finger is placed opposite the knife while the cartilage incision is made, and a watchful eye is kept for the white glistening perichondrium on the anterior surface, all will go well. This incision should be carried to the upper and lower limits of the main body of the auricular cartilage; otherwise, the procedure will fail since even a small area of intact cartilage in this area will interfere with the formation of the new antihelix. A slight curve in the incision is very desirable.

D The lateral leaf of the auricular cartilage must be so mobilized that the final stages of everting the two leaves forming the new antihelix are achieved virtually without reliance on the mattress sutures. However, the cartilage of the helix is not incised.

If the medial portion of the body of the auricular cartilage appears too wide, a small ellipse may be excised as shown by the dotted line. Again, it is desirable to have a slight wave in this incision so that the new antihelix thus formed will have a more graceful curve.

(*Text continued on page 392.*)

Plate 164   The Ear

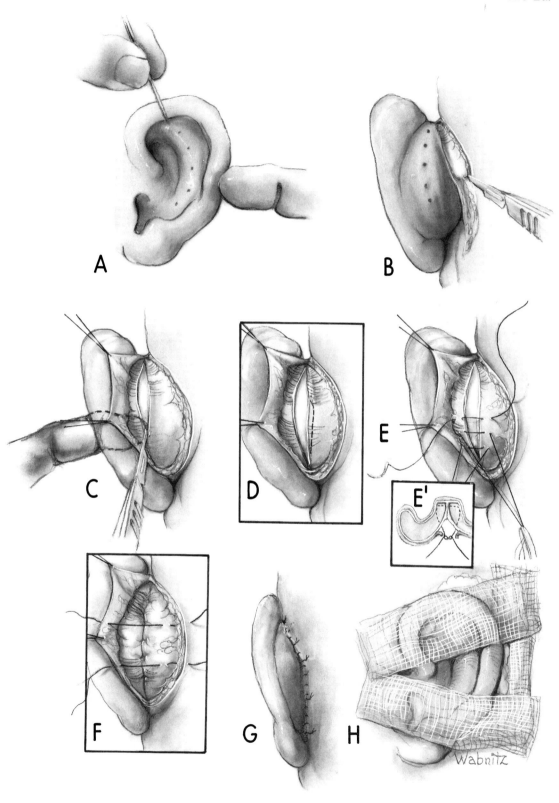

E
E¹ The two leaves of auricular cartilage are now approximated with inverting mattress sutures, using 4-0 white silk. A cross section of the position of the sutures and the inverted edges of cartilage is shown in E^1. All the sutures, usually five to seven, are placed before any are tied. A fine, multitoothed forceps may be used on the anterior surface of the inverted cartilage (the new antihelix) to maintain the desired position while the sutures are tied.

F
G The skin is approximated with four interrupted 5-0 Dermalene sutures by including the tissue over the mastoid bone deep in the cephaloauricular sulcus. This prevents bridging of the skin closure across this sulcus. A continuous suture may be used to approximate any gaping skin edges.

H The dressing is important. Absorbent cotton soaked with Furacin solution is painstakingly used to fill the concavities of the auricle. A small amount is placed posteriorly. Across the auricle, two or three strips of gauze soaked with flexible collodion are used for immobilization. Over this, a four-inch stockinette is pulled as a protecting night cap. Small windows are cut in the stockinette to visualize the color of the helix. Ten days elapse before the collodion strips are removed. Thereafter, the stockinette alone may be used for an indeterminate period, especially during sleep.

Complications

1. Sharp edge of antihelix.
2. Protrusion of upper or lower portion of auricular cartilage.

Plate 164 Repeated   The Ear

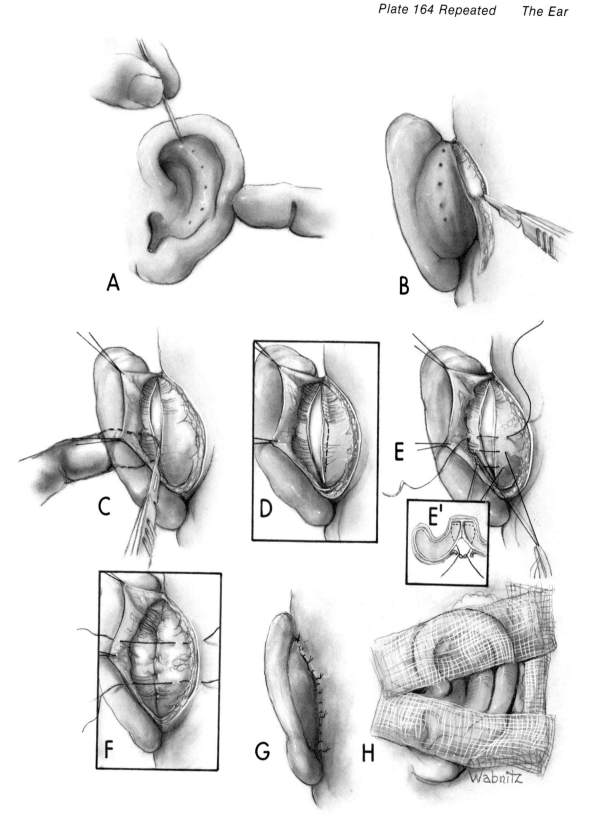

A

B

C

D

E

E'

F

G

H

Wabnitz

MATTRESS SUTURE TECHNIQUE (CORRECTION OF PROMINENT OR DEFORMED EARS) (After Mustardé, 1963)

One of the main criticisms of the Luckett technique in which an incision is made through the cartilage of the new antihelix (see previous plate) is the tendency to form a sharp edge along the new antihelix. A definite contraindication to this cartilage incision technique is a very soft and thin cartilage. Mustardé obviates this undesirable result by the use of horizontal mattress sutures without a cartilage incision. On the other hand, this mattress suture technique may result in too prominent "a roll" of the new antihelix. Converse, Stark and Saunders use abrasion or shaving of the medial aspect of the cartilage to reduce this roll or bulk of the folded cartilage. Holmes achieves a similar result by using multiple minute incisions ("fish scale"). In addition, other associated or isolated deformities may exist, such as prominence due to a deeply cupped concha with or without normal antihelix. Both Mustardé and Furnas have modifications of the mattress suture technique to correct this latter deformity. Hence, combinations of procedures are sometimes necessary to achieve a pleasing and satisfactory result.

Highpoints

1. Mattress sutures rather than cartilage incisions are the mainstays of the correction.
2. These mattress sutures encompass both layers of perichondrium.
3. Use a minimum of three sutures. The number is varied depending on the extent of the deformity; however, a superior suture is almost always necessary and an inferior suture is necessary if the lobule is prominent.
4. The position and tension of the sutures may likewise be varied depending on the deformity.
5. Distance between the sutures should not exceed 4.0 mm.
6. Rarely does a portion of the antitragus or thickened cartilage of the posterior surface of the lobule require excision if too prominent.

A   Demonstration of cartilage anatomy composing a normal ear.

B   Deformity is absence of antihelix. The ear is folded back to form the new antihelix. This is now marked on the skin with a sterile solution of methylene blue dye. Following this curved line, both medially and laterally being at least 7 mm from the curved line, through and through punctures are made by a hypodermic needle stained with a similar dye. These marks indicate the placement of the mattress sutures.

C   An eclipse of skin 0.5 to 1.5 cm wide is excised on the posterior aspect of the auricle. Skin and subcutaneous flaps are elevated to expose the dye marks through the perichondrium. Mattress sutures of 4-0 plastic material are now placed along the dye marks. These sutures pass through both posterior and anterior layers of perichondrium as well as cartilage but, of course, not through the skin. A noncutting edge needle is best to avoid slashing the cartilage. As each suture is placed, it is temporarily snugged down and the effect on the antihelix is surveyed to be sure the result is pleasing without any folds between the helix and antihelix. If not correct, the suture is removed and replaced. Spacing should not exceed 4.0 mm. The number, position and tension vary depending on the deformity and the desired result. It is not necessary to firmly approximate the posterior layers of the perichondrium (steps *F* and *G*).

D   A variation of the staining technique is depicted. The puncture marks are made along the new antihelix.

E   Similar mattress sutures are placed paralleling the dye marks. The same precautions, trials and placements are performed as under step *C*.

F   Coronal section depicts the placement of sutures through both layers of perichondrium and cartilage but not the skin.

(Text continued on opposite page.)

Plate 165   The Ear

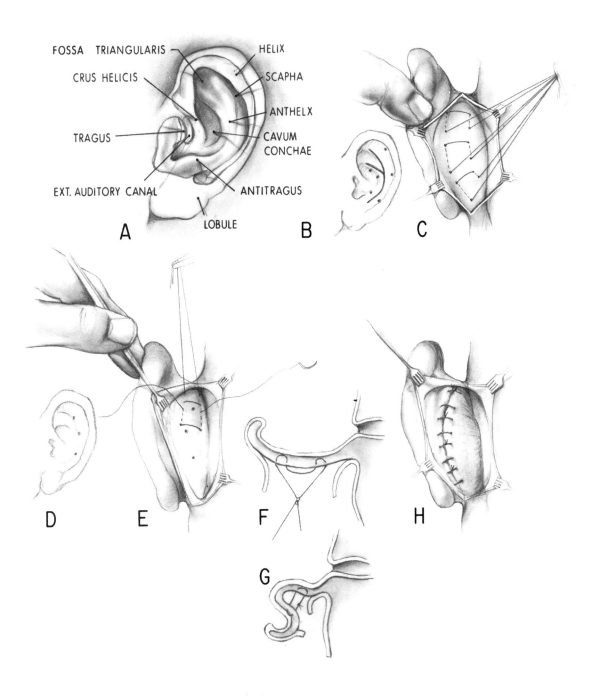

A

FOSSA TRIANGULARIS
CRUS HELICIS
TRAGUS
EXT. AUDITORY CANAL
LOBULE

HELIX
SCAPHA
ANTHELX
CAVUM CONCHAE
ANTITRAGUS

B

C

D

E

F

G

H

G   Coronal section depicts the sutures tied. It is not necessary to approximate the posterior layer of perichondrium. Tension depends on the desired results.

H   The completed mattress suture line. If the concha is too cup-shaped, it is sutured to the periosteum of the mastoid bone (step *O*).

MATTRESS SUTURE TECHNIQUE (CORRECTION OF PROMINENT OR DEFORMED EARS) (*Continued*)

I   If the superior portion of the helix has a tendency to fold out, a tacking suture is placed through the perichondrium and cartilage into the periosteum of the adjacent temporal bone as depicted.

J   By the same token, if the lobule protrudes, a similar type of suture is placed inferiorly.

K   Prominence of the ear may be due to a deeply cupped concha. Depicted is a relatively normal antihelix with a deep concha.

L   Mustardé corrects this by repositioning the antihelix with mattress sutures. Coronal section depicts the deformity. The arrow indicates the existing antihelix. The suture is placed so that the concha cupping is reduced and the antihelix repositioned medially.

M   The completed correction in coronal section. Again, the arrow depicts the original antihelix with the new antihelix depicted by *X*.

N   Furnas (1968) corrects this deeply cupped concha with a normal antihelix by transecting the posterior auricular muscle and then placing mattress sutures through the auricular cartilage secured to the exposed periosteum and fascia overlying the mastoid bone. Two mattress-type sutures are used. Exact positioning of these sutures may require "trial and error."

O   Care must be used in the placement of these postauricular sutures to avoid pulling the concha forward. Depicted is correct placement.

P   Placement of sutures is incorrect, pulling concha forward, thus narrowing the external auditory canal orifice.

    The dressing is similar to that shown in plate 165, step *H*.

Plate 166   The Ear

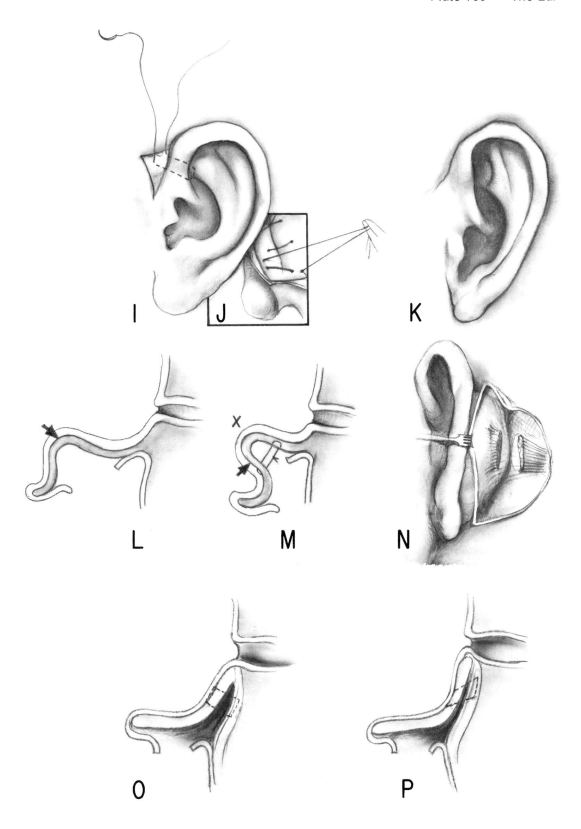

I

J

K

L

M

N

O

P

SURGICAL TREATMENT OF HEMATOMA OF THE
AURICLE—"CAULIFLOWER EAR"

Highpoints

1. Following aspiration conforming pressure, dressing is necessary.
2. Careful follow-up to be sure hematoma does not recur and progress to fibrous deposits and chondritis.
3. Repeated aspirations are often necessary—if repeated more than two or three times, one or two mattress sutures over dressing are usually necessary.
4. In any dressing, keep the outside edge of the helix exposed to check blood supply.

A   Aspiration of hematoma.

B   Absorbent cotton (genuine cotton, not rayon) is soaked with liquid Furacin and molded to the contour of the auricle. It is held in place with strips of plain one half inch packing gauze soaked with collodion.

C   If aspiration and Furacin cotton dressing fails, one or two mattress sutures through the scapha and fluffed gauze with buttons or Silastic guards fore and aft are used. This situation is rare if the initial aspiration was complete and Furacin cotton dressing firmly applied.

D   If a hematoma or repeated hematomas are not treated and proceed to fibrous deposits, aspiration is worthless. A shaving procedure is then necessary. Depicted is the line of incision of the skin flap.

E   The flap is elevated and retracted with extreme care. The skin can easily be fragmented. The excess fibrous tissue and portion of thickened cartilage if present are removed.

F   If excess bleeding is present, a small polyethylene tube can be inserted through the cartilage and this connected to gentle suction. An alternative is to follow the method depicted in step *C*.

G   Closure with fine 6-0 nylon sutures. The tubing is removed in several days when no additional drainage is obtained.

Plate 167   The Ear

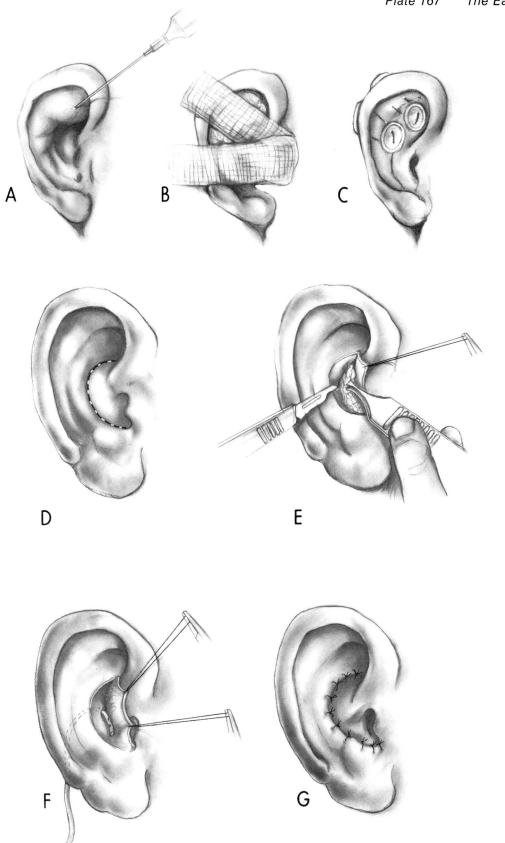

A

B

C

D

E

F

G

Z-PLASTY FOR STENOSIS OF EXTERNAL
AUDITORY CANAL

When possible this procedure is preferred to the operation of excision and intermediate split skin graft over a stent. The operation microscope may be of aid.

A
B   The stenotic area of the external auditory canal, which may be congenital or the result of trauma or burn.

C   The edge of the stenotic opening is excised or incised. The presenting skin surface is marked into quadrants.

D   Elevation of the presenting skin surface is begun by inserting a small right-angled knife between the inner and outer layers of skin at the stenotic site.

E   As the dissection proceeds, the outer presenting skin surface is divided into quadrants and care is taken not to incise the inner or hidden layer of skin. These four flaps are elevated to the normal canal wall.

F   The inner or hidden layer of skin is now incised in quadrants with the incisions bisecting the bases of the outer flaps. Again four flaps of skin are dissected to the normal canal wall. If any thick scar or subcutaneous tissue remains between the two layers of skin, this is excised.

G   The inner and outer flaps are interposed, the inner flaps **Y** turned outward while the outer flaps **X** are turned inward. Sutures of 5-0 or 6-0 Dermalene are placed where necessary. One fourth inch gauze soaked with liquid Furacin or impregnated with an antibiotic ointment is used as a dressing.

H   A lateral view showing the interposed flaps of skin.

Complications

1. Friability of skin flaps.
2. Recurrent cicatrix.

Plate 168   The Ear

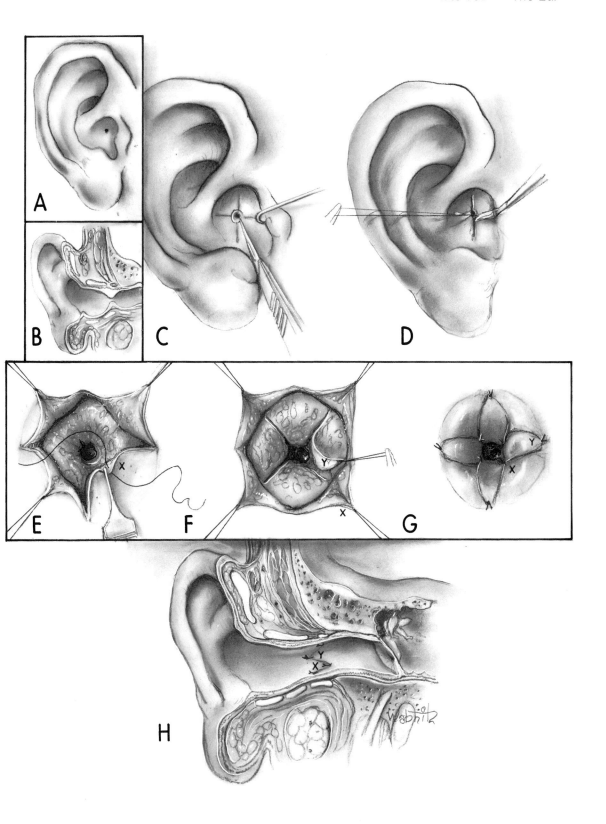

EXCISION OF SMALL MALIGNANT TUMOR OF OUTER PORTION OF EXTERNAL AUDITORY CANAL

Highpoints

1. This procedure is limited to small (less than 1.0 cm) tumors which have not reached inner half of external auditory canal nor have involved bone nor involved the typanic membrane. If bone is involved, a temporal bone resection is usually indicated.
2. Immediate skin graft.

A The area excised is depicted by the solid line. The periosteum of the adjacent mastoid bone may be removed. The entire cartilaginous canal is resected along with a portion of bony canal. A radical mastoidectomy may be necessary, and, if so, an attempt is made to preserve the facial nerve. If the bone is involved, not only is the facial nerve sacrificed but usually a temporal bone resection is indicated (plates 171 and 172, or technique of Bocca).

B An incision is made surrounding the external auditory canal. A postauricular approach may be necessary to increase the exposure.

C The split thickness skin graft in place.

D Around a section of polyethylene tubing, cotton soaked with Furacin liquid maintains pressure on the graft.

Complications

1. Recurrent disease in which too large a lesion is resected by this limited procedure.
2. Cicatricial stenosis of reconstructed canal.

EXCISION OF HEMANGIOMA OF FACE INVOLVING LOBULE OF EAR

E The skin with the hemangioma is excised from the ear lobule and the preauricular area region.

F An infra- and postauricular skin flap is mobilized and rotated to cover the bare area on the lobule. The preauricular defect is closed by the technique of a face lift in which the skin of the face is mobilized, staying superficial to the parotid fascia.

G The closure.

Plate 169   The Ear

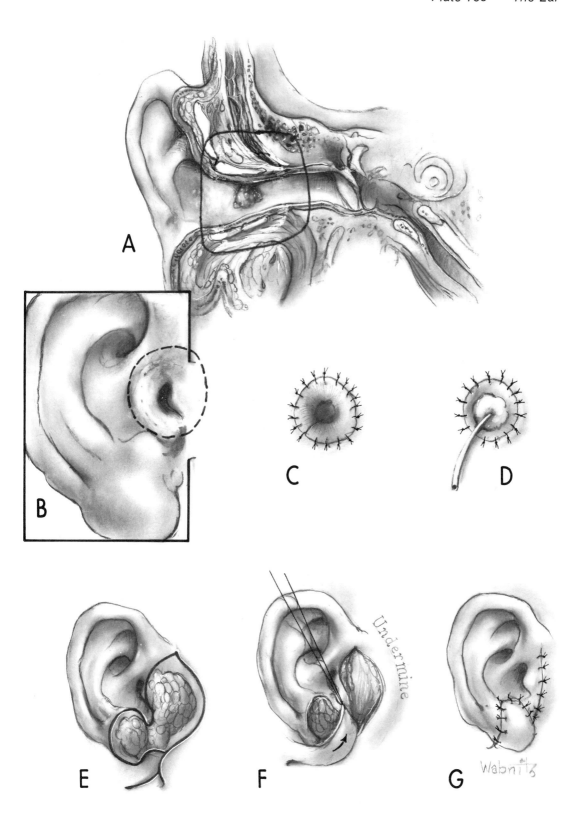

A

B

C

D

E

F

Undermine

G

Wabnitz

EXCISION OF MALIGNANT TUMORS OF AURICLE

Highpoints

1. Resect with adequate margins.
2. Resection of all layers – through and through – is preferred.
3. When using postauricular skin flaps for reconstruction, avoid hair-bearing skin.

A   A simple, **V**, full thickness excision is ideal for small tumors limited to the helix.

B   Primary closure results in minimal deformity.

C   When the tumor involves both the helix and the crura of the antihelix, a larger triangular, full thickness area must be excised.

D   Immediate reconstruction is performed with the use of a postauricular full thickness skin flap. The flap is severed along the dotted line in three to four weeks, leaving sufficient length to roll the end on itself to form a new helix and serve as cover for the posterior aspect of the flap.
   The donor site is closed either by advancing the edges or by split thickness skin graft.

E   With small tumors limited to the midregion of the auricle, e.g., the antihelix, an island is resected through and through in the shape of an ellipse.

F   The defect.

G   Primary closure following the natural curve of the antihelix. The helix will appear distorted and pinched.

H   Larger tumors in the region of the antihelix may require a postauricular skin flap for a more acceptable cosmetic result. A curved full thickness skin flap one-fourth to one-third wider than the defect is outlined with the base inferiorly. The entire flap need not be elevated at this initial stage. Elevation of the distal edge and lateral margins for approximation to the corresponding edges of the defect will usually suffice. This technique is suggested since occasionally complete elevation of the flap may require a delay of two weeks.

I   The flap turned into the defect.

J   The distal and lateral margins of the flap are sutured to the edges of the defect. The inferior edge of the defect is closed by approximation of the auricular skin edges. This area will be opened later to receive the skin flap when it is transected in three to four weeks. Any postauricular bare areas are covered with split thickness skin.

Plate 170   The Ear

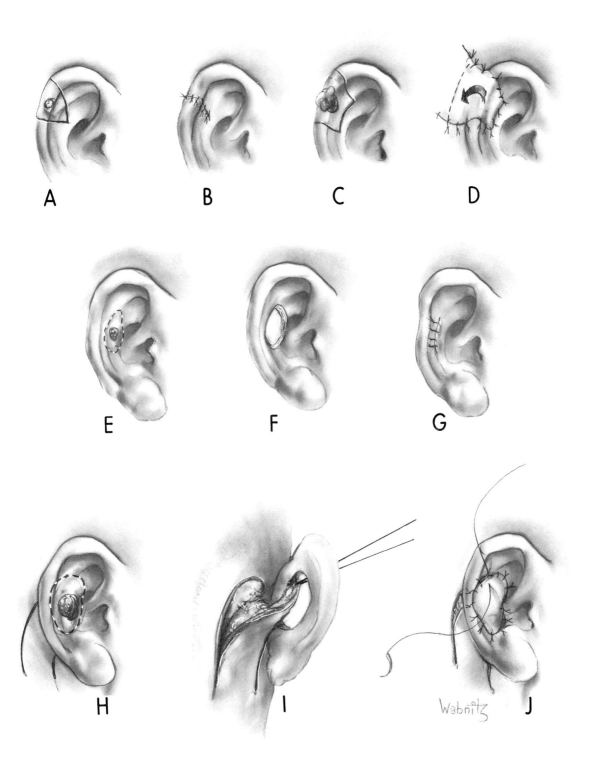

A

B

C

D

E

F

G

H

I

Wabnitz   J

TEMPORAL BONE RESECTION

By John S. Lewis, M.D.

Indication

Carcinoma involving the bony auditory canal, the middle ear or mastoid and extensive glomus jugulare tumors. In addition, the author feels that a partial temporal bone resection or radical mastoidectomy has been utilized in adenocystic carcinoma of the parotid salivary gland when the tumor has spread along the facial nerve.

Highpoints

1. Insertion of malleable spinal puncture needle in lumbar spinal canal for withdrawal of 30 to 40 cc of cerebrospinal fluid late in the procedure, allowing for exposure of the petrous pyramid.
2. Hypotensive anesthesia.
3. Through temporal craniotomy avoid trauma to temporal lobe and sigmoid and cavernous sinuses.
4. Cauterize superior and inferior petrosal sinuses and mastoid emissary vein and middle meningeal vessels if necessary.
5. At the skull base avoid injury to jugular vein, internal carotid artery, hypoglossal and vagus nerves. The facial nerve is sacrificed.
6. Lateral or sigmoid sinus tears are managed by proximal finger pressure and closure with atraumatic surgical silk or a temporal muscle plug. A large sinus tear at the jugular foramen level may be controlled with vaginal packing.

A   Skin incision with flap including pinna based superiorly with modification for neck dissection.

A¹   Skin incision based inferiorly with auditory meatus circumscribed.

A²   Skin incision to sacrifice diseased pinna with bony specimen. If the external ear is sacrificed or a large segment of dura removed, a posteriorly based scalp flap should be rotated to cover the defect.

B   Outline of extent of bony resection.

C   Diagram indicating extent of bony resection of squamosa and petrous pyramid.

D   Incision is carried through the auricularis and temporal muscles to expose the squamosa and mastoid with muscular attachments. Incision is made through the parotid gland, sacrificing the facial nerve, to the base of the zygoma and the ascending ramus of the mandible. The posterior facial and external jugular veins and superficial temporal artery are ligated and divided. The auditory canal is cored widely to be included with the specimen.

Plate 171   The Ear

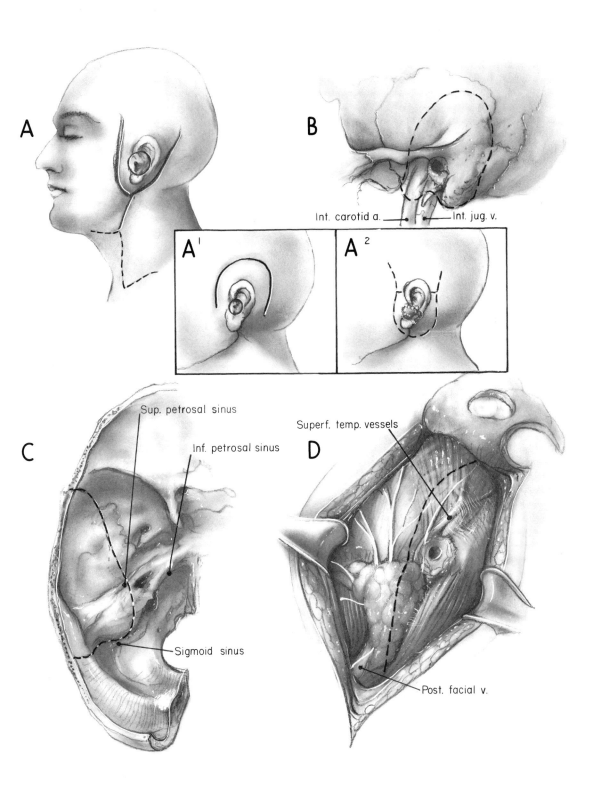

A

B

Int. carotid a.   Int. jug. v.

A¹

A²

C

Sup. petrosal sinus

Inf. petrosal sinus

Sigmoid sinus

D

Superf. temp. vessels

Post. facial v.

407

E   The zygoma is transected and the ascending ramus of the mandible is sectioned near the joint. The sternocleidomastoid muscle and posterior belly of the digastric are sectioned, exposing the internal jugular vein in the carotid sheath. The styloid process is transected with the stylohyoid muscle. A temporal craniotomy is performed mobilizing underlying dura of the temporal lobe of the brain. The lateral sinus and its sigmoid portion are carefully exposed.

F   Cerebrospinal fluid is withdrawn and the temporal lobe and sigmoid sinus are retracted from the petrous pyramid. A Stryker air drill saw with an orbital blade sections the anterior portion of the middle cranial fossa into the temporomandibular joint. The orbital blade makes the initial incisions on the three surfaces of the petrous near the junction of its medial and middle thirds. Chisels are directed transversely to complete the transections. When dura is involved, it is freed from the petrous pyramid with the electrocautery knife, the bony resection is completed and then the dura removed and replaced with temporal fascia. It may be necessary to ligate the lateral sinus. This is accomplished by making an incision on either side of the sinus through the dura and then clamping and cutting through the sinus wall in stages. The opening is then closed with continuous 3-0 or 4-0 vascular silk.

G   Soft tissue attachments are transected and the bony specimen is removed at the level of the jugular foramen. The operative defect, including brain and dura, petrous remnant, carotid and jugular vessels, hypoglossal and vagus nerves, is shown.

H   The incision is closed in layers. The auditory meatal defect is lined in purse fashion with a split thickness skin graft.

Complications

1. Hemorrhage is usually from lateral sinus or petrosal vessels. Median blood loss is 2500 cc.
2. Infection is usually in postirradiated cases and often is caused by *Pseudomonas aeruginosa*. The use of systemic colistimethate (Colymycin) and local acetic acid and acriflavine dressings is most effective.
3. Cerebrospinal otorrhea from dural tears. This can be prevented by the use of temporal muscle flaps to cover exposed dura and by rotation of the scalp flap to cover the defect. If postoperative leak lasts for more than five days, the wound should be reopened and the dura repaired and splinted with muscle tamponade.
4. Complete loss of facial nerve function. A face lift type of procedure can easily be performed at the initial procedure if the operator so desires. A lateral tarsorrhaphy will help prevent corneal ulceration.
5. Vertigo lasts from five to 15 days and there may be a period of unsteadiness for several months.
6. Hearing loss is complete.
7. Carotid artery thrombosis has occurred in two cases from trauma and is perhaps the most serious complication.

Operative mortality equals 10 per cent.
Results of temporal bone resection:

Total Experience (1951–1965)	— 92 cases
Five year cure	— 26 cases (26 per cent)
Squamous carcinoma	— 81 cases
Five year cure	— 20 cases (25 per cent)

Plate 172   The Ear

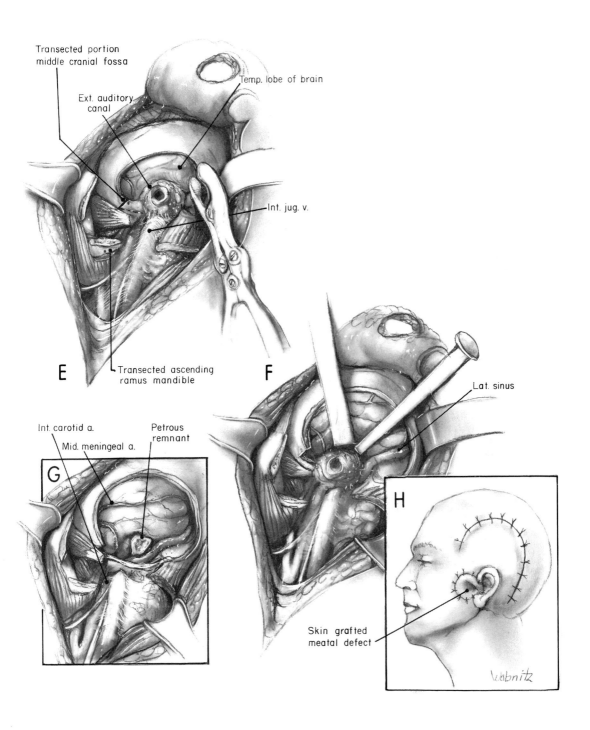

Transected portion
middle cranial fossa

Temp. lobe of brain

Ext. auditory
canal

Int. jug. v.

E

Transected ascending
ramus mandible

F

Lat. sinus

Int. carotid a.

Petrous
remnant

Mid. meningeal a.

G

H

Skin grafted
meatal defect

Wabnitz

409

BIBLIOGRAPHY

Adams, G. L., Paparella, M. M., and El Fiky, F. M.: Primary and metastatic tumors of the temporal bone. Laryngoscope *81*:1273–1285, 1971.

Argamaso, R. V., and Lewin, M. L.: Repair of partial ear loss with local composite flap. Plast. Reconstr. Surg. *42*:437–441, 1968.

Brown, J. B., Fryer, M. P., and Morgan, L. R.: Problems in reconstruction of the auricle. Plast. Reconstr. Surg. *43*:597–604, 1969.

Coleman, C. C., Jr.: Removal of the temporal bone for cancer. Amer. J. Surg. *112*:583, 1966.

Conley, J. J., and Novack, A. J.: The surgical treatment of malignant tumors of the ear and temporal bone. Arch. Otolaryng. *71*:635, 1960.

Dowling, J. A., Foley, F. D., and Moncrief, J. A.: Chondritis in the burned ear. Plast. Reconstr. Surg. *42*:115–122, 1968.

Ely, E. T.: An operation for prominence of the auricles. Arch. Otol. *10*:97, 1881.

Farrior, R. T.: Otoplasty for children. Otolaryng. Clin. N. Amer. *3*:365–374, 1970.

Fields, W. S., and Alford, B. R.: Neurological Aspects of Auditory and Vestibular Disorders. Springfield, Illinois, Charles C Thomas, Publisher, 1954.

Furnas, D. W.: Correction of prominent ears by concha-mastoid sutures. Plast. Reconstr. Surg. *42*:189–193, 1968.

Goode, R. L.: Mattress suture otoplasty. Trans. Amer. Acad. Ophthal. Otolaryng. *72*:427–434, 1968.

Goode, R. L., Proffitt, S. D., and Rafaty, F. M.: Complications of otoplasty. Arch. Otolaryng. *91*:352–355, 1970.

Holmes, E. M.: A further evaluation of the Gouge technique in changing the shape of ears. Laryngoscope *72*:915–924, 1962.

Holmes, E. M.: A new procedure for correcting outstanding ears. Arch. Otolaryng. *69*:409–415, 1959.

House, W. F., and Hitselberger, W. E.: Endolymphatic subarachnoid shunt for Ménière's disease. Arch. Otolaryng. *82*:144–146, 1965.

Kaplan, H. L., Norris, J. E., Freeman, B. S., and Brown, W. G.: Relapsing polychondritis. Report of a case. J.A.M.A. *180*:164–166, 1962.

Katz, A. D.: Preauricular sinuses. A congenital hereditary anomaly. Amer. J. Surg. *110*:612–614, 1965.

Lewis, J. S.: Tumors of the external ear and temporal bone. Otolaryngology *2*:(Chapter 26), 1971.

Lewis, J. S., and Page, R.: Radical surgery for malignant tumors of the ear. Arch. Otolaryng. *83*:114, 1966.

Lewis, J. S., and Parsons, H.: Surgery for Advanced ear cancer. Annals Otol. *67*:364, 1958.

Luckett, W. H.: A new operation for prominent ears based on the anatomy of the deformity. Surg. Gynec. Obstet *10*:635–637, 1910.

Mladick, R. W., Horton, C. E., Adamson, J. E., and Cohen, B. I.: The pocket principle. A new technique for the reattachment of a severed ear part. Plast. Reconstr. Surg. *48*:219–223, 1971.

Mustardé, J. C.: The correction of prominent ears using simple mattress sutures. Brit. J. Plast. Surg. *16*:170–176, 1963.

Myers, E. N., Stool, S., and Weltschew, A.: Rhabdomyosarcoma of the middle ear. Ann. Otol. *77*:949–958, 1968.

Nelson, W. R., Kell, J. F., Jr., and Kay, S.: Temporal bone resection and radical neck dissection for basal cell carcinoma with metastases. Surg. Gynec. Obstet. *115*:585–592, 1962.

Pack, G. T., Conley, J., and Oropeza, R.: Melanoma of the external ear. Arch. Otolaryng. *92*:106–113, 1970.

Parsons, H., and Lewis, J. S.: Subtotal resection of the temporal bone for cancer of the ear. Cancer *7*:995, 1954.

Passe, E. R. G.: Sympathectomy in relation to Ménière's disease, tinnitus and deafness. Proc. Roy. Soc. Med. *44*:760, 1951.

Pearson, C. M., Kline, H. M., and Newcomer, V. D.: Relapsing polychondritis. New Eng. J. Med. *263*:51–58, 1960.

Rogers, B. O.: Ely's 1881 operation for correction of protruding ears. A medical "first." Plast. Reconstr. Surg. *42*:584–586, 1968.

Rothfeld, I. D.: Suture technique of otoplasty. Arch. Otolaryng. 89:883–886, 1969.

Shambaugh, G. E., Jr.: Surgery of the Ear. 2nd ed. Philadelphia, W. B. Saunders Company, 1967.

Singleton, G. T.: Cervical sympathetic chain block in sudden deafness. Laryngoscope 81:734–736, 1971.

Spira, M., McCrea, R., Gerow, F. J., and Hardy, S. B.: Correction of the principal deformities causing protruding ears. Plast. Reconstr. Surg. 44:150–154, 1969.

Tardy, M. E., Jr., Tenta, L. T., and Pastorek, N. J.: Mattress suture otoplasty: Indi-cations and limitations. Laryngoscope 79:961–968, 1969.

Ward, G. E., Lock, W. W., and Lawrence, W., Jr.: Radical operation for carcinoma of the external auditory canal and middle ear. Amer. J. Surg. 82:169, 1951.

Wilmot, T. J.: Sympathectomy for Ménière's disease — A long-term review. J. Laryng. 83:323–331, 1969.

Wright, J. W., Jr., and Taylor, C. E.: Tomography and the facial nerve. Trans. Amer. Acad. Ophthal. Otolaryng. 72:103–110, 1968.

10. FRACTURES OF FACIAL BONES

REDUCTION OF FRACTURED NOSE

Highpoints

1. Early reduction within 24 hours if feasible despite edema, unless massive.
2. Clinical evaluation far more important than x-ray films.
3. Topical or local anesthesia except in unmanageable child.
4. The simpler the method of reduction, the better.

Anesthesia

Topical anesthesia using four tampons of cotton with 10 per cent cocaine and a vaso-constrictor. Two inserted in each side of the nose for 10 to 15 minutes usually is sufficient. In the presence of marked or even moderate edema of the mucosa, the superiorly located tampons are carefully inserted somewhat higher after five minutes. If necessary, additional anesthesia is achieved by local injection of a suitable agent, e.g., 1 per cent xylocaine without adrenalin into the tissue at the base of the columella, glabella and the infraorbital nerve at its foramen at the infraorbital rim. General anesthesia is seldom necessary except in unmanageable children.

DEPRESSION OF RIGHT NASAL BONE WITH LATERAL DISPLACEMENT OF LEFT NASAL BONE

A The elevator is inserted in the right nares with the narrow edge facing forward and the broad surface alongside nasal septum. This instrument must not have any sharp edges. Ideally it measures 8 mm × 3 mm × 180 mm.

B The narrow edge of the elevator is placed high in the nasal pyramid. It must not be inserted so far as to injure the cribriform plate of the ethmoid.

C With counter pressure on the laterally displaced left nasal bone, the elevator is moved in an outward, forward and lateral direction. Prying with a fulcrum motion must be avoided. Reduction will be accompanied by a snapping sound. Nasal packing usually is not necessary. The use of an external splint depends on the degree of impaction following reduction.

DEPRESSION OF NASAL (FRONTAL) PROCESS OF RIGHT MAXILLA

D The elevator is inserted in right naris with broad surface against lateral nasal wall.

E The elevator is low in the nasal pyramid. The thrust is in an outward and lateral direction. Again prying is to be avoided; no counter pressure on the nose is indicated.

   The nasal septum is almost always displaced in fractures of the external bony framework. Maintenance of reduction is difficult since the cartilage tends to snap out of position much as a piece of spring sheet metal. Packing may be of help in such instances. Eventually many of these patients require submucous resection of the septum or septoplasty if the nasal obstruction is severe. Internal splinting with Teflon or Silastic can be of some help (see plate 66, step *F*). Although some surgeons utilize an Asch forceps to realign the septum, the author believes that the instrument can cause mucosal damage to the septum.

F Reduction of the nasal septum using the elevator with the broad side against the convex deformity. Medial pressure is exerted. Ash-type forceps are not recommended.

G Nasal packing using one half inch gauze strip soaked with liquid Furacin or antibiotic ointment is placed in one naris to overcorrect the deformity. Such packing is also used in severely comminuted fractures of the external bony vault.

H An aluminum, foam rubber-covered splint or dental molding compound is used when severe comminution is present or when there is a possibility of misalignment. External sheets of lead and silicone with through and through sutures are rarely needed (see plate 158, step *F*).

Plate 173   Fractures of Facial Bones

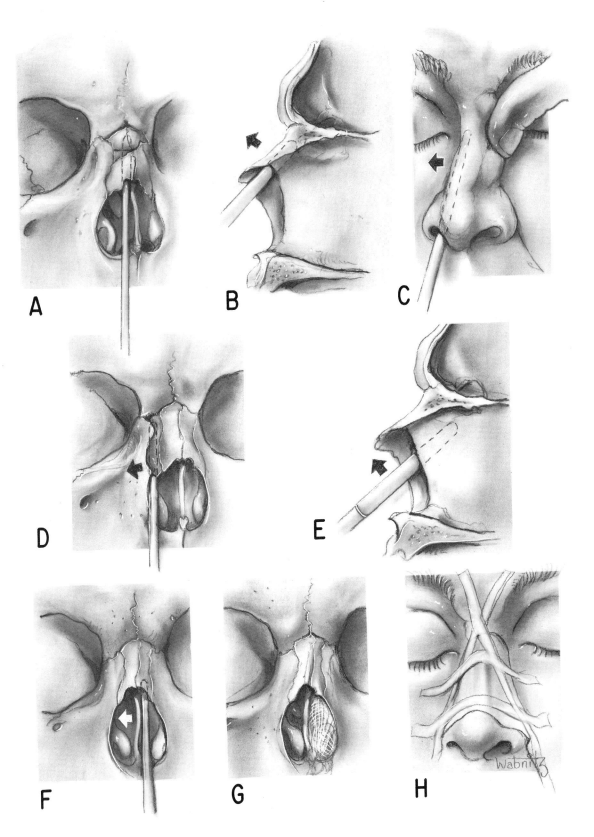

A

B

C

D

E

F

G

H

FRACTURES OF MANDIBLE

Highpoints

1. Evaluate the supraglottic airway; severely comminuted, multiple fractures may have extensive soft tissue injury involving the floor of the mouth and the tongue posteriorly. Such injuries require a tracheostomy.
2. For uncomplicated fractures, the simplest treatment method is the use of Erich arch bars (step G) or a form of interdental wires if sufficient teeth are present.
3. Never wire upper and lower jaws together immediately following injury. Aspiration of vomitus with obstruction to airway from blood and edema is always a possibility.
4. Proper occlusion of upper and lower jaws is the keynote of treatment.
5. If reduction with arch bars or interdental wiring fails, some type of internal fixation is necessary. This is specifically required in the edentulous patient.

A A Barton-type bandage is an excellent temporary support. It allows oral suction easily and can be released quickly if necessary. Kling is an admirably suited material for the bandage. The anterior extension over the chin is avoided if there is danger of posterior displacement.

B Interdental wire 25 cm in length is used. The material may be either Angle's standard brass ligature wire (0.508 mm) or stainless steel wire size #24 or #26.

Using a single wire, multiple loops are formed around four teeth starting with the first or second molar and working forward. The wire is placed around the molar with the shorter end lying along the outer surface of the teeth. The longer end is passed below and then above this outer wire forming a small loop of sufficient length to allow for final twisting and the formation of a hook. The short outer end of the wire is raised forward each time the long interdental end is first placed between the teeth. This aids in the placement of the interdental end in the under and over positions. The same procedure is repeated on the maxillary teeth and on the opposite side.

C Small pointed pliers or a heavy needle holder is used to twist the loops. The loops are first pulled forward and outward before twisting is begun. The loops on the mandible are bent downward and the loops on the maxilla are bent upward to form hooks around which rubber bands are placed (G).

D Intramedullary fixation with a Kirschner wire. The neural canal is to be avoided when drilling the holes. Exposure of the fracture site is similar to that depicted on plate 175.

E After the Kirschner wire is inserted, malleable silver or stainless steel wire is inserted through drill holes to maintain approximation. This type of internal fixation is left in place permanently. If a Kirschner wire is not used, the interosseous wire should be in the form of a figure eight pattern or two wires should be used.

F Another method of fixation with a Kirschner wire is to insert the wire through a small stab wound in the chin and use a Kirschner wire drill to pierce the thick cortical bone and thence through the medullary canal.

G The Kirschner wire in position. It may be used in conjunction with Erich arch bars when necessary to maintain proper reduction and occlusion. The Kirschner wire may be removed or left *in situ* when the fracture heals.

FRACTURE OF CONDYLAR PROCESS

By and large the consensus in fractures of the condylar process is conservative closed manipulation under analgesia or general anesthesia. This is followed by fixation, using arch bars connected with rubber bands or interdental wires (steps B,

(Text continued on opposite page.)

Plate 174   *Fractures of Facial Bones*

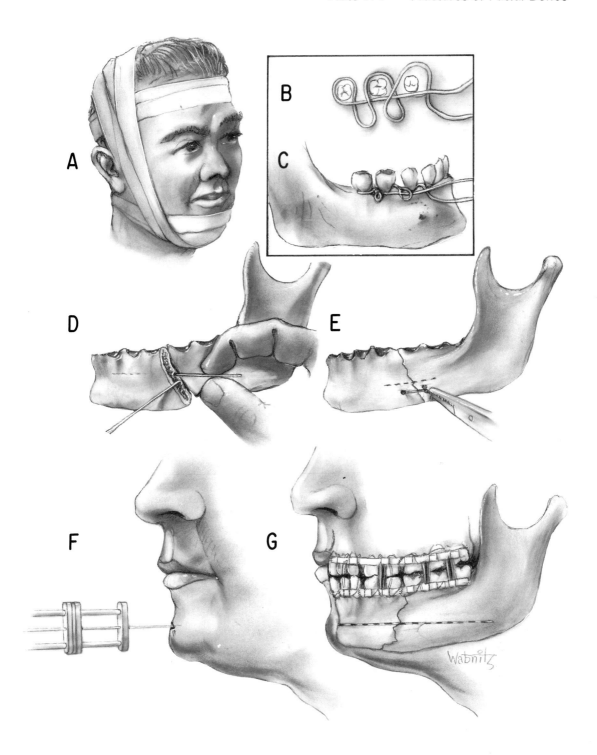

C and *G*). In children there may be a question regarding interference with the growth center and some surgeons suggest open reduction. This is performed through a preauricular incision taking extreme care not to injure the facial nerve. Intraosseous wires through drill holes proximally and distally are then inserted. These wires must be heavy enough to avoid subsequent breaking of the wires.

OPEN REDUCTION OF FRACTURED MANDIBLE USING A PLATE

Highpoints

1. Avoid injury to mandibular and cervical branches of facial nerve.
2. Maintain proper occlusion.
3. All drill holes should avoid the neural canal if possible.

Indications

1. Failure of Erich arch bars or interdental wiring.
2. Edentulous jaws.
3. Malunion.

Arch bars or interdental wires are not usually necessary for proper occlusion with this open reduction technique if there is a single fracture. On the other hand, with multiple and comminuted fractures, arch bars or interdental wires (see plate 174) are a great aid in obtaining and maintaining proper occlusion. These arch bars or wires are placed prior to the open reduction and removed one to two weeks following the internal fixation.

A   A horizontal incision following a natural skin crease is made 3 to 4 cm below the lower border of the horizontal portion of the mandible.

B   The skin incision is carried through the platysma muscle and its fascial envelope but not through the layer of the cervical fascia which invests the submaxillary salivary gland.

C   The upper skin flap is developed carefully in order to identify and preserve the mandibular branch of the facial nerve. This nerve may lie as much as 2 cm below the lower border of the horizontal ramus of the mandible in a plane deep to the platysma muscle and its investing fascia and superficial to the external maxillary artery and anterior facial vein. Its course may be compared to a hammock hanging from the mandible. The cervical branch innervates the platysma muscle, and its injury may be a factor in causing upward displacement of the lower lip.

After the mandibular branch of the facial nerve has been identified, the upper skin flap is further mobilized to expose the fracture site. Either a Cushing-type vein retractor or simple stay sutures through the platysmal muscle are used to hold the flaps apart. Depending on the location of the fracture, the external maxillary artery and facial vein may require either ligation and division or retraction to one side or the other. The periosteum may be either elevated or left intact. Displacement depends primarily on the masseter muscle which draws the posterior fragment upward. The pterygoid process adds to this displacement, while the suprahyoid and infrahyoid muscles tend to pull the anterior fragment downward and slightly inward.

D   After reduction, a Conley mandibular bar is held in place with bone-holding forceps. Again, care must be exercised to avoid damage to the mandibular nerve. At least two screws must be on either side of the fracture site. If a hole in the bar is near the fracture site, a diagonally drilled hole across the fracture site is used for the insertion of supporting wire.

E   A No. 30 malleable silver wire or braided stainless steel wire is inserted and either twisted or tied at the inferior edge of the mandible. The ends are turned in.

F   When the fracture site is further posterior, double wire fixation may be the procedure of choice because of the proximity of the masseter muscle. The external maxillary artery and facial vein are doubly ligated and divided. The mandibular nerve again crosses the operative field and must be protected. Its emergence from the tail of the parotid gland is usually visualized. Transection of a portion of the masseter muscle is necessary to expose the fracture site. Drill holes are placed obliquely across both fragments. A No. 30 malleable silver wire is then inserted, twisted and the ends turned in. Repair of the masseter muscle is not necessary if only 1 to 2 cm has been transected.

Plate 175   Fractures of Facial Bones

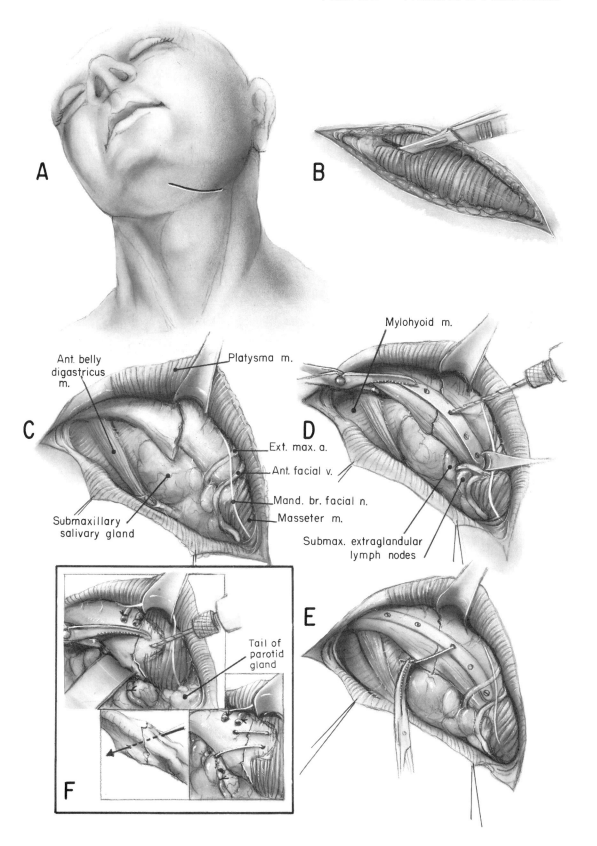

A

B

C

Ant. belly
digastricus
m.

Platysma m.

Ext. max. a.

Ant. facial v.

Mand. br. facial n.

Masseter m.

Submaxillary
salivary gland

D

Mylohyoid m.

Submax. extraglandular
lymph nodes

E

F

Tail of
parotid
gland

OPEN REDUCTION OF DEPRESSED FRACTURE OF ZYGOMATIC ARCH WITH OR WITHOUT FRACTURE OF BODY OF ZYGOMA (GILLIES' TECHNIQUE)

Highpoints

1. The earlier the reduction, the better—usually within 48 hours.
2. Use temporal muscle as guide for placement of elevator.
3. Slightly overcorrect the depressed fragments.

A
B   Although the extended or exaggerated Waters x-ray view, which is the basic standby for most facial bone fractures, is suitable, the Titterington position is one of the specific x-ray views for depressed fractures of the zygomatic arch. This position is indicated in the drawings with the arrows showing the direction of the x-ray tube.

C   The incision is made above the hairline and slightly oblique. Beneath the skin and superficial temporal fossa is encountered the superior auricularis muscle, which is separated in the direction of its fibers. If the hairline is low and the incision made lower, the fibers of the auricularis anterior are exposed. These fibers are more horizontal than the auricularis superior and are thus separated in a horizontal plane. Deep to these muscle fibers lies the heavy deep temporal fascia.

D   The deep temporal fascia is then incised, exposing the temporalis muscle. This fascia may have two closely adherent layers. The entire layer(s) of the fascia must be incised, and the temporal muscle is used as a guide for the placement of the elevator.

E   A blunt sturdy elevator is inserted between the deep temporal fascia and the temporalis muscle. The instrument then slips easily and directly under the zygomatic arch.

F   A cutaway illustration showing the skin incision and the position of the elevator superficial to the temporalis muscle and deep to the depressed zygomatic arch and deep temporal fascia. With a gauze roll protecting the upper skin edge and acting partially as a fulcrum, the depressed arch is elevated and slightly overcorrected. The left hand is best used as an actual fulcrum to avoid undue pressure on the skull.

G   When there is an associated fracture of the body of the zygoma, this fracture is reduced through the same approach (see plate 177).

Closure consists of three or four sutures to approximate the deep temporal fascia. The skin is then closed. A 4″ × 4″ gauze sponge is folded three times and used as a pressure pad over the incision.

Rarely does this type of fracture require interosseous wiring, unless there has been undue delay in the reduction (see plate 177, step *F*).

Plate 176   Fractures of Facial Bones

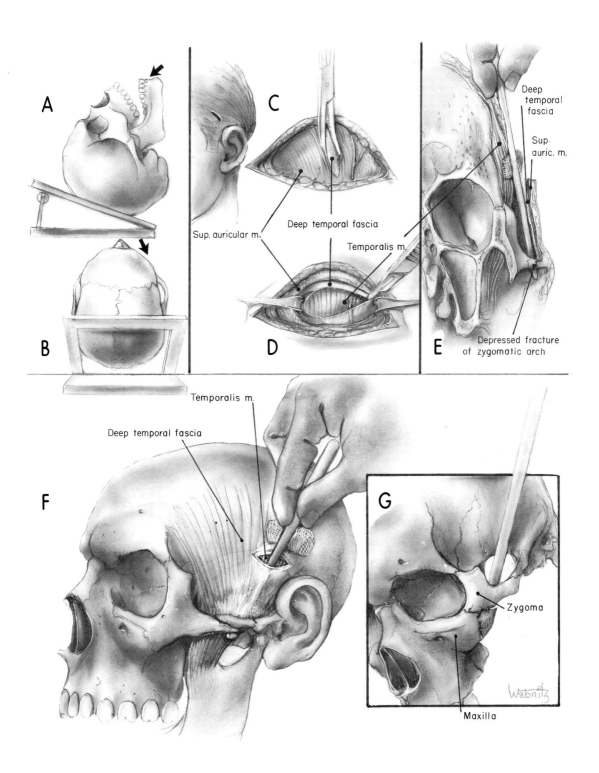

A

B

C

Deep temporal fascia

Sup. auricular m.

Temporalis m.

D

Deep temporal fascia

Sup. auric. m.

Depressed fracture of zygomatic arch

E

Temporalis m.

Deep temporal fascia

F

G

Zygoma

Maxilla

OPEN REDUCTION OF DEPRESSED FRACTURE OF ZYGOMA AND PORTION OF MAXILLA

EARLY REDUCTION

Highpoints

1. The earlier the reduction, the better—usually within 48 hours.
2. Use temporal muscle as guide for placement of elevator.
3. Slightly overcorrect the depressed fragments.
4. Combined maneuver of elevation of depressed segments and downward pressure on raised infraorbital rim.
5. Evaluate presence or absence of fracture of floor of orbit and treat accordingly (see plate 184).

A
B Views of the fracture. The anterolateral wall of the maxilla is depressed and comminuted as is the body of the zygoma. The fracture line extends through the infraorbital foramen with upward rotation of the lateral portion of the infraorbital rim. The zygomatic arch may or may not be depressed. There is associated hypoesthesia of the skin of the cheek and upper lip, trismus, malocclusion, epistaxis and a cosmetic deformity characterized by a depression over the body of the zygoma and maxilla. Diplopia may be present.

C
D Using the same approach (Gillies') as for simple depressed zygomatic arch fractures (plate 176), a blunt elevator is inserted in the plane deep to the deep temporal fascia. The elevator is placed under the body of the zygoma and lateral wall of the maxilla (*E*). An outward motion is applied to the elevator, while the thumb of the opposite hand exerts downward pressure (arrows) on the raised lateral portion of the infraorbital rim. The depressed zygomatic arch, if present, is elevated as in plate 176. Slight overcorrection is usually desirable.

E If the posterolateral wall of the maxilla is severely comminuted, entrance into the antrum via this temporal approach is possible. Thus, the entire anterior wall of the maxilla may be elevated. However, severe comminution of the anterior wall may preclude postreduction impaction of the fragments, and it is then necessary to resort to the canine fossa approach with packing (plate 178).

LATE REDUCTION

F If the reduction has been delayed and the alignment of the fragments cannot be achieved or maintained, open reduction at one or all fracture sites is necessary. Depicted is an intraosseous wire placed through drill holes in the zygomatic arch. Extreme care must be taken not to injure branches of the facial nerve. This can be achieved by separating all subcutaneous tissue by blunt dissection down to the fracture site. The twisted wire is bent so as not to project against the skin or the temporalis muscle. Ideally the periosteum is closed over the wire.

Plate 177   Fractures of Facial Bones

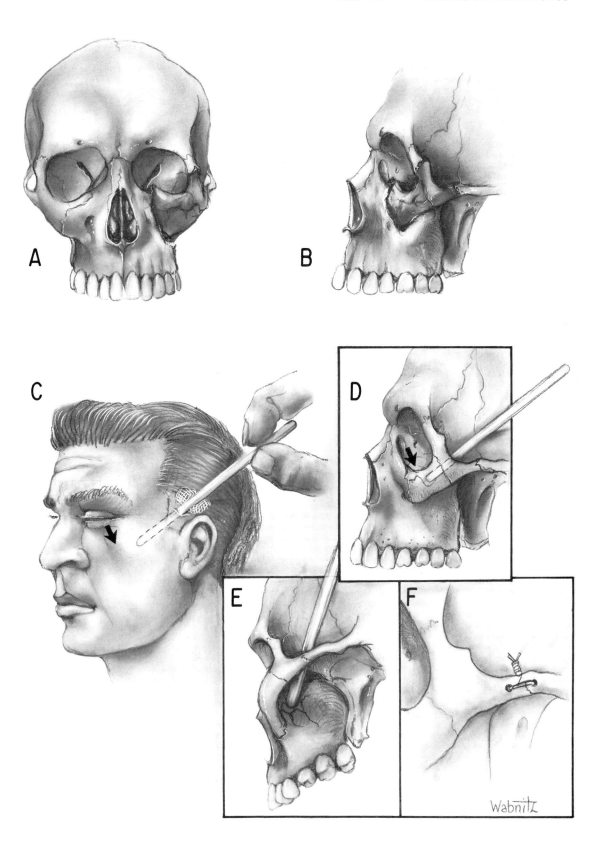

EARLY REDUCTION OF DEPRESSED COMMINUTED FRACTURE OF ANTERIOR WALL OF MAXILLA

Highpoints

1. This method is usually only effective in the early reduction of such fractures— within 24 to 48 hours. Later than this, interosseous wiring is necessary to maintain reduction (see plate 178, step A).
2. Edema and hemorrhage may mask a severe cosmetic deformity.
3. Antral packing is almost always necessary.
4. Always perform intranasal antrostomy for drainage and close canine fossa incision without drainage.
5. Evaluate presence or absence of fracture of the floor of orbit and treat accordingly (see plate 184).

A
B Views of fracture. The main fracture line usually extends through the infraorbital foramen with downward depression of the lateral infraorbital rim. The anterior wall of the antrum is comminuted. There is associated hypoesthesia of the skin of the cheek and upper lip, trismus, malocclusion, epistaxis and usually diplopia. The cosmetic deformity may or may not be apparent, depending on the degree of edema or hemorrhage.

C A small incision is made in the canine fossa. The details of the approach are similar to that for a Caldwell-Luc operation (plates 28 and 29).

D The anterior wall of the antrum is exposed, demonstrating some of the comminuted fragments. A small elevator is then inserted into the antrum through the site of comminution. Clotted blood is removed by suction and with the elevator the depressed fragments are raised by pressure from within the antrum. Any free fragments of bone are removed. An evaluation of the roof of the antrum (floor of orbit) is now made (see plate 185).

E An intranasal antrostomy through the inferior meatus is performed (plate 27, steps A and A¹).

F The antrum is packed with one half inch gauze soaked in liquid Furacin or with antibiotic ointment with one end drawn out through the intranasal antrostomy. The other end is left in the antrum. This packing maintains the position of the comminuted fragments. The canine fossa incision is closed without drainage. Removal of the packing through the nose is started on the fifth to seventh day. Complete removal is accomplished over several days. Antibiotics are necessary with antral packing.

Complication

Injury to optic nerve causing blindness due either to pushing fragment of bone upward against optic nerve, or to too much pressure from packing causing thrombosis of vessels in orbital contents.

Plate 178   Fractures of Facial Bones

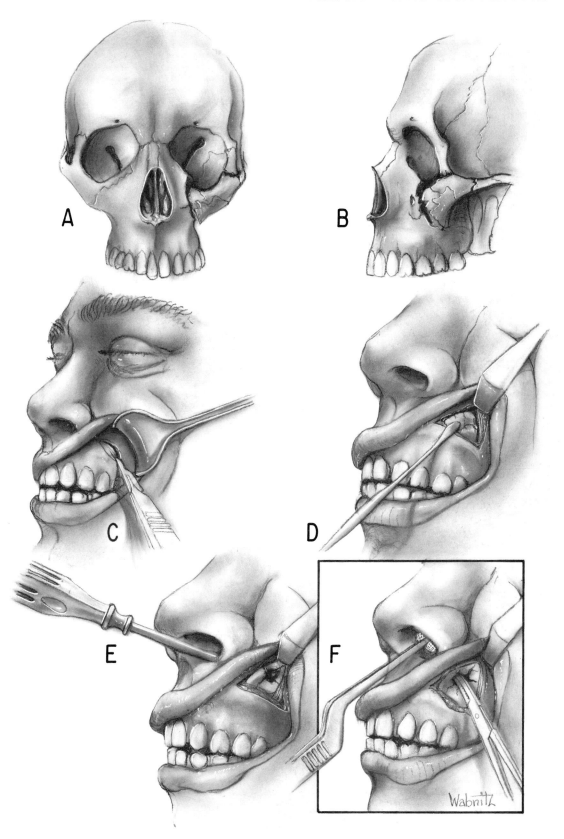

INTRAOSSEOUS WIRING FOR FACIAL FRACTURES

When reduction is delayed beyond 48 to 72 hours or when there is marked separation of the fracture sites, wiring across the fracture site through drill holes is necessary to maintain reduction.

Highpoints

1. Incisions follow natural skin crease.
2. Small incision as possible. Retract skin edges gently.
3. Use blunt dissection in subcutaneous tissue and muscle to avoid injury to branches of facial nerve.
4. Periosteum is usually elevated and then is closed over the wire and fracture site.
5. Exposure at infraorbital region affords exploration of orbital floor (see plates 185 and 186) for herniation of orbital contents into antrum. Treat according to findings.
6. Drill holes should be as small as feasible. Always take extreme care of structures behind drill hole sites and angulate direction of holes accordingly.
7. Bend twisted wire so that surrounding soft tissue is not irritated.

A
B Fracture sites depicted. Extension into the floor of the orbit is very probable. The zygomatic arch may be fractured in more than one location. If the arch is depressed, it can usually be elevated through the brow incision which is used for the approximation of the zygomaticofrontal fracture. If not satisfactory, a separate approach is made through the temporal region (Gillies') (see plate 176). The fracture along the infraorbital rim is most often through the infraorbital foramen. Any fragments of bone infringing on the infraorbital nerve should be disengaged.

C The various types of skin incisions are depicted. The exposure in zygomaticofrontal area can be either through the lateral aspect of the brow (solid line) or along a natural skin crease lateral to the lateral canthus of the eye. In either event, never shave the hair of the brow. The infraorbital incision is along a natural skin crease. If this incision is too long, edema of the lid will persist for months. The lids may be temporarily sutured closed to protect the cornea. Separation of the subcutaneous tissue and muscle fibers is by blunt dissection to avoid injury to branches of the facial nerve, especially if the lateral canthal incision is used.

D The periosteum has been incised (the incisions pictured are large for clarity) and is now being gently elevated, exposing the fracture site. Exploration of the lateral orbital rim can be performed through the incision by extending the subcutaneous plane. Through this incision an elevator can at times be inserted deep to the zygomatic arch for elevation of depressed fractures of this bony structure. If not feasible, a separate incision can be utilized in the temporal region (Gillies') (see plate 176).

E Small drill holes are then made about 6 to 7 mm from the edge of the fracture on each side. A malleable retractor or other suitable instrument is inserted medially to protect the orbital contents. The drill holes are directed posterolaterally to avoid entering the orbit and the cranial cavity. This is most important.

F Stainless steel wire (0.35 mm in diameter) is then passed through the drill holes and twisted posteriorly to the fracture site. The wire is then cut, leaving a twisted section of 7 to 9 mm which is bent in behind the bone.
   A similar exposure, drill holes and intraosseous wiring have been performed along the intraorbital rim fracture. Through this incision, the floor of the orbit is explored for fracture and herniation of orbital fat or inferior rectus and inferior oblique muscles into the antrum. If so, treatment is as shown on plates 184, 185 and 186. Again, extreme care is exercised when drilling the holes with a malleable retractor protecting the globe.
   Intraosseous wiring may be required for reduction of the zygomatic arch (see plate 177, step *F*). Not all fracture sites may require intraosseous wiring. The decision rests with the evaluation of the total result of reduction. Even after all fracture sites are wired, depression of the malar bone may still be present. Outward and upward traction is then necessary. It is a simple matter to attach a wire from the infraorbital rim to a

Plate 179   Fractures of Facial Bones

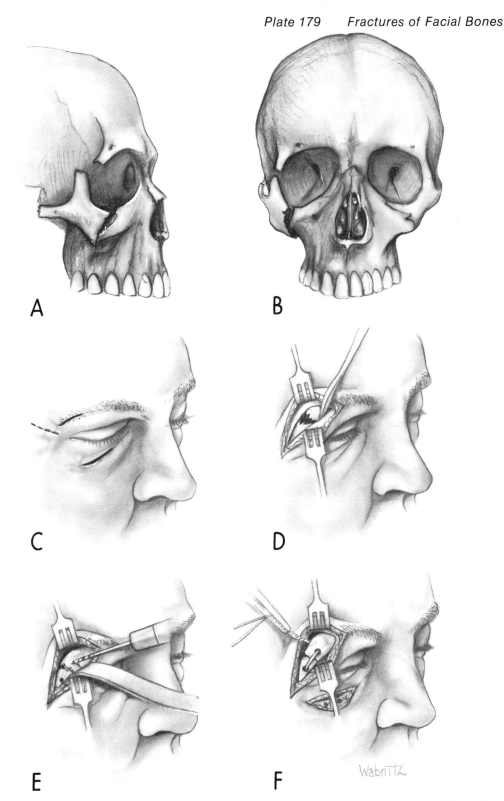

A

B

C

D

E

F

Lane plate secured with tibial bolts to the zygomatic process of the frontal bone (see plate 187).

Closure consists of approximation of periosteum, muscle, where necessary, and skin. Some extra time and care at this juncture will result in a barely visible scar if the surgeon has been mindful that his assistant has not pulled too hard on the skin retractors. Stay sutures rather than retractors or skin hooks may be preferred.

"TENT PEG" METHOD OF REDUCTION AND FIXATION OF FACIAL BONE FRACTURES (STRAITH, 1958)

Indication

Occasionally a fracture in the zygomatic frontal region of the orbital rim is so high and the superior edge of the fracture is so close to the cranium itself that intraosseous wiring through drill holes would require that the twisted ends of the wire be placed within the orbit. To avoid this, small sections of Kirschner wire inserted in an angle serve as pegs around which the intraosseous wire is secured. This method is seldom referred to, yet it is worthwhile to keep in one's armamentarium.

Highpoints

1. Insert pegs at angle with distal or projecting end away from fracture site.
2. Projecting end of peg need be only 0.5 cm long.
3. Be sure that at least one peg is in bone that is not displaced in the fracture complex.
4. Keep in mind structures that are deep to the site of the peg insertion.
5. One must have a steady hand when inserting the peg; otherwise, it will become loose and slip out – a drawback against the procedure.

A
B Views of fracture. The fracture involves the zygoma with the infraorbital and lateral orbital rim and arch. The clinical picture is similar to other fractures of the zygoma except that a cosmetic deformity may not be apparent at the time of injury. Reduction cannot be maintained by the temporal approach.

C A small incision is made over the fracture site of the lateral orbital rim. Fibers of the orbicularis oculi muscle are separated, taking care not to injure either sensory or motor nerve fibers. Using a Kirschner drill, a Kirschner wire is inserted through a previously made stab wound into the cortex of the bone above the fracture site. The depth of insertion is from 0.5 to 1.0 cm. The wire is placed so that the buried end is at an angle toward the fracture site and the projecting end away from the fracture site. The wire is cut with about 1.5 cm projecting beyond the skin surface.

D Stainless steel wire #0 is looped around the peg and drawn into the wound with a clamp. If desired, the wire may be drawn through with a needle at each free end.

E Another peg of Kirschner wire is inserted in the bone below the fracture site. In this case, the original incision may afford sufficient exposure to eliminate another stab wound. The stainless steel wire is then looped around this second peg. While the assistant maintains the reduction, the wire is twisted and tightened. The excess length of both pegs is now cut off, leaving only about 0.5 cm projecting beyond the surface of the bone.

F The two pegs and wire are in place.

G The wound is closed, completely covering the pegs and wire.

The pegs are usually removed in four to six weeks, since they project into the subcutaneous tissue, another drawback against the technique.

Plate 180   Fractures of Facial Bones

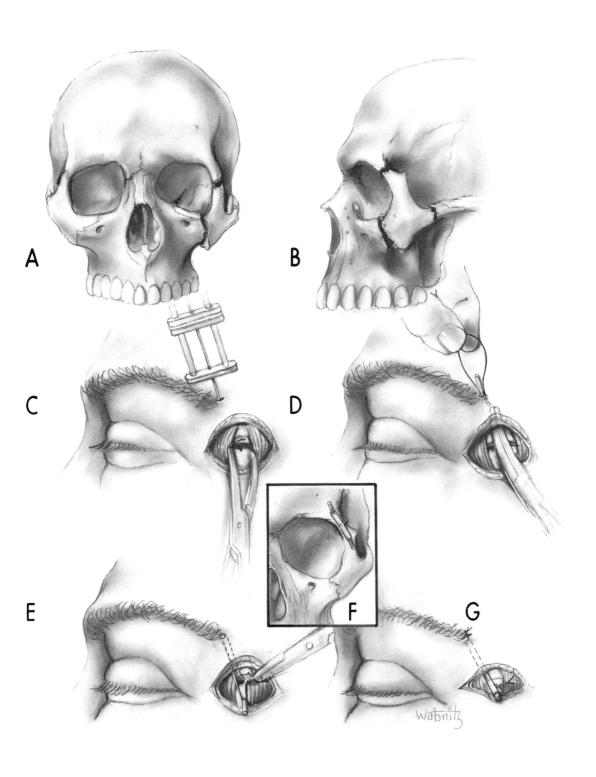

OPEN REDUCTION OF COMPLETE FRACTURE OF
UPPER DENTAL ARCH OF MAXILLA
(LE FORT I OR GUÉRIN)

There are a number of methods of reduction and immobilization of this type of fracture. Depicted are two methods:
1. Suspensory wires (steps *C* through *F*)
    a. From infraorbital rim
    b. From lateral orbital rim
2. Direct intraosseous wiring (step *G*)

Highpoints

1. Be certain that bone to which suspensory wires are attached is not displaced or mobile as a result of another fracture.
2. Interdental fixation using arch bars or interdental wiring is often required to permit malocclusion.
3. If fracture is bilateral (as pictured), fixation must be bilateral.
4. Depending on associated intraoral and pharyngeal injuries, tracheostomy may be necessary.
5. Evaluate and correct any injury to the nasal septum.

A Views of fracture. The fracture line extends through the base of both maxillae, dis-
B lodging the upper dental arch. Displacement is downward and usually posterior. This type of fracture is called a Le Fort I or Guérin.

SUSPENSORY WIRE TECHNIQUE

C Depicted are two types of suspension wires. Both types are not usually required in
D any one patient. The more anterior suspension wire (22 to 25 gauge stainless steel) is secured to the infraorbital rim in a drill hole through the rim avoiding the infraorbital nerve. This wire is looped over the rim and passes into the region of the canine fossa. A needle may be necessary to guide the two ends of the wire along the anterior wall of the maxilla into the mouth. The displaced fracture is then reduced and held in place by an assistant, with upward pressure on the mandible closing the mouth. The two ends of the wire may be secured to either a lower arch bar or an upper arch bar. When secured to a lower arch bar, occlusion is immediately achieved and maintained when the mandible is intact. The main caution is the fact that the jaw is wired closed and this should not be performed while the patient is under general anesthesia because of the danger of aspiration.

If the more posterior suspensory wire is utilized, this passes behind the zygoma. A needle may be used to pass the wire (step *C*) or a fine dental-type hook may be used to draw the wire superiorly (step *D*). The criticism of this maneuver is the possible contamination of the wire and the hook from oral bacteria.

These wires may tend to displace the fracture posteriorly.

E The completion of the procedure. The posterior suspensory wire is either secured to a tent peg, E^2, or passed through a drill hole, E^3, in the lateral orbital rim with a pull-out wire.

E¹ The suspensory wire is attached to the upper arch bar or the lower arch bar as described previously.

F A composite drawing showing the location of each type of suspensory wires.

DIRECT INTRAOSSEOUS WIRING TECHNIQUE

G In patients who are edentulous, direct intraosseous wiring can be utilized. By and large, if good adaptation is achieved, occlusion will be of little concern, thus obviating the use of Gunning-type splints (plate 194, step *C*) which otherwise might be necessary to achieve good occlusion.

Plate 181   *Fractures of Facial Bones*

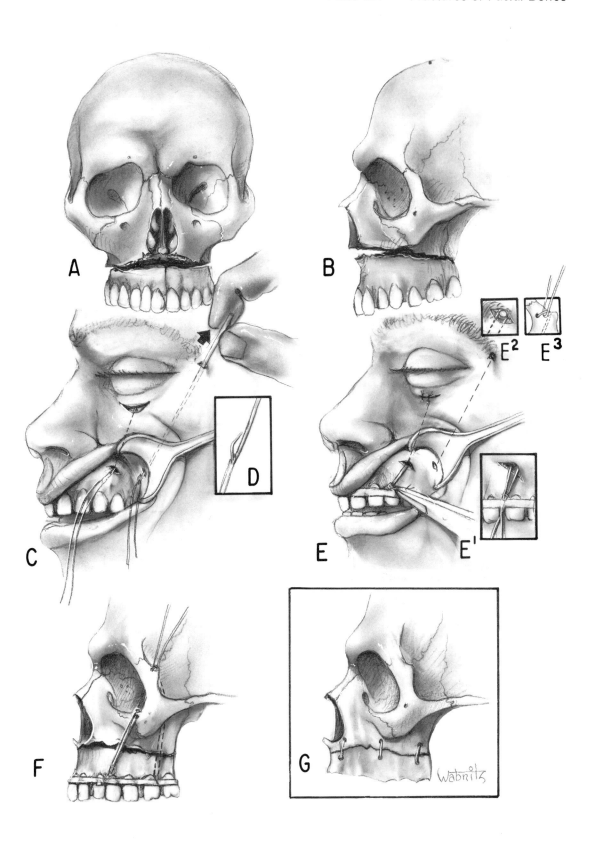

INTERNAL FIXATION OF FRACTURE THROUGH MIDDLE THIRD OF MAXILLA (LE FORT II OR PYRAMIDAL FRACTURE)

Fractures of this type and variations thereof may well be treated by the same methods described for Le Fort I and III type fractures, i.e., suspensory wires connected to an arch bar or direct intraosseous wiring (see plates 181, F, and 183).

Another method of treatment of the Le Fort II type is by the insertion of a Kirschner wire through each side of the stable molar bones and through the superior portion of the floating pyramidal fracture.

Highpoints

1. Malocclusion must be corrected and proper occlusion maintained, usually with arch bars or interdental wires.
2. Sites of entry and exit of the through and through Kirschner wire must not be involved in the fracture—these sites must be stable and attached to the cranium.
3. Extreme care must be utilized so that the Kirschner is in an exact horizontal plane so that the orbit is not entered.
4. Tracheostomy usually is indicated.

A Views of fracture. The fracture involves the body of both maxillae extending into
B the antra. Displacement is downward and usually posterior. A number of types of variations are possible, with some extending slightly more superiorly as depicted by the dotted line as well as through the infraorbital foramina. Injuries to the nasal septum are much more common than with the Le Fort I. The important feature is that the fracture, as with Le Fort I, passes inferior to the body of the malar bone which remains attached to the rest of the facial skeleton.

C With the arch bars in place, the assistant carefully maintains correct reduction and correct occlusion. A Kirschner wire is then inserted through a portion of the zygoma which is stable and not involved in the fracture. If a nasotracheal anesthesia tube is used, be certain that the wire does not pierce the tube. This method of administering general anesthesia must be performed with extreme care, since the introduction of a nasotracheal tube crosses the fracture lines and may cause additional damage. Usually there are severe accompanying soft tissue injuries intraorally and a tracheostomy is preferred. The introduction of the Kirschner wire must be in an exact horizontal plane and must penetrate a sufficient amount of the apex of the pyramidal fracture. It is for these reasons that this method is not widely utilized.

D The wire is driven through and through, catching the fractured central portion of the maxilla. The point of exit must be through stable bone attached to the cranium. The arch bars or interdental wires of the upper and lower dental arch are connected by rubber bands or wire (plate 174). The Kirschner wire may be cut flush with the skin or allowed to project about 1.0 cm and covered with antibiotic ointment and pad or cork. The wire can be removed in four to six weeks.

E The cross mark indicates the site of entrance or exit of the Kirschner wire.

Complications

1. Misdirection of wire.
2. Injury to orbital contents.

Plate 182   Fractures of Facial Bones

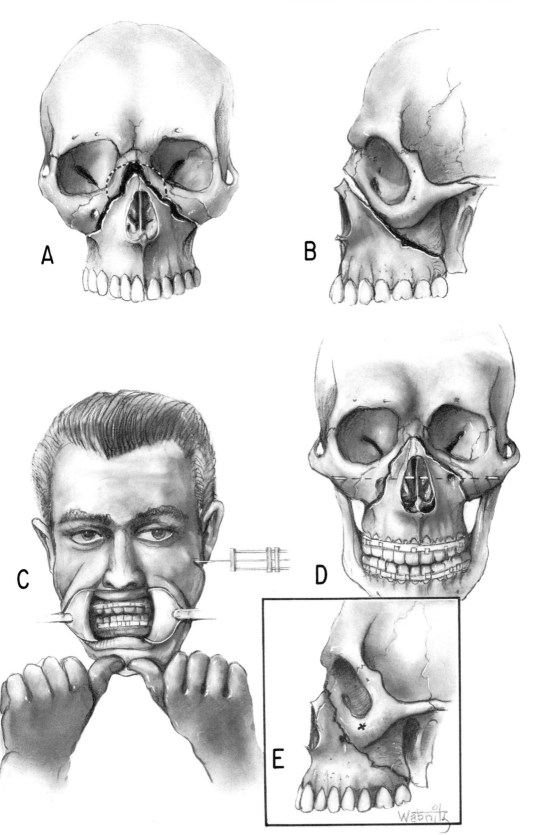

OPEN REDUCTION OF FRACTURES THROUGH GLABELLA, ORBIT AND ZYGOMATIC ARCH (LE FORT III OR CRANIOFACIAL DISJUNCTION)

The important, unfortunate feature of this type of fracture is the possible damage to the cribriform plate of the ethmoid bones, laceration or tearing of the dura and subsequent cerebrospinal rhinorrhea. Danger of infection with meningitis is always present. Fortunately, the bone in the immediate region of the optic foramen is quite dense and hence injury to the optic nerve is not as common as one might expect. On the other hand, this fracture may be the result of being thrown through the windshield. Fragments of glass thus have been seen to penetrate the fracture line and fatally injure the globe and optic nerve. X-ray films of this fracture and its variations must be carefully evaluated for foreign material.

Highpoints

1. Malocclusion is corrected and maintained with arch bars or interdental wires only after the danger of aspiration is over.
2. Eye injuries must be completely evaluated and treated early.
3. Tracheostomy.
4. Be certain that posterior displacement is corrected. The basic principle is elevation and forward reduction of the floating midfacial component.

A
B Views of fractures demonstrating the typical dishpan deformity. The fracture lines involve the glabella, medial and lateral walls of the orbit, portion of the orbit floor and zygomatic arch. The cribriform plate of the ethmoid may be fractured. Variations may occur which can extend into the maxillary antra. A skull fracture is always a possibility. Displacement is downward and usually more posterior than in Le Fort I or II. Concomitant intracranial injuries further complicate the management as well as the injury to the globe and serious hemorrhage. Drainage of the orbit is performed through a small stab wound inferiorly or laterally if bleeding continues and pressure on the globe is increased.

C The basic principle in reduction is the use of a number of intraosseous wires and suspensory wires, depending on a complete assessment of all fractures. After suitable intraosseous wires have been placed (see plate 179, step *F*), suspensory wires (22 to 24 gauge stainless steel) are passed through a hollow needle which has had its base removed. This guide needle is inserted behind the zygoma and passed into the alveolar labial region. The suspensory wires are thus fed into the mouth and the guide needle removed through the mouth.

C[1] Close-up views which detail the course of the wire through the drill holes.

D The completed reduction and fixation. Arch bars with rubber band traction is a must. At times the operative intervention is delayed because of associated intracranial injuries. With a protracted delay, fibrous tissue has proliferated and adequate reduction, especially in regard to the correction of the posterior displacement, is not entirely satisfactory. To correct the resulting dishpan deformity, some type of external traction will be necessary. Various types of devices have been described, including the halo frame, the Crawford appliance, the Erich appliance, plaster skull caps and traction with weights. A method using tibial bolts and a Lane plate is described on plate 187.

D[1] Demonstrates the placement for the pullout wires after the fracture has healed.

Plate 183   Fractures of Facial Bones

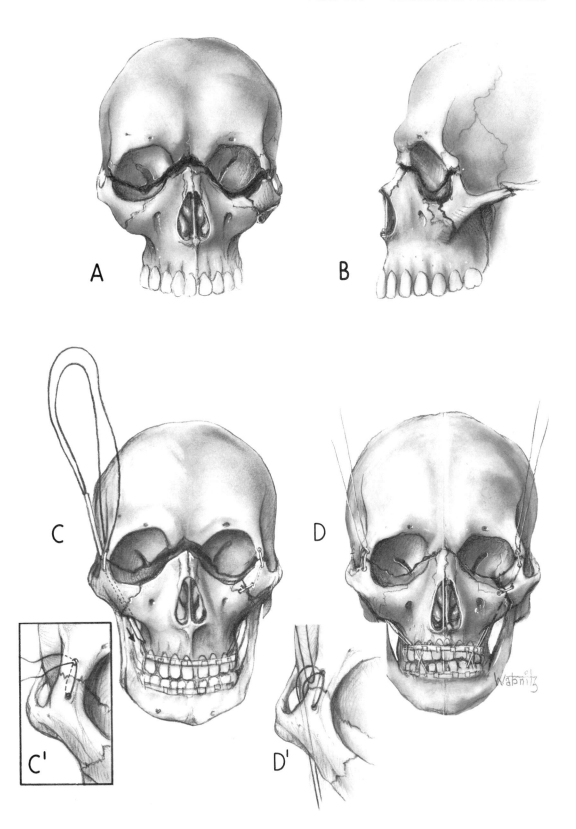

FRACTURES OF FLOOR OF ORBIT

Fractures of the floor of the orbit may be divided into two main types—indirect and direct—depending on the point of contact of the traumatic force associated with absence or presence of a fracture of the infraorbital rim.

1. *Indirect* (step D) "classical blowout" (Converse and Smith, 1960) or depressed (Dingman, 1964) fracture of the orbital floor is due to blunt trauma to the globe resulting in increased intraorbital pressure. This, in turn, causes a fracture of the thin portion of the bony floor anterior to the inferior orbital fissure. Orbital fat, the inferior rectus and inferior oblique muscle are very apt to herniate into the antrum. The relatively thick infraorbital rim is not fractured. The floor of the orbit is thus fractured downward in an indirect fashion by a referred or transmitted force.

2. *Direct* (step E) fracture of the orbital floor is due to trauma to the infraorbital rim causing an immediate fracture of this rim; hence, a fracture of the orbital floor by direct extension of the force. Herniation of fat and muscle downward into the antrum may or may not occur.

Dingman has reported one patient sustaining an injury to the infraorbital rim and maxilla resulting in an upward herniation of the floor of the orbit—a so-called blow-in fracture.

Signs and Symptoms—Variable

1. Diplopia.
2. Enophthalmos. (Exophthalmos may occur with elevated or blow-in type.)
3. Ecchymosis and edema.
4. Paresthesia over distribution of infraorbital nerve with direct type.

Less common:
5. Epistaxis—early.
6. Narrowing of palpebral fissure after immediate edema has subsided as a late finding.
7. Pupil dilated and fixed—late.
8. Loss of vision.

A   Depicted is the typical picture of a fracture of the left orbital floor characterized by:
1. Enophthalmos.
2. Downward displacement of the globe.
   (The elevated or blow-in fracture has just the reverse type of findings.)
This downward displacement of the globe can also be due to a fracture of the lateral rim of the orbit, allowing the lateral canthal ligament to drop.

B   With an upward gaze, the affected eye is fixed because of impaction of either or both the inferior rectus and inferior oblique muscles.

C   Diagnosis is aided by x-ray examination with Water's view and planograms. Instillation of air into the antrum is dangerous because of the possibility of inducing air embolism. The traction test as depicted confirms the impaction and incarceration of the inferior rectus muscle. This test consists in grasping the tendon of the muscle and applying slight traction. It differentiates the diplopia caused by impaction of the inferior rectus from weakness or paralysis of the superior rectus. Local anesthesia is necessary.

Types of Fractures of the Orbital Floor

D   *Indirect* (blowout). A blunt object, larger than the bony orbit, pushes the globe inward and downward with herniation of the inferior rectus muscle or the inferior oblique muscle with or without the nerve supply to the inferior oblique muscle. If the object causing the trauma is smaller than the orbital bony framework, there may be irreparable damage to the globe with or without fracture.

436

Plate 184   Fractures of Facial Bones

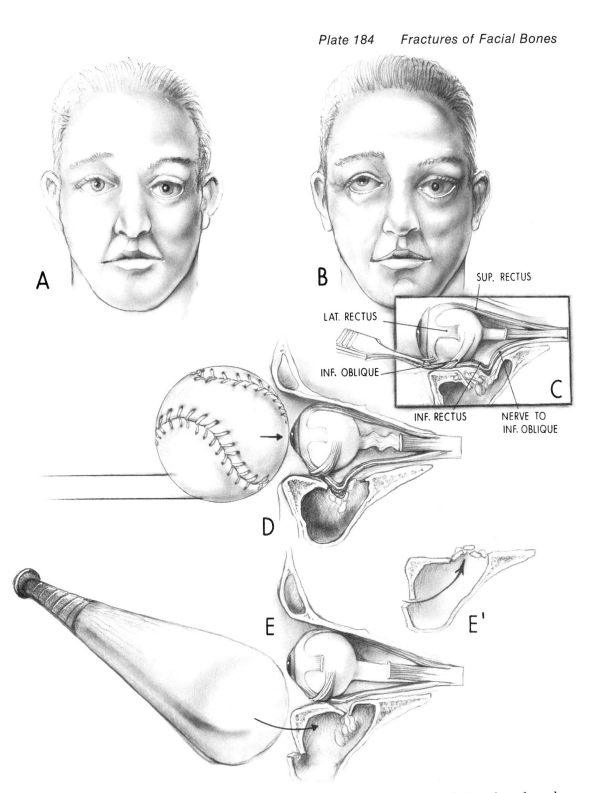

A

B

SUP. RECTUS

LAT. RECTUS

INF. OBLIQUE

INF. RECTUS

NERVE TO
INF. OBLIQUE

C

D

E

E'

E   *Direct.* The force of trauma is received directly on the infraorbital rim, thus directly fracturing the floor of the orbit. Associated fracture of the maxilla, zygoma and other parts of the orbital framework occurs in varying degrees and extent.

E¹   The blunt force is received by the maxilla, causing an elevated or blow-in fracture of the orbital floor.

FRACTURES OF FLOOR OF ORBIT (*Continued*)

Technique of Operation

Exploration of antrum is usually indicated in early treatment, especially when impaction of muscles is absent or minimal. At times, all that is required to maintain reduction is packing the antrum with antibiotic impregnated gauze. The approach is via a Caldwell-Luc operation (see plates 28 and 29). When performed, opening should be large enough to insert a finger to palpate the roof of the antrum. The bone from the anterior inferior wall of the antrum thus removed should be saved if possible for use as a bone graft to the floor of the orbit if support for the globe becomes necessary.

Highpoints

1. Do not injure orbital septum (steps *G* and *H*) or lacrimal sac (see plate 143).
2. Subperiosteal elevation along floor of orbit.
3. Completely free any impaction of inferior rectus or inferior oblique muscles, especially posteriorly, and accompanying nerves.
4. Check muscle mobility at close of operation using the traction test.
5. Do not hesitate to employ combined approach: antrum and infraorbital.
6. Autogenous bone graft preferred.

F A choice of three incisions is shown. The highest one has the advantage of minimal lid edema but can cause minimal ectropion which is usually transient. The two lower incisions through natural creases are somewhat more direct to the superior aspect of the infraorbital rim but are very apt to cause lid edema. The lid edges may be temporarily sutured together with 6-0 silk to protect the cornea.

G Cross-sectional view depicting relationship of incisions to orbicularis oculi muscle and orbital septum (palpebral fascia). The muscle is split along its fibers; the orbital septum is used as a guide to the periosteum to which it is continuous.

H The superior aspect of the infraorbital rim is exposed. An incision is made through the periosteum along the dotted line.

I The periosteum is then elevated using blunt dissection. This exposes the fractures and the impaction of the inferior rectus or inferior oblique muscles. It is important to carry the periosteal elevation sufficiently posteriorly to free the entire extent of the impaction. Avoid injury to the nerve to the inferior oblique muscle and, most importantly, the optic nerve.

Plate 185   Fractures of Facial Bones

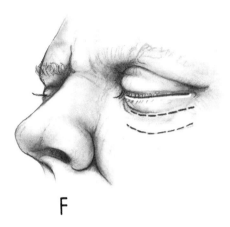

F

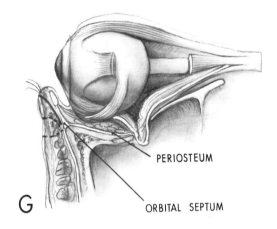

G

PERIOSTEUM

ORBITAL SEPTUM

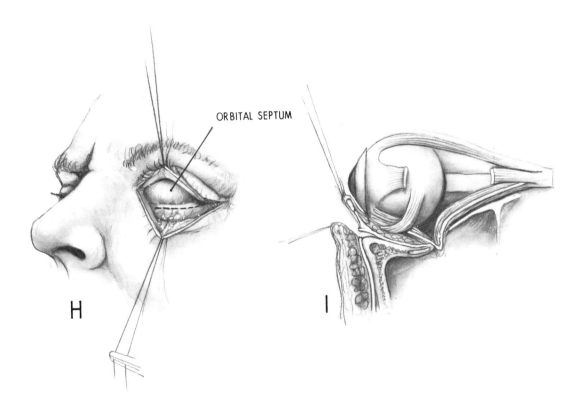

ORBITAL SEPTUM

H

I

FRACTURES OF FLOOR OF ORBIT (*Continued*)

J   Insertion of autogenous bone graft to defect in the floor of the orbit. This bone may come from the anterior wall of antrum if a Caldwell-Luc operation has been performed. The bone fragment is excellent since it is thin and concave, if it is large enough. Otherwise, an iliac bone graft is used. Plastic sheets of Silastic (or molded Silastic), Teflon or Supermin can also be utilized. The autogenous bone is preferred. Care must be taken that the graft is inserted sufficiently posteriorly and is reasonably secure before the wound is closed. Occasionally using a combined approach, especially if the operation is performed within 24 to 48 hours of the injury, antral packing may suffice to hold the depressed fragments of bone in position. The problem, however, may be adhesions which may develop between fracture healing sites and the muscles.

K   Cross section showing the graft in place. The bony fragments are not usually reducible unless the antrum is explored.

L   With direct-type fractures of the floor of the orbit which are associated with one or more fractures of the orbit rim and zygomatic arch, various types of additional interosseous wires may be necessary. Depicted are fractures which are approximated and fixed with independent interosseous wires. The wire through the fracture of the zygomatic arch may or may not be necessary. This is left until last. The fracture of the floor of the orbit is handled as previously described.

M   Occasionally the floor of the orbit fractures of the direct type as depicted in step *L* will require additional outward traction to maintain reduction of the depressed malar bone. This is accomplished using the "tibial bolt" method of traction (see plate 187).

Complications

1. Bone graft or plastic material may slide forward.
2. Ectropion or edema of lower lid resulting from skin incision.
3. Increased intraorbital pressure due to hemorrhage and edema possibly endangering vision. Decompress stat.
4. Glaucoma or predisposition to glaucoma.
5. Hyphema—accumulation of blood in the anterior chamber of the globe.
6. Cataract formation.
7. Injury to optic nerve.

Plate 186   Fractures of Facial Bones

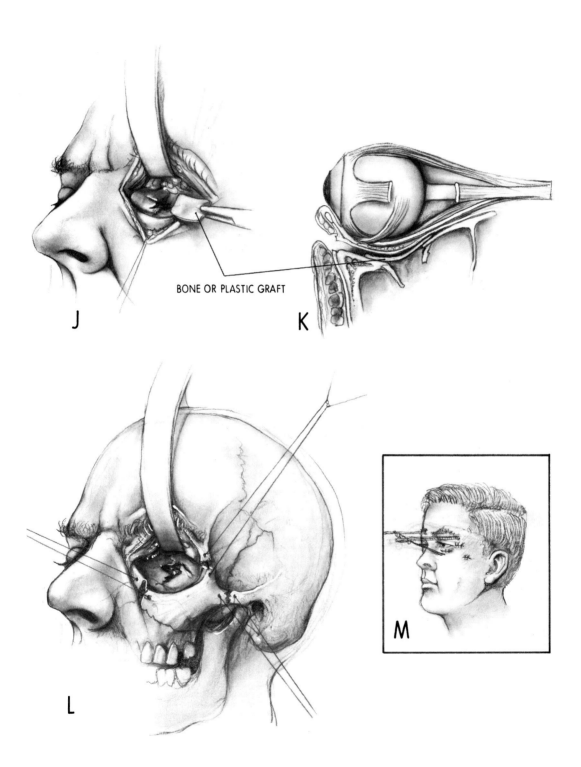

BONE OR PLASTIC GRAFT

J

K

L

M

EXTERNAL TRACTION FOR DEPRESSED FACIAL FRACTURE

Occasionally there is a need to maintain forward external traction in the management of a depressed facial fracture. Plaster head caps and various other frames and devices have drawbacks not the least of which is discomfort for the patient. Depicted is a technique utilizing tibial bolts and an eight-hole Lane plate, equipment readily available in most operating rooms.

Two situations arise when such external traction is helpful. One is when there is severe comminution of the fragments, making a point of forward fixation difficult to maintain. This is demonstrated in steps *A* and *B*. The other situation is in a delayed reduction for a midface fracture, e.g., Le Fort II or III when reduction, although achieved, cannot be satisfactorily maintained as in steps *C, D* and *E*.

Highpoints

1. The equipment needed consists of two tibial bolts, each with three nuts and one eight-hole Lane plate.
2. Be sure holes drilled for tibial bolts are several sizes smaller than the diameter of the bolts—3 to 4 mm depth hole suffices.
3. Holes must be placed so that they do not perforate the inner table of the skull which is being drilled in the lowest portion of the zygomatic processes of the frontal bone.

Basic Technique

1. Small incisions are made at the lateral edge of both brows over the stable portion of the zygomatic processes of the frontal bone.
2. A drill hole is made 3 to 4 mm deep in the lower portion of each zygomatic process of the frontal bone with a drill several sizes smaller than the diameter of the tibial bolts.
3. Tibial bolts with three nuts are then screwed tightly into the drill holes. One nut is used as a lock nut to secure the tibial bolt to the bone. The head (distal end) of the tibial bolt is cut off.
4. An eight-hole Lane plate is then slipped over the ends of the tibial bolts with one nut above and one nut below the plate. Both tibial bolts are bent slightly to the midline to accommodate the plate. The two nuts are then tightened on each bolt securing the plate in position. The ends of the bolts are guarded with sections of plastic or rubber tubing.
5. The Lane plate now serves as the point of external traction to which wires and rubber bands may be secured.
6. Traction is continued for about three weeks.

A View of fracture. There is a comminuted fracture of the left infraorbital rim with depression of the left malar bone and separation of the left frontomaxillary suture line and zygomatic arch. Owing to the comminution of the medial portion of the infraorbital rim, it is not possible to maintain adequate reduction despite the usual wiring methods. External traction is necessary.

B The tibial bolts and Lane plate are in position. Through a small incision over the infraorbital rim, 1-0 wire is secured through drill holes to the major depressed fragment. The wire is brought out through the skin and secured to the Lane plate. Other wires may be necessary to correct medial or lateral displacement.

C A midface fracture of the Le Fort type II is depicted with inward and downward displacement causing a dishpan deformity. There is an associated fracture of the malar bone with fracture of the zygomatic arch. Since the fracture is over two weeks old, adequate forward reduction cannot be maintained by the usual suspension and intraosseous wires. These wires, although very effective in the correction of the downward displacement, are ineffective in maintaining the forward reduction necessary to correct the dishpan deformity. These suspension wires actually may tend to pull the floating fragment posteriorly. Anterior, forward and outward tractions are necessary.

(Text continued on opposite page.)

Plate 187   *Fractures of Facial Bones*

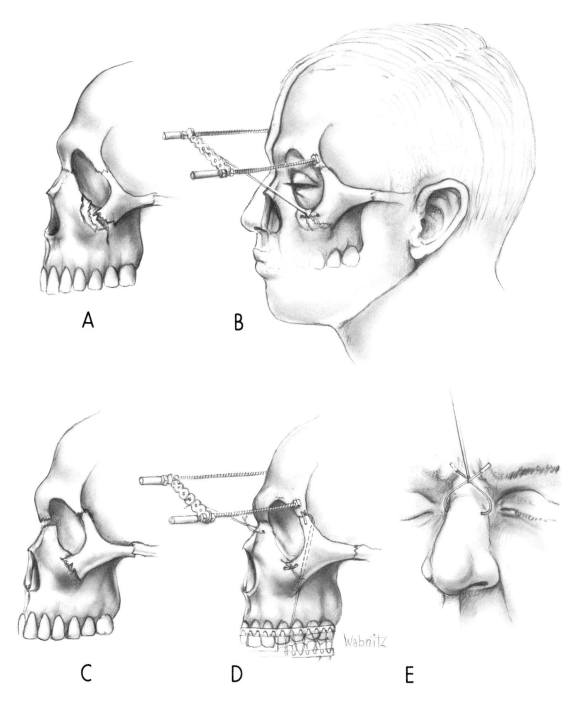

A   B

C   D   E

Wabnitz

D   After the suspending wires are secured to the upper dental arch bar and the other fracture sites are reduced and wired as depicted, the midface fragment cannot be maintained in a forward position. The tibial bolts and Lane plate are then utilized, forming a purchase site for external traction. A Kirschner wire is passed through the frontal processes of each maxilla and bent in triangular fashion. The Kirschner wire is then connected with 1-0 wire or heavy rubber bands to the Lane plate. To aid in correct occlusion, the upper dental arch bar is approximated to the lower dental arch bar.

E   Anterior view of the bent Kirschner wire through the nose.

INTERNAL FIXATION OF FRACTURED HARD PALATE

Highpoints

    1. Avoid unnecessary removal of teeth.
    2. Maintain correct occlusion; if arch bars or interdental wires are necessary, they should be connected only after the danger of aspiration is over.
    3. Tracheostomy may be necessary if there are severe lacerations of tongue.
    4. Reduce nasal fractures concomitantly.

There is a fracture through the nasal floor and hard palate with a lateral extension into the antrum. Soft tissue injury and nasal fractures are usually extensive. Careful evaluation of lacerations of the tongue is mandatory for repair and usually elective tracheostomy is the safer step.

A   Two through and through angulated drill holes are placed one on either side of the fracture site. These are located anteriorly as high as possible to avoid injury to the roots of the teeth. The drill holes exit in the hard palate. It is important that reduction be maintained during the placement of the second drill hole.

B
C   Stainless steel wire #0 or malleable silver wire #30 is then inserted through the drill holes with the loop placed anteriorly. The free ends are pulled tight and twisted intraorally.

    If there is any question of malocclusion, arch bars or interdental wires are used and connected with rubber bands (plate 174).

Plate 188   Fractures of Facial Bones

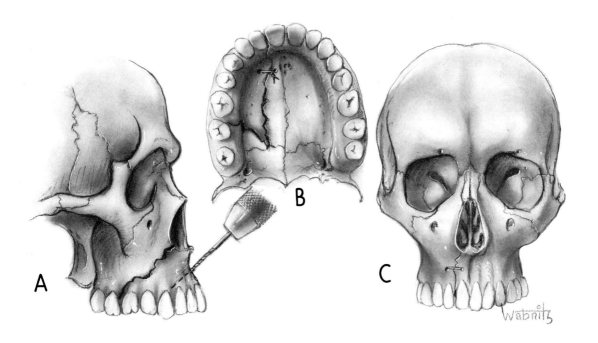

BIBLIOGRAPHY

Aiello, L. M., and Myers, E. N.: Blow-out fracture of the orbital floor. Arch. Otolaryng. 82:638–648, 1965.

Bailey, B. J., and Barton, S.: Management of mid-facial fractures. Laryngoscope 79:694–713, 1969.

Bernstein, L.: Delayed management of facial fractures. Laryngoscope 80:1323–1341, 1970.

Briggs, R. M., and Wood-Smith, D.: A simple technique for intermaxillary fixation. Surg., Gynec. Obstet. 129:1271–1274, 1969.

Butler, R. M., Morledge, D., Holt, G. P., and Kreiger, A. E.: A system of surgical approaches to orbital floor fractures. Trans. Amer. Acad. Ophthal. Otolaryng. 75:519–525, 1971.

Converse, J. M.: Reconstructive Plastic Surgery. Vol. II. Philadelphia, W. B. Saunders Company, 1964.

Converse, J. M., and Smith, B.: Blowout fracture of the floor of the orbit. Trans. Amer. Acad. Ophthal. Otolaryng. 64:676, 1960.

Converse, J. M., and Smith, B.: Enophthalmos and diplopia in fractures of the orbital floor. Brit. J. Surg. 9:265, 1957.

Crawford, M. J.: Selection of appliances for typical facial fractures. Oral Surg. 1:442–451, 1948.

Crewe, T. C.: A halo frame for facial injuries. Brit. J. Oral Surg. 1:147–149, 1966.

Danforth, H. B.: Mandibular fractures: Use of acrylic splints for immobilization. Laryngoscope 79:280–287, 1969.

Dingman, R. O.: The management of facial injuries and fractures of the facial bones. In Converse, J. M. (ed.): Reconstructive Plastic Surgery. Vol. II. Philadelphia, W. B. Saunders Company, 1964.

Dingman, R. O.: The use of iliac bone in the repair of facial and cranial defects. Plas. Reconstr. Surg. 6:179–195, 1950.

Emery, J. M., von Noorden, G. K., and Schlernitzauer, D. A.: Orbital floor fractures: Long-term follow-up of cases with and without surgical repair. Trans. Amer. Acad. Ophthal. Otolaryng. 75:802–812, 1971.

Erich, J. B.: Treatment of fractures of the zygoma and floor of the orbit. Amer. J. Surg. 112:432–435, 1966.

Failla, A.: Operative management of injuries involving the frontal sinuses. A study of eighteen operated cases. Laryngoscope 78:1833–1852, 1968.

Fink, W. H.: Anatomical study of the orbital fascia—With special emphasis on its relation to the extrinsic muscles. Published as a Supplement to the Trans. Amer. Acad. Ophthal. Otolaryng., September-October 1959.

Fryer, M. P., Brown, J. B., Davis, G., Morgan, L. R., and Sthienchoak, M.: Evaluation of internal wire pin fixation of mandibular fractures. Surg. Gynec. Obstet. January 1971.

Furnas, D. W.: Transverse maxillary osteotomy for malunion of maxillary fractures. Case report. Plast. Reconstr. Surg. 42:378–383, 1968.

Gillies, H., and Millard, D. R., Jr.: The Principles and Art of Plastic Surgery. Vols. I and II. Boston, Little, Brown and Company, 1957.

Gould, H. R., and Titus, C. O.: Internal orbital fractures: The value of laminagraphy in diagnosis. Amer. J. Roentgen. 97:618–623, 1966.

Gwyn, P. P., Carraway, J. H., Horton, C. E., Adamson, J. E., and Mladick, R. A.: Facial fractures—Associated injuries and complications. Plast. Reconstr. Surg. 47:225–230, 1971.

Hand, W. L., and Sanford, J. P.: Posttraumatic bacterial meningitis. Ann. Intern. Med. 72:869–874, 1970.

Hardin, J. C., Jr.: Frontomaxillary suspension of comminuted type III facial fractures. Plast. Reconstr. Surg. 40:450–452, 1967.

Hoffmeister, F. S.: Facial trauma—Errors in management. New York J. Med. 71:1076–1078, 1971.

Hoopes, J. E., Wolfort, F. G., and Jabaley, M. E.: Operative treatment of fractures of mandibular condyle in children. Plast. Reconstr. Surg. 46:357–362, 1970.

Huffman, W. C., and Bernstein, L.: Immediate replacement of the zygomatic compound. Arch. Otolaryng. 83:368–371, 1966.

Irby, W. B., and Rast, W. C., Jr.: Extracranial

fixation of the facial skeleton: Review and report of case. J. Oral Surg. 27:900–908, 1969.

Ivy, R. H.: Evaluation of advances in the treatment of fractures of the jaws since 1941. Preliminary survey. Plast. Reconstr. Surg. 42:472–476, 1968.

Khedroo, L. G.: External pin fixation for treatment of mandibular fractures: A reappraisal. J. Oral Surg. 28:101–108, 1970.

Lockey, M. W., Hahn, G. W., and Corgill, D. A.: Mandibular fractures. Metallic implant fixation using vitallium mesh. Arch. Otolaryng. 84:451–456, 1966.

Loré, J. M., Jr., and Zingapan, E.: External traction for depressed facial fractures. New York J. Med. 72: February 15, 1972.

Mandarino, M. P., and Salvatore, J. E.: Polyurethane polymer (Ostamer): Its use in fractured and diseased bones. Surg. Forum 9:762–765, 1958.

May, M., Ogura, J. H., and Schramm, V.: Nasofrontal duct in frontal sinus fractures. Arch. Otolaryng. 92:538, 1970.

McGovern, F. H.: Facial nerve injuries in skull fractures: Recent advances in management. Arch. Otolaryng. 88:536–542, 1968.

Panuska, H. J., and Dedolph, T. H.: Extraoral traction with halo head frame for complex facial fractures. J. Oral Surg. 23:212–221, 1965.

Perry, J., and Nickel, V. L.: Total cervical-spine fusion for neck paralysis. J. Bone Joint Surg. (Amer.) 41:37–60, 1959.

Rowe, N. L., and Killey, H. C.: Fractures of the facial skeleton. 2nd ed. Baltimore, The Williams & Wilkins Company, 1968.

Saviano, M. F., and Alonso, W. A.: Blow-out fractures of the orbit. Laryngoscope February 25, 1970.

Shumrick, D. A., et al.: Symposium: Maxillofacial trauma. Trans. Amer. Acad. Ophthal. Otolaryng. 74:1044–1092, 1970.

Smith, B., and Valauri, A. J.: The orbit. *In* Converse, J. M. (ed.): Reconstructive Plastic Surgery. Vol. II. Philadelphia, W. B. Saunders Company, 1964.

Straith, R. E.: Facial bone fixation by tent-stake method. Film Presentation at American Society of Plastic Reconstructive Surgery, 1958.

Tessier, P.: Total osteotomy of the middle third of the face for faciostenosis or for sequelae of Le Fort III fractures. Plast. Reconstr. Surg. 48:533–541, 1971.

Thompson, H.: The "Halo" traction apparatus. A method of external splinting of the cervical spine after injury. J. Bone Joint Surg. (Brit.) 44:655–661, 1962.

Thomson, H. G., Farmer, A. W., and Lindsay, W. K.: Condylar neck fractures of the mandible in children. Plast. Reconstr. Surg. 34:452–463, 1964.

Tipton, J. B.: Semiopen method for the treatment of fractures of the mandible. Surg. Gynec. Obstet. 130:865–868, 1970.

Valvassori, G. E., and Hord, G. E.: Traumatic sinus disease. Seminars Roentgen. 3:160–171, 1968.

Vinik, M., and Gargano, F. P.: Orbital fractures. Amer. J. Roentgen. 97:607–613, 1966.

Wilde, N. J.: The tolerance of the temporomandibular joint to fracture, dislocation, and associated injury. Plast. Reconstr. Surg. 25:574–583, 1960.

11. CYSTS AND TUMORS INVOLVING THE MANDIBLE

EXCISION OF CYSTS OF MANDIBLE

Cysts of the mandible are similar to the odontogenic cysts of the maxilla (see plate 45). They are benign, arising from embryonic epithelial roots or remnants and hence have an epithelial lining.

Highpoints

1. Preserve teeth and mandibular nerve if resection of cyst wall is not compromised.
2. Attempt to remove cyst intact.
3. Scrupulously remove all remnants of cyst wall if the wall fragments. Use electrocautery if all else fails.
4. Devitalized teeth require root canal therapy.

RADICULAR CYST

A radicular cyst (dental root or dentoperiosteal) may occur as the result of an apical abscess or at the site of a previous extraction. As the cyst enlarges, it may decompress through a small perforation in the most prominent portion. With the large radicular cyst, there is considerable bone absorption and danger of fracture. They may be either entirely filled with liquid or semisolid.

A   An elliptical incision is made over the most prominent portion to include, if present, the drainage site. With large cysts, there is usually no overlying bone in this region. If bone is present, it is removed with fine forceps. If no drainage site is present, the incision is then made over juxtaposed normal bone, developing a mucoperiosteal flap as depicted in A^1. Preserve, if possible, the neurovascular bundle; however, the bundle is sacrificed if necessary. Avoid medial dissection, if possible. In any event, do not injure the lingual nerve A^2). If the approach depicted in A^1 is used, the thin overlying bone is resected to facilitate removal of the cyst.

B   The mucous membrane is left intact at the drainage site, but medially and laterally it is separated by blunt dissection using a fine nasal freer.

C   If traction is necessary, the cyst is grasped with blunt forceps at the ellipse of the mucous membrane left attached to the cyst wall. Dissection is continued with the freer. If the cyst is reasonably symmetrical, it can be removed intact; if it is large and irregular, it usually fragments. Diligent and meticulous dissection is necessary in order to remove all these fragments of the cyst wall. The cyst wall is made up of epithelial cells and any remaining in the bony defect will tend to cause a recurrence.

D   A half inch gauze strip soaked with liquid Furacin is inserted in the bony defect. If necessary, sutures of nylon are placed over the gauze strip to keep it in place. The wound heals by secondary intention. If the approach depicted in A^1 is utilized, the mucosa is approximated over the surgical defect and the drain is brought out in a more dependent portion of the wound (D^1).

Plate 189   Cysts and Tumors Involving the Mandible

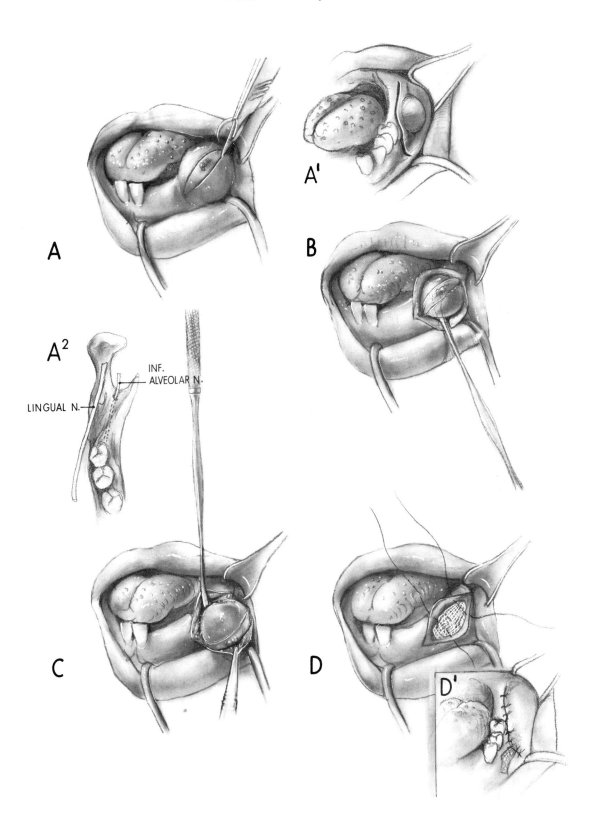

A

A'

A²

INF.
ALVEOLAR N.

LINGUAL N.

B

C

D

D'

EXCISION OF CYSTS OF MANDIBLE (*Continued*)

DENTIGEROUS CYST

A dentigerous cyst represents an anomaly of the teeth and hence, on x-ray, teeth in various stages of development are noted within the cystic cavity.

Highpoints

1. Preserve teeth and mandibular nerve if resection of cyst wall is not compromised.
2. Attempt to remove cyst intact.
3. Scrupulously remove all remnants of cyst wall if the wall fragments. Use electrocautery if all else fails.
4. Devitalized teeth require root canal therapy.

A A horizontal incision is made at the most dependent level of the tumefaction. The overlying bone is removed with fine bone forceps, or if very thin it may be undermined and outfractured with a nasal freer.

B The edges of the bony defect are trimmed with rongeurs, taking care not to break the cyst wall.

C Using a fine nasal freer, the cyst wall is separated from the bony cavity. If the cyst wall fragments, every remnant must be carefully removed. The wound is packed with one half inch strip gauze soaked with Furacin liquid. If possible, the mucosa is approximated with nylon and the gauze strip drain is brought out through the most dependent portion of the wound, attempting more primary healing. Otherwise, the healing is by secondary intention, requiring up to four months depending on the size of the defect.

D Depicted is the neurovascular bundle which, if feasible, is preserved; however, the bundle is sacrificed if necessary.

Complications

1. Fracture of mandible.
2. Recurrence.
3. Injury to viable teeth.

Plate 190 Cysts and Tumors Involving the Mandible

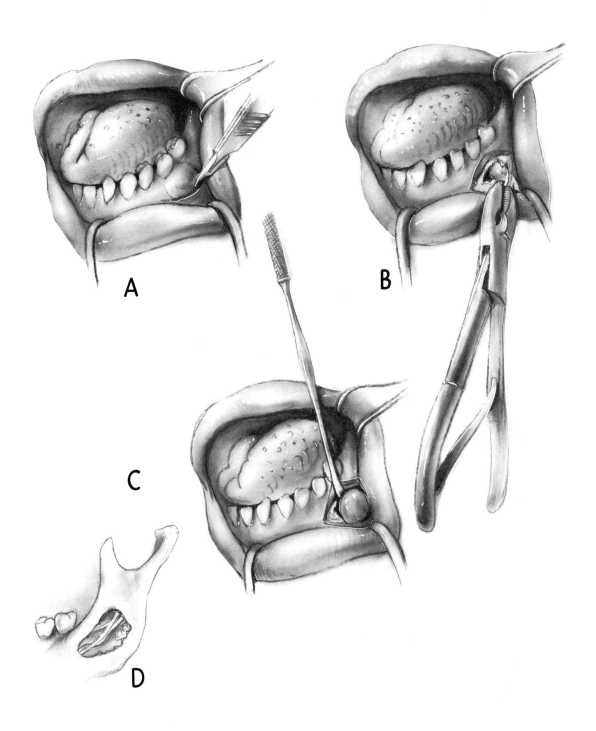

A

B

C

D

MARGINAL SEGMENTAL RESECTION OF MANDIBLE

Highpoints

1. Procedure suitable for moderately sized benign lesions of the mandible when curettage has failed or is not indicated. (Not usually performed for cysts.)
2. Not suitable for malignant bone lesions.
3. Preserve mandibular and cervical branches of the facial nerve.

A   Cross section of mandible in vicinity of second molar tooth depicting underlying mandibular lesion. Although adamantinoma (ameloblastoma) is considered benign in that it rarely metastasizes, it is locally invasive. Care must be exercised that adequate resection be performed. Radiographs do not show the full extent of these tumors since they extend at least 1.3 cm beyond the positive findings on the x-ray. For larger ones, resection of the entire ascending ramus and a portion of the body of the mandible to the mental foramen is required. This encompasses the entire neurovascular canal along which such tumors may spread.

B   An oblique or horizontal slightly curved upper cervical incision is made 2 to 3 cm below the angle of the mandible. Extreme care must be taken to avoid injury to the mandibular branch and, if possible, to the cervical branch of the facial nerve. This latter nerve may also play a part in depressing the lower lip through its innervation of the platysma muscle. This muscle is continuous with and more or less blends with some of the other muscles, connected to the lower lip, especially the depressor anguli oris (triangularis) (Hollinshead, 1954).

C   Upper lower skin flaps containing the platysma and possibly a portion of the triangularis are elevated. The external maxillary artery and anterior facial vein are doubly ligated and transected. The mandibular branch of the facial nerve crosses these vessels and is best carefully retracted superiorly with the distal cut ends of the vessels. The cervical branch of the facial nerve is retracted inferiorly. The anterior two thirds of the masseter muscle is transected, thus exposing the region of the angle of the mandible. The tail of the parotid and a portion of the submaxillary salivary gland are likewise exposed. The dotted line depicts the incision to be made in the oral mucosa in the molar region.

D   The oral cavity is entered, exposing the second molar tooth. The third molar tooth has been previously removed.

E   Diagrammatic representation of the lesion which is within the mandible and the bone to be resected. The x-ray films of the mandible are used as a guide to map out the area to be resected, keeping in mind that an adamantinoma extends beyond the x-ray delineation. An estimated 1.5 to 2.0 cm of normal bone is used for the margins. Using a sagittal plane saw, the block of mandible including the second molar tooth is resected. Small portions of bone are curetted along the three margins on the remaining mandible. These specimens are sent for a histological evaluation for adequacy of resection if the lesion is an adamantinoma. Bleeding from the mandible is controlled with cautery. If the remaining strut of bone is extremely thin, support can be achieved with an inlay iliac bone graft (see plate 193).

F   Since there may not be a sufficient oral mucous membrane to line the resulting defect in the bone, the cavity is packed with strip gauze impregnated with Furacin or an antibiotic ointment. The edges of mucous membrane partially cover the packing and the end of the packing brought out into the oral cavity. The transected portion of the masseter muscle is repaired. The platysma and triangularis muscles are reapproximated and the skin closed without drainage.

Plate 191   Cysts and Tumors Involving the Mandible

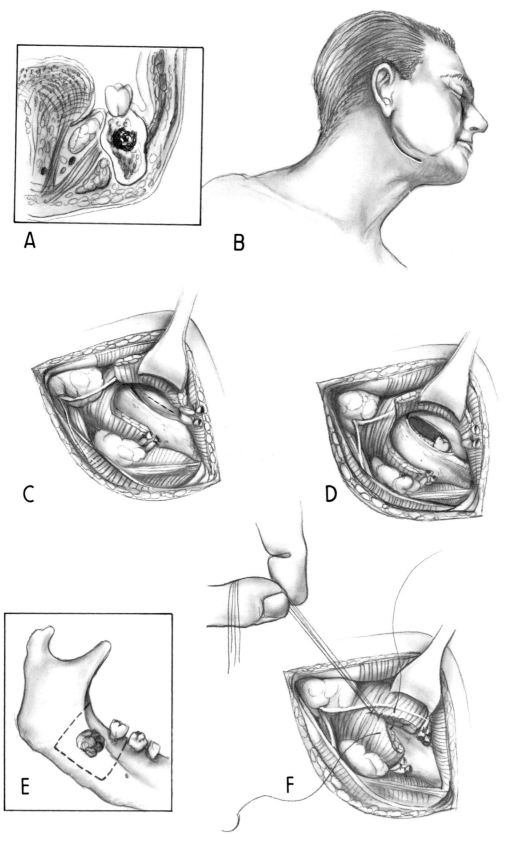

A

B

C

D

E

F

RESECTION OF LARGE BENIGN TUMORS OF MANDIBLE

Highpoints

1. Segmental resection of mandible is usually indicated in any large benign tumor.
2. Immediate reconstruction of mandible is performed if there is sufficient soft tissue for coverage of graft; otherwise, secondary bone graft is preferred.
3. Preserve continuity of mandibular division of facial nerve in cheek flap.
4. Although rare, an adamantinoma can be malignant and a complete histological evaluation must be made.

A   The lower lip is split in the midline by an incision which crosses the chin and then swings laterally and horizontally in a natural skin crease. This horizontal extension must be at least 4 cm below the edge of the horizontal portion of the mandible to avoid injury to the mandibular division of the facial nerve, which hangs like a hammock below the ramus. An alternate incision is a visor-type flap similar to that depicted on plate 231, step *I*, in which the lip is not split.

B   A sectional view depicting the local invasive characteristics of an adamantinoma. The area resected is outlined by the dotted line.

C   The full thickness cheek flap is turned laterally by incising the gingivobuccal gutter and the attachments of the buccinator muscle to the mandible. The external maxillary artery and anterior facial vein are ligated and divided as close to the capsule of the submaxillary gland as possible. This preserves the mandibular division of the facial nerve, since the nerve is superficial to these vessels. The insertion of the masseter muscle on the mandible requires sectioning, depending on the extent of the tumefaction.

D   Depending on the nature of the lesion, a satisfactory margin of normal bone is left with the specimen. In an adamantinoma 2 cm is considered safe. The horizontal portion is transected with a Gigli saw near the angle, with partial transection of the masseter muscle. A lower incisor tooth has been removed to facilitate transection anteriorly. Any teeth that are fragmented are removed.

Plate 192   Cysts and Tumors Involving the Mandible

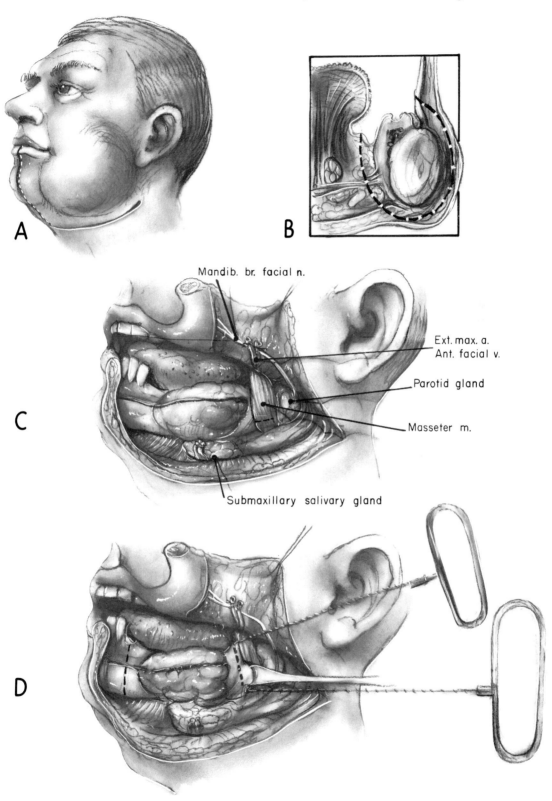

A

B

C

Mandib. br. facial n.

Ext. max. a.
Ant. facial v.

Parotid gland

Masseter m.

Submaxillary salivary gland

D

RESECTION OF LARGE BENIGN TUMORS
OF MANDIBLE (*Continued*)

E The horizontal portion with tumefaction has been removed by an incision through the floor of the mouth transecting the origin of the mylohyoid muscle from the inside of the mandible along the mylohyoid line.

If there is encroachment of the adamantinoma on the submaxillary or sublingual salivary gland, these are excised with the section of mandible.

It is not wise to insert a primary bone graft for reconstruction having entered the oral cavity resulting in a contaminated wound. Hence stabilization if desired is achieved by one Kirschner wire bent and fixed with tie wires as depicted in plate 194, step C^1 or two wires as in step C^2 or utilizing a tibial bolt locked in position with nuts and wire (Mladick, 1972). As a secondary stage, a bone graft from iliac crest or rib can be utilized.

RECONSTRUCTION OF MANDIBLE

A graft is obtained from the sixth or seventh rib laterally (see plate 22). The lateral curve of the rib is used to replace the anterior curve of the horizontal portion of the mandible. It is important that the correct occlusion of the remaining portion of the mandible be maintained during the insertion and fixation of the graft.

F A short section of Kirschner wire is used as an intramedullary support at both ends of the graft.

G Fixation is completed with the use of Conley vitallium mandibular plates.

H When a marginal segmental resection results in a thin cortical layer of bone, support is achieved with an inlay iliac bone graft. A Conley plate is used for fixation.

I Depicted is another type of autogenous bone graft stabilized by tie wires and one or two Kirschner wires.

Complications

1. High percentage loss of immediate bone grafting if oral cavity is entered is due to osteomyelitis of bone graft.
2. Recurrence of adamantinoma if the resection is inadequate.

There is a high percentage of loss of immediate bone grafting if the oral cavity is entered owing to osteomyelitis of the bone graft.

Other types of reconstruction are on plates 194 and 196.

Recently, very impressive mandibular reconstruction has been demonstrated by using bank bone, cored out and then packed with autogenous bone marrow from the iliac crest. The cortex of the bank bone evidently acts as a strut and encasement for the autogenous bone marrow, protecting the latter from invasion of fibrous tissue. The use of a millipore filter and tantalum trough packed with autogenous marrow serves a similar purpose (DeFries, Marble and Sell).

Plate 193   *Cysts and Tumors Involving the Mandible*

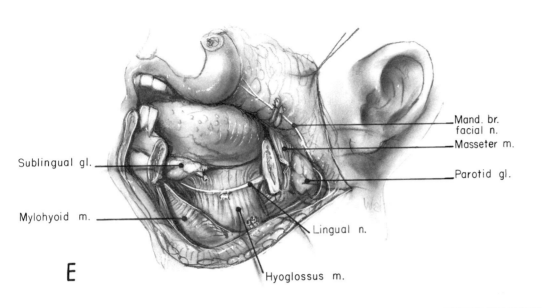

Mand. br.
facial n.

Masseter m.

Parotid gl.

Sublingual gl.

Mylohyoid m.

Lingual n.

Hyoglossus m.

E

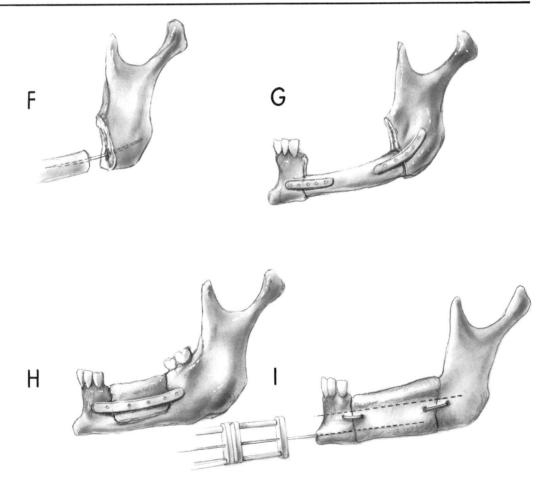

F

G

H

I

RESECTION AND RECONSTRUCTION OF ANTERIOR PORTION OF MANDIBLE USING ILIAC BONE GRAFT

Highpoints

1. Do not compromise extent of ablative surgery to facilitate reconstruction phase.
2. Place incision (usually horizontal cervical type) so that forehead flap or delto-pectoral flap may be utilized if necessary to fill in floor of mouth defect or chin defect.
3. Incision should not overlie planned location of Kirschner wire.
4. Avoid ligation of superficial temporal artery, posterior auricular artery or one lingual artery if at all possible.
5. Always stage the procedure—a minimum of six to eight weeks.
6. Immobilization of mandibular fragments to maxilla is necessary if internal fixation not stable and should be continued to the time of the reconstruction phase.
7. Keep use of hardware to minimum.
8. The oral cavity must not be entered at the reconstruction stage.
9. Make template for iliac bone graft at second stage prior to the shaping of the graft.
10. An adequate amount of autogenous cancellous bone appears to be the vital factor in bone graft regeneration.
11. Tracheostomy is necessary.

A Carcinoma arises from the alveolar process with invasion of the anterior portion of the mandible and the adjacent floor of the mouth. The dotted line depicts the area of resection which is combined with a radical neck dissection in the predominate side and a suprahyoid dissection on the opposite side. This suprahyoid dissection is a virtual necessity because of the extent of the resected mandible.

B The neck dissection incisions are of the horizontal type (MacFee, 1960), with or without the vertical limb. The upper horizontal incision is carried across to the opposite side and is placed well below the chin so as not to overlie the Kirschner wire and reconstructed mandible. The upper chin flap is then raised as a visor without transecting the lip (refer to plates 195 and 231, step *I*).

C Following the ablative surgery, the free ends of the mandible are spaced and locked with a Kirschner wire bent in the manner depicted (*C¹*). A groove is cut in each end of the mandible for the vertical limb of the Kirschner wire. Small tie wires through drill holes help keep this in position. An alternate method is the use of two Kirschner wires bent in a simple arch (*C²*) (MacDougall, 1965).

Depicted is an edentulous patient in whom Gunning-type splints are fixed to the mandible and maxilla. Circumferential wires fix the lower splint to the mandible. A Rowe-type perialveolar introducer is being inserted through the alveolar process of the maxilla to facilitate wire fixation for the Gunning splint.

(Text continued on page 462.)

Plate 194   Cysts and Tumors Involving the Mandible

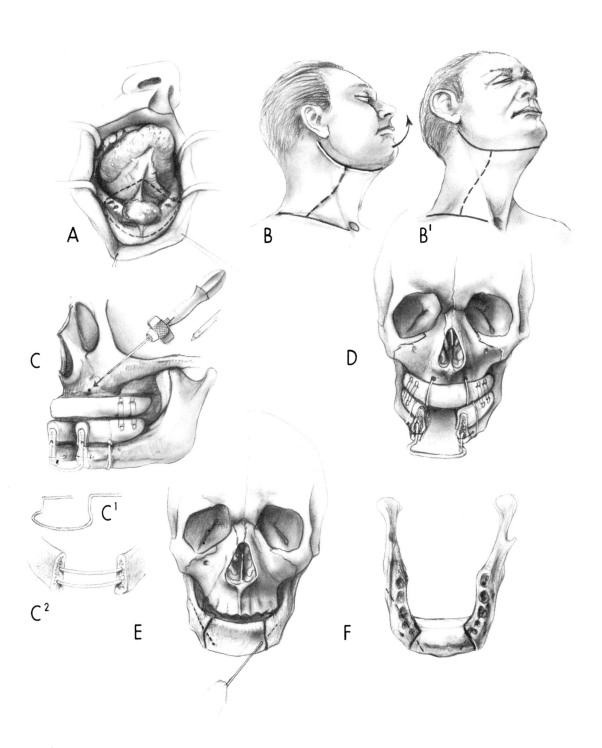

A

B   B'

C

C¹

C²   E   D

F

RESECTION AND RECONSTRUCTION OF ANTERIOR
PORTION OF MANDIBLE USING ILIAC
BONE GRAFT (*Continued*)

D   The upper splint is now secured to the lower splint with the use of wire attached to the hooks in the splint. In this manner, there is complete immobilization of the two mandibular fragments to the maxilla in reasonably good occlusion.

   If the area resected is such that the remaining tongue and lip can be utilized for closure, care must be taken so that the so-called oral cripple does not result from a tongue fixed to the floor of the mouth or mandible. All suture lines must avoid tension. Plastic suture material is used throughout. Avoid placing any suture line directly over the Kirschner wire.

   If, on the other hand, adequate tensionless closure cannot be achieved with local tissue, the oral defect will require a transposed flap. Apron, forehead or deltopectoral flaps may be used (refer to plates 114, 118 and 108). These phases of reconstruction have priority over any contemplated bone graft and must precede a bone graft as a separate stage.

   Occasionally wound breakdown occurs or pressure over the Kirschner wire causes skin breakdown. If the Kirschner wire has been in place for four to five weeks, enough fibrosis has occurred and relative fixation of the mandibular fragments has been achieved. The hardware is then removed through skin breakdown and reconstruction is begun two weeks after complete wound healing. The problem with this complication is skin contracture and, if severe, it may require a transposed flap.

E   After a minimum of six to eight weeks, reconstruction may be performed. All wounds must be well healed. If the original lesion appeared to be aggressive or nodes were positive, a delay of three to six months is preferred.

   The upper horizontal cervical incision is opened. The ends of the mandible are exposed and the Kirschner wire is removed. Extreme care must be used to avoid entrance into the oral cavity. Such an inadvertent opening could cause doom to the bone graft because of possible infection and fistula formation.

   With the fixation of the mandible to the maxilla undisturbed, the mandibular defect is measured, or, better yet, a template is cut from sheet plastic. An iliac bone graft is removed as depicted in plate 22.

   The graft is shaped as shown in step *F*. Kirschner wires or Steinman pins are inserted through the graft into the mandibular fragments, one on each side (see plate 174, *F*). Rib reconstruction is shown in plate 196.

F   A view from above shows the iliac bone graft in position. The mortise configuration of the graft yields excellent support and an interlocking effect which increases strength. It is quite easy to shape if a previous template is cut and fitted. At this time, the upper chin flap is tried for size over the template. Skin closure must not be under tension. If a template is not used, shaping the bone graft can be tedious and haphazard. A sagittal plane saw and bone-holding forceps are used for shaping.

   If the closure of the original wound at the first stage requires a transposed flap, its pedicle is transected at this stage unless a significant orocutaneous fistula exists. If such a fistula is present, and could communicate with the operative wound of this stage, transection of the pedicle and closure of the fistula should be performed at a previous separate stage.

   Closure of the cervical incision is performed without tension. The main problem in closure may be some dead space inferior to the bone graft. This must be carefully closed by suturing the under layer of the skin flap to the surrounding soft tissue deep below the graft.

Complications

   1. Absorption of bone graft.
   2. Breakdown of overlying skin.
   3. Wound infection.
   4. Asymmetry of reconstructed mandible.

Plate 194 Repeated   *Cysts and Tumors Involving the Mandible*

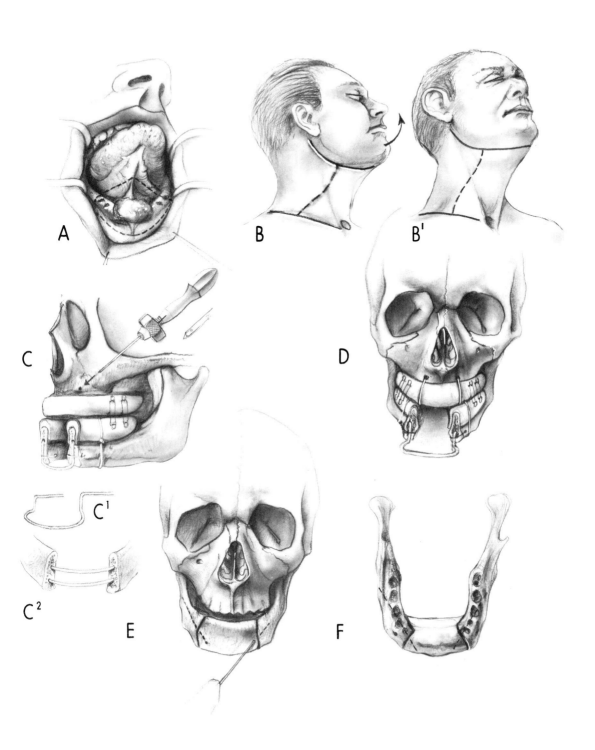

A

B

B'

C

C¹

C²

D

E

F

RESECTION AND RECONSTRUCTION OF MAJOR PORTION OF BODY OF MANDIBLE

Highpoints

(Review *Highpoints* on page 460.)

1. Do not compromise extent of resection for ease of reconstruction.
2. When there is invasion of the inferior alveolar canal, the tumor can spread along the inferior alveolar canal with the inferior alveolar nerve.
3. The forehead flap may be delayed or not delayed. If possible, delay the flap since loss of the distal end of this long flap can occur. Always delay the flap when preoperative radiation has been used.
4. Preserve, if possible, ipsilateral superficial temporal and posterior auricular arteries which supply the flap. It is best to preserve the external carotid artery from which these vessels arise, although some surgeons feel that this vessel may be sacrificed (MacGregor, 1963).
5. Do not extend the inferior incision of the forehead flap below a horizontal imaginary line extending from the lateral canthus of the eye in order to avoid injury to the zygomatic branch of the seventh nerve which supplies the orbicularis oculi muscle.
6. Avoid compression of a forehead flap pedicle either by zygomatic arch or by Kirschner wire.
7. Immobilize mandibular remnants with Kirschner wire.
8. Use extreme care to approximate the oral mucosa surrounding the mandibular remnants to the edges of the forehead flap.
9. At the reconstructive stage, performed six weeks or later, the following is accomplished:
   a. Forehead flap is divided and the pedicle is returned to the donor site.
   b. Orocutaneous fistula is closed.
   c. If there is sufficient soft tissue present and if the wound is not contaminated by the orocutaneous fistula, reconstruction of the mandible can be performed at this time; otherwise, it is delayed until a later stage. Additional soft tissue can be obtained from a deltopectoral flap.
10. Mandibular reconstruction can be accomplished by one of the following methods:
    a. Iliac bone graft (plate 194).
    b. Bent rib graft is skewered on Kirschner wire (Millard).
    c. Frozen bone bank mandible is hollowed and packed with autogenous cortical bone (Defries et al., 1971).
    d. Millipore filter with tantulum trough packed with autogenous cortical bone.
    e. Plastic replacement.
11. Two of the most important dicta for mandibular reconstruction are the *noncontaminated wound* and adequate *immobilization* of any type of bone graft. Immediate reconstruction using bone graft is usually not successful.
12. Do not shave scalp hair in the region of the distal portion of the forehead flap which will be used for the reconstruction, thus avoiding hair-bearing tissue in the flap.

A   Horizontal skin incisions are utilized for the radical neck dissection, thus forming a type of visor flap over the mandible. Thus the lower lip is not transected in a vertical plane. The base of the forehead is depicted with a posterior extension to include the posterior auricular artery as well as the superficial temporal artery. The inferior incision of the forehead flap does not extend below the level of the lateral canthus of the eye, thus sparing the zygomatic branch of the seventh nerve to the orbicularis oculi muscle.

A¹   Anterior view of the extended forehead flap. The utilized portion of the flap should be nonhair-bearing. A delay of two weeks is recommended, especially if the patient has had preoperative radiation therapy, since the blood supply of the remaining tissue in the ablative area may be poor.

B   Depicted is the lesion which extends across the midline with direct involvement of

(*Text continued on opposite page.*)

Plate 195   *Cysts and Tumors Involving the Mandible*

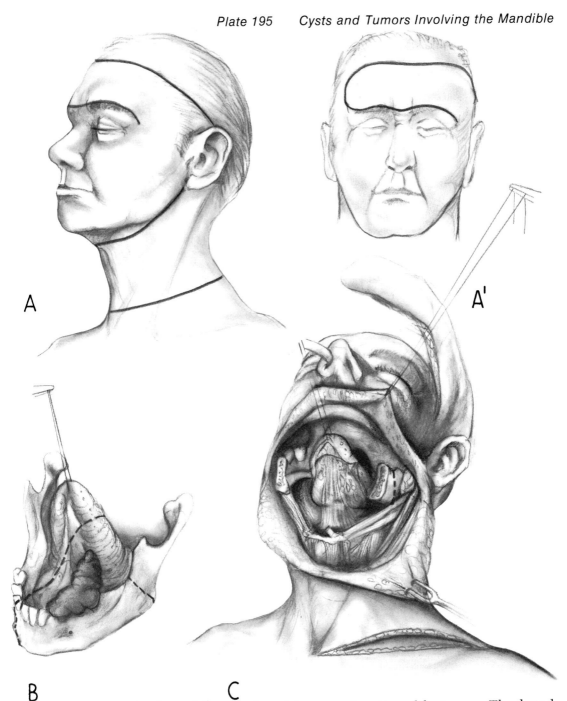

A

A'

B

C

the mandible, the floor of the mouth and the ventral portion of the tongue. The dotted lines indicate the lines of resection.

Extension of the resection to include a portion of the base of the tongue and tonsillar region can be performed and the defect closed very satisfactorily with the forehead flap when it is delivered into the oral cavity via the subzygomatic approach (refer to plate 118).

C   The operative site following the ablative surgery which consists of a left radical neck dissection, right suprahyoid neck dissection, resection of major portion of body of mandible, floor of mouth and partial ventral glossectomy. The chin visor flap is elevated upward and the forehead flap is mobilized.

(*Text continued on page 466.*)

465

RESECTION AND RECONSTRUCTION OF MAJOR PORTION
OF BODY OF MANDIBLE (*Continued*)

D   A bent Kirschner wire has been inserted to stabilize the mandibular remnants following the technique depicted in plate 194.

   The forehead flap is sutured in place using continuous 4-0 plastic sutures for the mucosa to skin layer. Interrupted second and third layer sutures are placed for additional support. The forehead flap enters the wound at the posterior end of the upper horizontal cervical incision (Millard). The inferior margin of the flap now becomes superior or anterior and is sutured to the mucosa of the lower lip. The superior margin of the flap now becomes the inferior or posterior margin and is sutured to the remaining portion of the tongue, the floor of the mouth, if any remains, and the mucosa overlying the ends of the mandible. It is this latter area in which extreme care is necessary for watertight closure without tension. Two Hemovac suction systems are advised as well as a firm dressing to aid immobilization of the mandible. If breakdown does occur, proper local care will usually result in satisfactory healing.

   The donor area is covered with one continuous split thickness skin graft taken, if feasible, from the anterior chest wall, if nonhair-bearing, or from the thigh. A word of caution regarding the entrance of the forehead flap through the upper cervical incision—if the flap crosses the Kirschner wire or it is in any way kinked, it is safer to bring the flap into the oral cavity via the subzygomatic approach, as depicted in plates 118 and 197.

E   Closure of wound showing the entrance of the flap and the small orocutaneous fistula (arrow). A split thickness skin graft from the thigh is used as a temporary dressing over the exposed pedicle of the flap.

F   *Reconstruction Stage* (after Millard). Six weeks later, a rib bone graft with a strip
G   of the periosteum has been notched on its concave surface. A medium-sized Kirschner wire is bent to conform to the mandibular defect and inserted through the rib. The original Kirschner wire used for stabilization has been removed. Step *F* is a view of the rib graft above its concave surface; step *G* is an anterior view.

   The upper cervical flap is elevated, the flap pedicle divided, the temporary skin graft removed and the flap pedicle returned to the donor site. The orocutaneous fistula is closed. The rib bone graft with Kirschner wire is inserted into the mandibular defect. The rib ends and mandibular ends are slotted and then wired to afford fixation. If at all possible, additional immobilization can be achieved by fixation of the mandibular fragments to the maxilla as described in plate 194. The oral cavity must not be entered at this stage, in order to maintain a noncontaminated wound; otherwise, the bone graft will fail. If an adequate lower alveolar ridge and buccal sulcus for denture placement is absent owing to an inadequate width of the forehead flap, a buccal gutter is formed. This is achieved by separating the lower lip from the cheek and lining the new sulcus with a dermal graft over a gutta-percha mold. This should be done at a separate stage to avoid the possible contamination of a bone graft. A serious drawback to this rib graft is total absorption of the graft. It is believed that the paucity of cancellous bone is the cause (Rappaport).

   If there is marked deficiency of the soft tissue bed for the rib graft, a deltopectoral flap is utilized.

H   Depicted is the use of vitallium mesh formed in the shape of a trough or cage. Within the trough are packed portions of medullary bone taken via a trephine (2 to 2.5 cm) opening made in the iliac bone. Richter, Sugg and Boyne (1968) suggest the use of a millipore filter (cellulose acetate with a poke size of 0.45 micron) to line the trough to prevent the invasion of fibroblasts into the fragments of the medullary bone. Fixation of the vitallium mesh to the remnant ends of the mandible must be firm with adequate immobilization of all portions of the mandible. Cuts in the mesh are made in unopposing fashion to facilitate contouring the mesh. Small screws are placed at each end of the mesh into the remaining stumps of the mandible. This type of reconstruction, as all types, should be performed as a second stage through an external incision which does not violate the oral cavity. There must be a sterile field. Immobilization of the reconstructed mandible must be complete. A serious drawback is the breakdown of overlying skin.

Plate 196   Cysts and Tumors Involving the Mandible

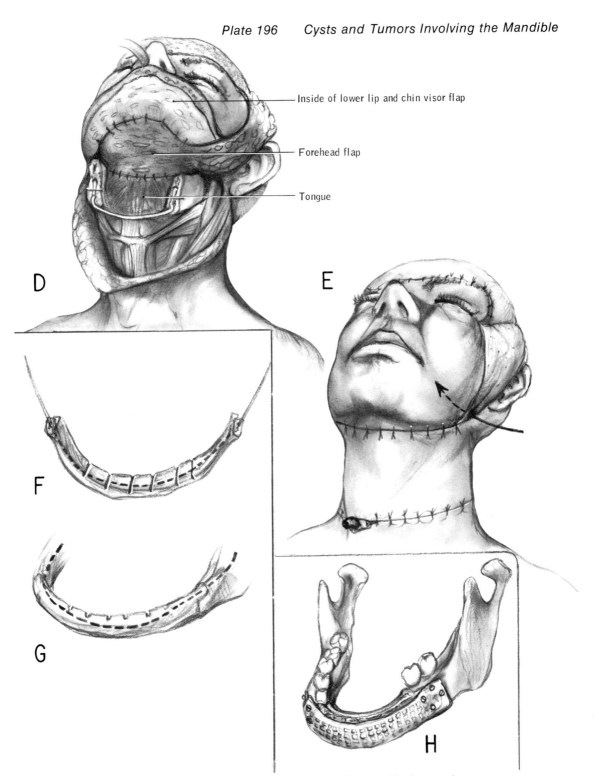

Inside of lower lip and chin visor flap

Forehead flap

Tongue

D

E

F

G

H

Corgill and Hahn have introduced preformed mandibular replacement sections of vitallium mesh for mandibular reconstruction. Conley has devised vitallium mandibular bars with flanged ends for fixation to the transected ends of the mandible.

Additional experiences with mandibular reconstruction have been reported by Sako and Marchetta (1962); MacDougall (1965); Anlyan (1965); Cook, Walker and Schewe (1965); McQuarrie (1970); Brown (1970); Catania and Molinari (1970); and Cislaghi and Catania (1970).

RESECTION OF HEMIMANDIBLE, LATERAL OROPHARYNGEAL WALL AND PORTION OF SOFT PALATE AND HEMIGLOSSECTOMY WITH RECONSTRUCTION USING A FOREHEAD FLAP

Highpoints

Refer to pages 460 and 464.

A The tumor extends from the soft palate, the tonsilar region along the lateral border of the tongue and the floor of the mouth, with direct involvement of the mandible. The dotted line depicts the area resected with disarticulation of the mandible.

B The resection of the primary lesion with radical neck dissection. The lip has been split to develop a large cheek flap. This affords excellent exposure of the oropharyngeal and palatal area, as well as exposure for mandibular disarticulation. Adequate resection of the contents of the pterygoid space must be performed, especially if trismus is present.

   The forehead flap is introduced deep to the zygomatic arch which has been transected in two locations and left attached to the overlying skin (refer to plate 118, step D). The arrow depicts the rotation of the flap so that the raw area is faced downward.

C The flap is sutured to the soft palate and remaining oropharyngeal mucosa. The distal end of the flap is sutured to the edges of the tongue and the cheek and the remaining floor of the mouth anteriorly. No attempt is made to reconstruct the mandible, since the line of resection does not cross the midline. Avoid creating an oral cripple.

D The completed closure. The dotted lines represent the course of the flap deep to the zygomatic arch and cheek. In six to eight weeks the forehead flap pedicle is returned to the donor site.

Complications

   1. Early recurrent disease with a large lesion.
   2. Lack of mobility of reconstructed area with pooling of saliva and food.

For deltopectoral flap reconstruction, see plate 113.

Plate 197   Cysts and Tumors Involving the Mandible

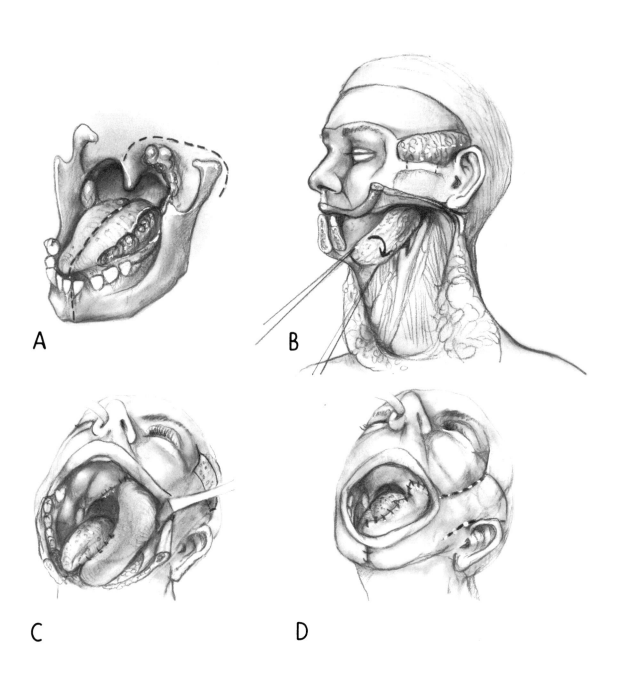

A

B

C

D

MARGINAL RESECTION OF MANDIBLE, PARTIAL GLOSSECTOMY AND RADICAL NECK DISSECTION FOR CARCINOMA OF FLOOR OF MOUTH

Discussion

The concept of marginal and total resection of the mandible has changed appreciably during the past decade. The evidence that the lymphatic channels draining the floor of the mouth and tongue pass directly into the periosteum of the mandible has been opened to question (Marchetta, Sako and Badillo, 1964). Hence it would appear that too many mandibles have been unnecessarily resected when the tumor has not directly invaded the periosteum. When the mandible itself is involved, there is no question that mandibular resection must be performed. It is the opinion of the author that when this has occurred a more extensive resection of the mandible should be performed, since spread of the tumor may well occur along the neurovascular bundle. The crux of the problem is what is adequate distance between gross disease involving the floor of the mouth and the periosteum of the mandible.

If there is any question, it still seems best to perform a marginal resection of the mandible. When there is an inadequate amount of local soft tissue present for closure, thus binding down the tongue and cheek, a transposed apron (plate 114), forehead (plate 118) or deltopectoral flap (plate 108) is definitely indicated to avoid creating an oral cripple.

In the past, possibly the resection of the entire body of the mandible was prompted by ease of closure of the operative defect rather than adequate ablative surgery.

When the mandible is preserved, a pull through procedure can be performed. The problem with the procedure is that there is restriction of exposure. It is usually better to transect the mandible and then to rewire the cut ends of the mandible.

Highpoints

1. Tracheostomy necessary.
2. Resect liberal portion of tongue.
3. Remove entire inner cortex and alveolar ridge of hemimandible.
4. Resect all tissue in continuity.
5. Remove all fragments of teeth with exposed roots.
6. Avoid creating an oral cripple by judicious use of transposed flaps and grafts.

A A tracheostomy is first performed under local anesthesia through a horizontal incision. A special anesthesia tracheostomy tube (Loré-Lawrence tube) #6 or #7 with bulky dressing extension is inserted. The patient is then put to sleep and the incision extended as in a standard radical neck dissection. The extension through the lower lip is not made until after the lower neck has been dissected. A variation of the incision is the performance of a lower lip visor flap as depicted on plate 231, step *I*.

B Cross-sectional view demonstrating the area of resected tissue at the level of the primary lesion in the floor of the mouth. A partial glossectomy is included. The marginal resection of the mandible includes the alveolar ridge and the entire inner cortex of the body of the mandible.

C Diagrammatic surface view showing that portion of the tongue, floor of mouth and alveolar ridge which is resected. Since the lesion is located anteriorly, the resection of the alveolar ridge extends beyond the midline.

D A standard radical neck dissection is performed as in plates 226 to 229, except that the structures in the digastric triangle are not disturbed at this stage. The lower lip is transected in the midline.

E The submental triangle is then dissected, removing all nodes and adipose tissue across the midline to the opposite anterior belly of the digastricus muscle. Separation of the cheek flap from the outer cortex of the mandible is begun, leaving the periosteum intact. This incision is made along the gingivobuccal sulcus.

Plate 198   Cysts and Tumors Involving the Mandible

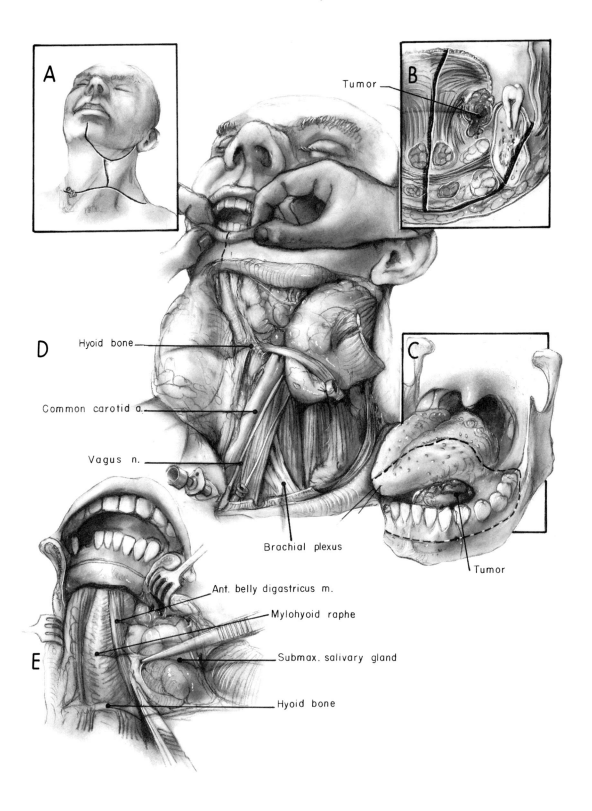

A

B

Tumor

D

Hyoid bone

Common carotid a.

Vagus n.

Brachial plexus

C

Tumor

E

Ant. belly digastricus m.

Mylohyoid raphe

Submax. salivary gland

Hyoid bone

MARGINAL RESECTION OF MANDIBLE, PARTIAL GLOSSECTOMY AND RADICAL NECK DISSECTION FOR CARCINOMA OF FLOOR OF MOUTH (*Continued*)

F   The insertion of the anterior belly of the digastricus is cut. One tooth is extracted at the site of transection of the mandible. A clamp is inserted through the floor of the mouth close to the mandible and the Gigli saw is drawn through.

G   With the Gigli saw, the upper half and inner half of the mandible is cut. The direction is then changed 90 degrees to the horizontal and the cut is extended across the midline as shown by the dotted line. An attempt is made to resect the inner cortex of the lower portion of the mandible which remains. If this is not possible, it is removed separately with a Stryker saw (G^1). Any tooth fragments are removed.

H   The tongue is split down the midline to the posterior third and then the incision is curved laterally. The mylohyoid muscles are separated along the raphe. The cheek flap is further mobilized to a point behind the last molar tooth.

Plate 199   Cysts and Tumors Involving the Mandible

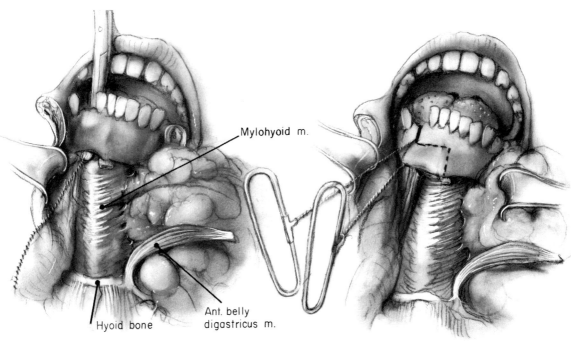

Mylohyoid m.

Hyoid bone

Ant. belly
digastricus m.

F

G

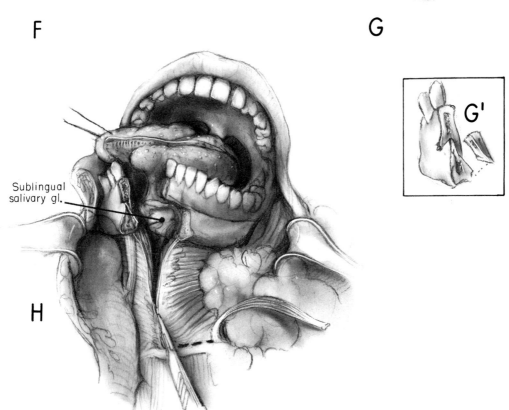

Sublingual
salivary gl.

H

G'

MARGINAL RESECTION OF MANDIBLE, PARTIAL GLOSSECTOMY AND RADICAL NECK DISSECTION FOR CARCINOMA OF FLOOR OF MOUTH (*Continued*)

I   A sagittal plane or coping saw is used to resect the inner cortex and alveolar ridge of the mandible. The coping saw is ideal since its flexibility permits it to follow the natural contour of the bone. The outer cortex is stabilized with a bone-holding forceps.

J
K   The angle and extent of the mandibular resection are shown in these schematic drawings of the mandible. In *J* the outer aspect is demonstrated; *K* is an end-on view;
L   *L* shows the inner aspect.

M   The incision is then carried across the posterior third of the tongue anterior to the circumvallate papillae. This incision reaches the saw cut behind the region of the last molar tooth.

    The remaining portion of the mandible is retracted outward, exposing the structures between the resected portion of the tongue and the inner resected portion of the mandible. These include the sublingual gland and adjacent muscles, i.e., the hyoglossus, genuglossus, genuhyoid and mylohyoid. All these structures are removed in continuity with the specimen by the standard neck dissection. The anterior and posterior bellies of the digastricus muscle as well as a portion of the stylohyoid muscle are likewise included with the contents of the digastric triangle, i.e., the submaxillary salivary gland and lymph nodes. The lingual and hypoglossal nerves are also sacrificed. All the previously mentioned muscles which are attached to the hyoid bone are resected close to the hyoid bone, leaving the bone intact.

N   Reconstruction is begun by stabilizing the mandible using a short section of a Kirschner wire inserted in either end of the exposed marrow cavity. A drill hole is in place in either side and a piece of stainless steel or malleable silver wire is passed through the holes and twisted tight.

Plate 200   Cysts and Tumors Involving the Mandible

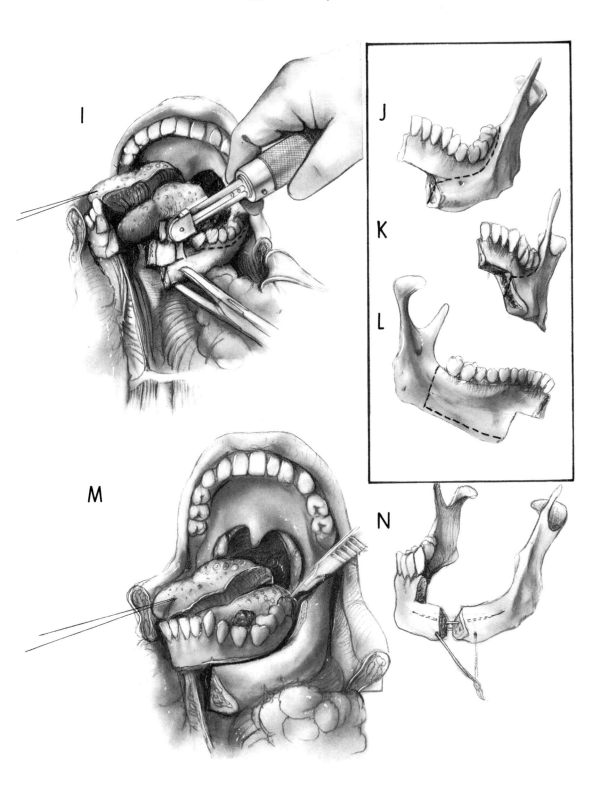

MARGINAL RESECTION OF MANDIBLE, PARTIAL GLOSSECTOMY AND RADICAL NECK DISSECTION FOR CARCINOMA OF FLOOR OF MOUTH (*Continued*)

O Three or four 2-0 chromic catgut sutures are used as the first layer of the soft tissue closure. These sutures pass through the muscles of the tongue, go under the mandible and include any soft tissue remaining above the hyoid bone and thence grasp the platysmal muscle in the skin flap. They are tied over the mandible. Refer to plates 114, 118 and 108 for closure using an apron, forehead or deltopectoral flap.

P A second layer of mattress sutures of 3-0 chromic catgut approximates the tongue musculature to the platysma. The exposed mandible is covered with this row of sutures by including a portion of the opposite skin flap and the floor of the mouth.

Q A third layer of mucosal sutures of 4-0 Dermalene or nylon completes the intraoral reconstruction.

   Before the lower lip is closed, 0.5 to 1.0 cm of the lower lip on the cheek flap is excised to tighten the lip reconstruction. This tends to prevent any drooling. The lower lip is approximated in three layers: mucosa, muscle and skin.

R The neck incisions are closed in two layers using continuous 4-0 chromic catgut for the platysmal muscle and 5-0 continuous nylon for the skin. Drains or suction catheters as used in the standard neck dissection complete the operation.

476

Plate 201   Cysts and Tumors Involving the Mandible

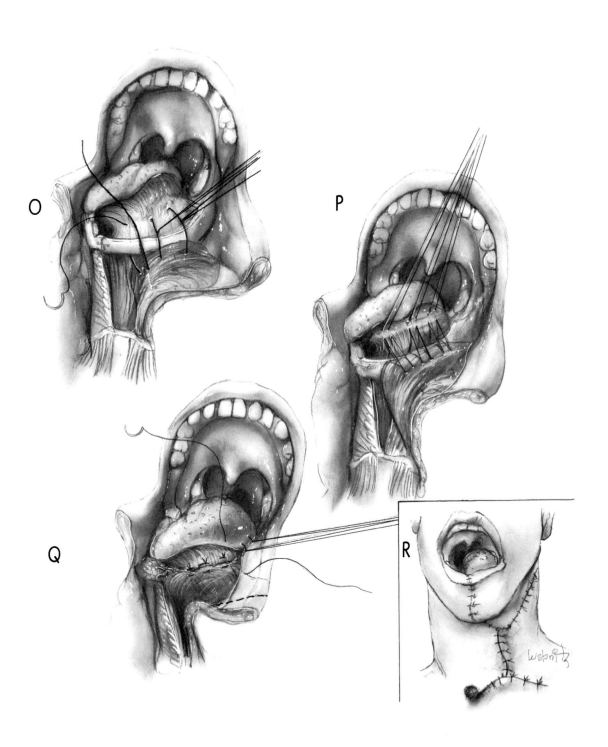

O

P

Q

R

COMBINED RADICAL NECK DISSECTION, HEMIGLOSSECTOMY AND HEMIMANDIBULECTOMY

Indications

This operation is performed for carcinomas of the floor of the mouth and tongue that involve the mandible or for primary carcinoma of the gingiva or the alveolar ridge of the mandible with or without extension to the upper alveolar ridge. Whether only the horizontal portion or both horizontal portion and ascending ramus are resected depends on the location and extent of the lesion. Another application is a large carcinoma of the tonsil with deep infiltration. A portion of the palate may be included as necessary.

In malignant tumors of the tongue in which an extended or hemiglossectomy is performed with preservation of all or part of the mandible, closure of the defect is achieved by an apron, forehead or deltopectoral flap (see plates 114, 118 and 108). Resection of the mandible is not indicated solely to facilitate ease of closure. The reader is referred to page 470 for a discussion of this problem.

Highpoints

1. Tracheostomy necessary.
2. Resect all tissue in continuity.
3. Resect liberal portion of tongue.
4. Resect portion of maxilla when necessary.
5. Remove all fragments of teeth with exposed roots.
6. Avoid creating an oral cripple by judicious use of transposed flaps and grafts. Flaps, however, are not as necessary or as warranted when the hemimandible is removed.

A The standard radical neck dissection incision is extended upward across the lower lip. A tracheostomy may be performed at the beginning or end of the operation. In either case, the hypopharynx is packed with gauze.

B Diagrammatic representation of the extent of resection for carcinoma of the tongue and the floor of the mouth involving the horizontal ramus of the mandible.

C Similar lesion viewed intraorally.

D The area of resection in this lesion, which involves the upper gingiva, includes a portion of the maxilla and palate.

E The standard neck dissection has been carried up to the level of the hyoid bone laterally. The submental area has been dissected and the lower lip is split in the midline.

E¹ A lower lip visor incision (plate 231, step *I*) can be used when the neoplasm is located anteriorly but not posteriorly. Exposure with this type of incision is inadequate for a posterior location of the neoplasm.

Plate 202   Cysts and Tumors Involving the Mandible

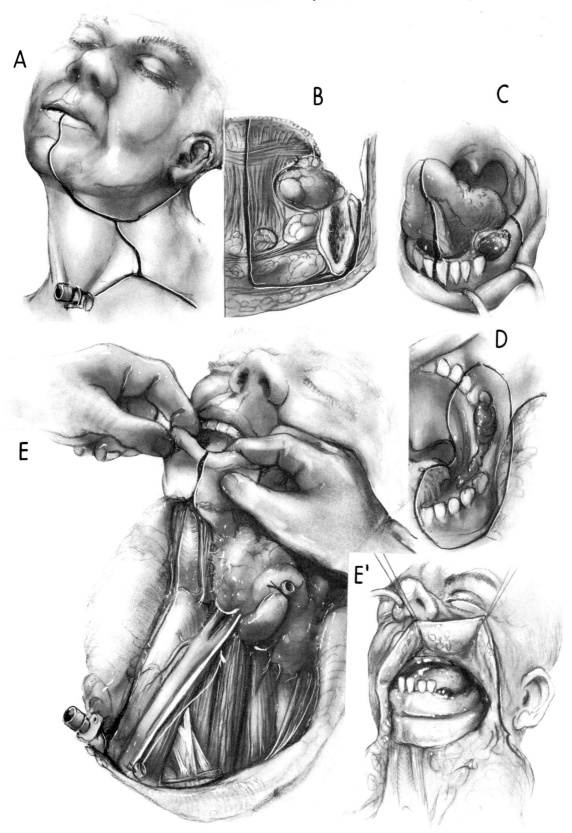

COMBINED RADICAL NECK DISSECTION, HEMIGLOSSECTOMY AND HEMIMANDIBULECTOMY (Continued)

F An incisor tooth, canine tooth or bicuspid (premolar) tooth is removed depending on the anterior extent of the tumor. A Gigli saw is inserted through the floor of the mouth and the mandible is sectioned. In this case, the origin of the anterior belly of the digastric muscle has been freed.

G The cheek flap is reflected laterally at least to the masseter muscle. Depending on the site of transection of the mandible, the mylohyoid muscle is sectioned. In this case it is transected at the raphe and along its insertion on the hyoid bone. In more lateral mandibular resections, the anterior belly of the digastric muscle and the median half of the mylohyoid are preserved. In either case, the submaxillary salivary gland and associated lymph nodes are left in continuity with the resected portion of mandible.

H The tongue is sectioned in the midline if the tumor location warrants a hemiglossectomy. Less tongue is removed in carcinoma of the gingiva. The incision is carried through the floor of the mouth and connected with the incision originating in the mylohyoid muscle. The sublingual gland is usually included in the resected specimen.

I Posteriorly, the tongue incision takes a wide sweep around the lesion and meets the inner aspect of the mandible well behind the grossly diseased area. If this incision reaches the molar area, the horizontal ramus is sectioned behind the last molar tooth with a Gigli saw or Stryker saw.

Plate 203   *Cysts and Tumors Involving the Mandible*

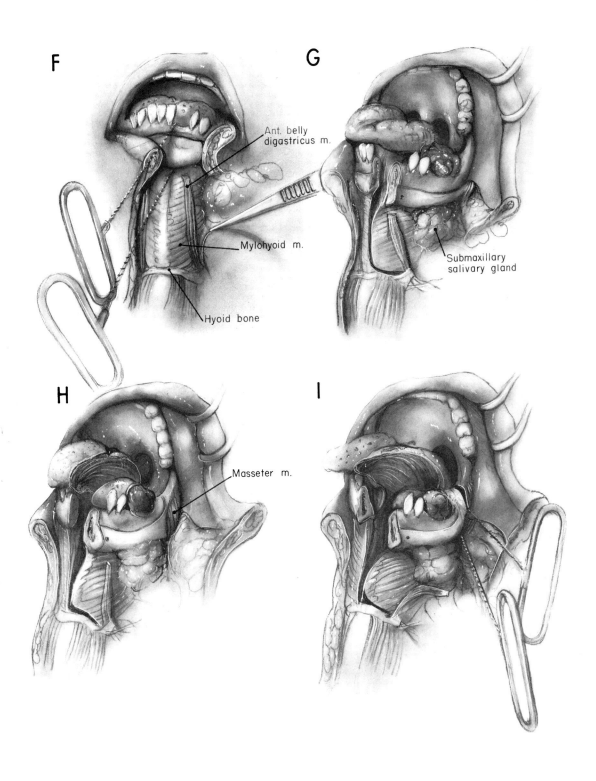

F

Ant. belly
digastricus m.

Mylohyoid m.

Hyoid bone

G

Submaxillary
salivary gland

H

Masseter m.

I

COMBINED RADICAL NECK DISSECTION, HEMIGLOSSECTOMY AND HEMIMANDIBULECTOMY (*Continued*)

J If the posterior tongue incision meets the region of the angle of the mandible, the ascending ramus is resected wholly or in part. In either case, the cheek flap includes virtually all soft tissue of the cheek. Thus, the facial nerve within the parotid is not injured. A variable amount of mucous membrane from the upper gingiva is removed depending on the extent of the resection. Depicted is an area resected for a tumor in the retromolar trigone. Involvement of the mandible requires an extention of the resection anteriorly.

K A diagrammatic oblique external view of the horizontal portion and ascending ramus of the mandible. The masseter muscle has been transected between its origin from the zygomatic process of the maxilla and zygomatic arch (not shown) and its insertion to the lateral surface of the ascending ramus and coronoid process. If the entire ascending ramus is resected this entails disarticulation, with transection of the attachments of the temporalis muscle to the coronoid process and the anterior border of the ascending ramus, of the external (lateral) pterygoid muscle to the condyle and joint capsule, and of the internal (medial) pterygoid muscle to the inner aspect of the angle of the mandible. If the ascending ramus is transected below the mandibular notch, the temporalis muscle and the external pterygoid muscle are left intact.

The major vessel in the area is the internal maxillary artery. This vessel or its branches will require ligation or occlusion with silver clips. Bleeding along with adequate exposure may be the problems in complete resection of the mandible.

L A view of the same region from below demonstrating the interrelations of the muscles and their insertions.

M When the tumor extends along the upper gingiva, the line of resection includes a portion of the upper alveolar ridge, which in turn requires resection of a portion of the floor of the antrum. A Stryker or sagittal plane saw with a small blade is used to resect the bone as depicted along the dotted line.

The primary lesion is now removed in continuity with the contents of the neck dissection. The structures included will vary slightly depending on the extent of the primary tumor. In the more extensive resections, this will include the sublingual gland and adjacent muscles, i.e., the hyoglossus, genioglossus, geniohyoid and mylohyoid. The anterior and posterior bellies of the digastricus muscle as well as a portion of the stylohyoid muscle are included, with the submaxillary salivary gland and adjacent lymph nodes. These muscles are detached along their attachments to the superior edge of the hyoid bone, which is left intact. The lingual and hypoglossal nerves are also included in the resected specimen when a significant portion or half of the tongue is resected. These nerves may otherwise be preserved.

N Depending on the operative defect, the wound is closed in one to three layers. If a defect exists along the upper alveolar ridge, the upper buccal mucosa is advanced across the defect. If possible, a two layer approximation is performed.

The musculature of the tongue is then approximated to the lower cheek flap using a two layer closure wherever possible.

O The third layer consists of the tongue mucosa sutured to the buccal mucosa. Transposed flaps, e.g., the deltopectoral, apron and forehead flaps, are utilized depending on the extent of the resection and the estimated crippling effect of using local tissue for closure.

Before the lower lip is approximated, 1 to 2 cm of lower lip along the dotted line is excised from the cheek flap. This tends to tighten the lower lip reconstruction and helps prevent drooling. The cut edges of the lower lip are approximated using three layer closure—mucous membrane, muscle and skin.

(Text continued on opposite page.)

Plate 204   *Cysts and Tumors Involving the Mandible*

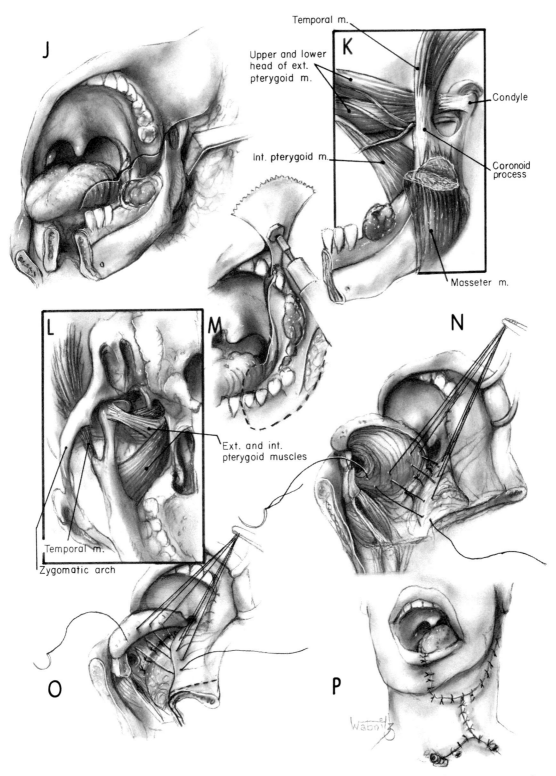

J

K

Temporal m.

Upper and lower head of ext. pterygoid m.

Int. pterygoid m.

Condyle

Coronoid process

Masseter m.

L

M

Temporal m.

Zygomatic arch

Ext. and int. pterygoid muscles

N

O

P

P   The neck incisions are closed in two layers using continuous 4-0 chromic catgut for the platysma muscle and 5-0 continuous nylon for the skin. Drains or suction catheters as used in the standard neck dissection complete the operation.

BIBLIOGRAPHY

Anand, S. V., Davey, W. W., and Cohen, B.: Tumours of the jaw in West Africa. Brit. J. Surg. *54*:901–917, 1967.

Anderson, R.: Prosthetic replacement of the hemisected Mandible. Cleveland Clin. Quart. *25*:18–20, 1958.

Anlyan, A. J.: Immediate reconstruction of mandibular defects with autogenous bone chip grafts. Amer. J. Surg. *110*: 564–567, 1965.

Arlen, M., Tollefsen, H. R., Huvos, A. G., and Marcove, R. C.: Chondrosarcoma of the head and neck. Amer. J. Surg. *120*: 456–460, 1970.

Boyne, P. J.: Regeneration of alveolar bone beneath cellulose acetate filter implants. J. Dent. Res. *43*:827, 1964.

Bromberg, B. E., Song, I. C., and Radlauer, C. B.: Surgical treatment of massive bony ankylosis of the temporomandibular joint. Plast. Reconstr. Surg. *43*: 66–70, 1969.

Brown, K. E.: Fabrication of implant supportive frame for autogenous bone marrow graph in mandibular reconstruction. Proceedings of the Tenth Annual Cancer Congress, Houston, Texas, May 1970.

Cantania, V., and Molinari, R.: Surgical removal of the mandible and prosthetic replacement of the lower jaw. Proceedings of the Tenth International Cancer Congress, Houston, Texas, May 1970.

Chambers, R. G., and Mahoney, W. D.: Osteogenic sarcoma of the mandible: Current management. Amer. J. Surg. *36*:463–471, 1970.

Cislaghi, E., and Catania, V.: Constructive evolution of the immediate mandibular prosthesis. Proceedings of the Tenth International Cancer Congress, Houston, Texas, May 1970.

Conley, J. J.: A technique for immediate bone grafting in treatment of benign and malignant tumors of the mandible and review of 17 consecutive cases. Cancer 6:568, 1953.

Cook, G. B., Walker, A. W., and Schewe, E. J., Jr.: The cerosium mandibular prosthesis. Amer. J. Surg. *110*:568–572, 1965.

DeFries, H. D., Marble, H. B., and Sell, K. W.: Reconstruction of the mandible. Use of a homograft combined with autogenous bone and marrow. Arch. Otolaryng. *93*:426–432, 1971.

Dingman, R. O., and Constant, E.: A fifteen year experience with temporo-mandibular joint disorders. Evaluation of 140 cases. Plast. Reconstr. Surg. *44*:119–124, 1969.

Dingman, R. O., Grabb, W. C., Oneal, R. M., and Ponitz, R. J.: Sternocleidomastoid muscle transplant to masseter area. Plast. Reconstr. Surg. *43*:5–12, 1969.

Fleming, I. D., and Morris, J. H.: Use of acrylic external splint after mandibular resection. Amer. J. Surg. *118*:708–711, 1969.

Furnas, D. W.: Tumbler flap for repair of large defects of the jaw. Amer. J. Surg. *118*:756–758, 1969.

Georigiade, N., Masters, F., Horton, C., and Pickrell, L.: The ameloblastoma (adamantinoma) and its surgical treatment. Plast. Reconstr. Surg. *15*:6, 1955.

Heck, W. E.: Odontogenic tumors and cysts. Laryngoscope 62:1097–1111, 1952.

Hollinshead, W. H.: Anatomy for Surgeons. Vol. I. The Head and Neck. New York, Hoeber-Harper, 1954.

Ju, D. M. C.: Localized anesthesia of the mental nerve. A significant sign of cancer of the mandible. Amer. J. Surg. *110*:573–579, 1965.

Lee, K. W., and Loke, S. J.: Squamous cell carcinoma arising in a dentigerous cyst. Cancer 20:2241–2244, 1967.

MacDougall, J. A.: Management of surgical mandibular defects. Amer. J. Surg. *110*: 562–563, 1965.

MacFee, W.: Transverse incisions for dissections. Ann. Surg. *151*:279–284, 1960.

MacGregor, I. A.: The temporal flap in facial cancer: A method of repair. Third International Congress of Plastic Surgery, 1963.

McQuarrie, D. G.: A simple prosthesis for immediate functional restoration of the mandible after surgical treatment for advanced oral cancer. Proceedings of the Tenth International Cancer Congress, Houston, Texas, May 1970.

Marchetta, F. C., Sako, K., and Badillo, J.:

Periosteal lymphatics of the mandible and intraoral carcinoma. Amer. J. Surg. 108:505–507, 1964.

Millard, D. R., Campbell, R. C., Stokley, P., and Garst, W.: Interim report on immediate mandibular repair. Amer. J. Surg. 118:726–731, 1969.

Millard, D. R., Dembrow, V., Shocket, E., Zavertnik, J., and Clinton-Thomas, C.: Immediate reconstruction of the resected mandibular arch. Amer. J. Surg. 114:605–613, 1967.

Millard, D. R., Garst, W. P., Campbell, R. C., and Stokley, S. P. H.: Composite lower jaw reconstruction. Plast. Reconstr. Surg. 46:22–30, 1970.

Millard, D. R., Jr., Maisels, D. O., and Batstone, J. H. F.: Immediate repair of radical resection of the anterior arch of the lower jaw. Plast. Reconstr. Surg. 39:153–161, 1967

Mladick, R. A., Horton, C. E., Adamson, J. E., and Carraway, J.: A simple technique for securing a K-wire to the mandible. Plast. Reconstr. Surg. 49:228–229, 1972.

Pankow, C.: Personal communication, 1969.

Rappaport, I.: Management of complications of head and neck cancer surgery. San Francisco, Fifty-Eighth Annual Clinical Congress, October 1972.

Richter, H. E., Jr., Sugg, W. E., Jr., and Boyne, P. J.: Stimulation of osteogenesis in the dog mandible by autogenous bone marrow transplants. Oral Surg. 26:396–405, 1968.

Roca, A. N., Smith, J., and Jing, B.: Osteosarcoma and parosteal osteogenic sarcoma of the maxilla and mandible: Study of 20 cases. Amer. J. Clin. Path. 54:625–636, 1970.

Rowe, N. L., and Killey, H. C.: Fractures of the Facial Skeleton. 2nd ed. Edinburgh, E. & S. Livingstone, Ltd., 1968.

Sako, K., and Marchetta, F. C.: The use of metal prostheses following anterior mandibulectomy and neck dissection for carcinoma of the oral cavity. Amer. J. Surg. 104:715–720, 1962.

Silverglade, L. B., Alvares, O. F., and Olech, E.: Central mucoepidermoid tumors of the jaws—Review of the literature and case report. Cancer 22:650–753, 1968.

Sharp, G. S., and Helsper, J. T.: Radiolucent spaces in the jaws. A new guide in diagnosis. Amer. J. Surg. 118:712–725, 1969.

Shramek, J. M., and Rappaport, I.: Panoramic radiography in head and neck pathology. Laryngoscope 80:1797–1808, 1970.

Stenström, S. J.: New technique for intraoral ramisection of mandible. Plast. Reconstr. Surg. 43:135–140, 1969.

Triedman, L. J.: Osteogenic sarcoma of the mandible. Amer. J. Surg. 110:580–584, 1965.

Ziegler, J. L., Wright, D. H., and Kyalwazi, S. K.: Differential diagnosis of Burkitt's lymphoma of the face and jaws. Cancer 27:503–514, 1971.

INDEX

Page numbers in **bold** refer to plates.